AF323985

Urologic Prostheses

UROLOGIC PROSTHESES

THE COMPLETE PRACTICAL GUIDE TO DEVICES, THEIR IMPLANTATION, AND PATIENT FOLLOW UP

Edited by

CULLEY C. CARSON III, MD

University of North Carolina School of Medicine, Chapel Hill, NC

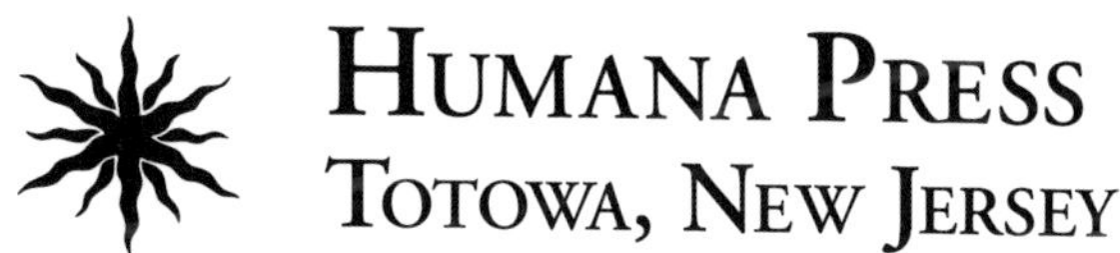

HUMANA PRESS
Totowa, New Jersey

Preface

Implanted man-made foreign bodies as substitutes for damaged or poorly functioning tissue structures have been a goal of physicians and surgeons for most of recorded history. The use of a foreign body for drainage of the urinary tract has been known and described for more than 5000 years. Metal bladder catheters introduced through the urethra were described by the Romans, evidence of which was found in Pompeii. Only in the past three decades, however, have materials been available for permanent implantation that are accepted by the body, infrequently extruded, and uncommonly affected by device infection. These materials, developed through research begun by the space program in the 1960s, have been fashioned into prostheses for use in plastic surgery, orthopedics, otorhinolaryngology, vascular surgery, cardiac surgery, and urologic surgery. Owing to the host acceptance of these materials and modern antibiotic prophylaxis to decrease the incidence of infection, urologic conditions can be treated with increasing success using these prosthetic devices. Use of prosthetic devices and material have now become an integral part of most surgical specialties, and continue to be more important in reconstructive substitute surgery in urology as well as for urinary drainage.

The first widely used and accepted prosthetics in urologic surgery were the testicular prostheses. Although currently there is some controversy about the long-term effects of silicone gel-filled and silicone foam-filled testicular prostheses designed similar to breast prostheses, a large number of testicular prostheses of various designs have been implanted with excellent cosmetic results and few reported complications. After a hiatus of almost a decade, these prosthetic devices are back, providing excellent prosthetic and cosmetic support for patients who have lost or not developed normal testes.

Prosthetic implants to restore erectile function were first attempted in the 1930s. Because of material difficulties, however, acceptable prostheses were not available until the 1970s. These devices are currently in worldwide use for restoring erectile function in patients with significant erectile dysfunction. Early prosthetic implants using rib cartilage and acrylic implanted beneath Buck's fascia were poorly tolerated and resulted in inadequate erectile function. These early prostheses were fraught with infection, extrusion, and pain, and functioned poorly in restoring the ability for patients to be sexually active. The creation of intracorporal cylinders of both semirigid and inflatable type in the early 1970s revolutionized the implantation of penile prostheses. With continued development and refinement, these prostheses are currently available in different forms. The modern penile implant can be expected to provide excellent function, satisfactory cosmetic results, and long-term reliability. Not only are these prostheses satisfactory for routine implantation, but they are also useful for penile reconstruction, the treatment of Peyronie's disease, priapism, and other complex penile conditions.

The use of prosthetic devices for the treatment of urinary incontinence has been long dreamed of. The introduction of several artificial urinary sphincters in the early 1970s has now narrowed to a single currently available inflatable artificial urinary sphincter as well as two injectable bulking agents. The refinement of this device over the past thirty years has resulted in a reliable, effective device for the management of intractable urinary continence from a variety of etiologies. The artificial urinary sphincter has been modified, refined, and perfected such that the reliability is excellent and the versatility of the device allows implanting surgeons to use the artificial urinary sphincter for incontinence in males and females of all ages, as well as in bladder reconstructive surgery. New uses in fecal incontinence are beginning to demonstrate effectiveness.

The cornerstone of prosthetic devices in the urinary tract, however, are those used for urinary drainage. Indwelling urinary stents have only been available for the past 20 years. Stents, modifications of the original urethral catheters, can now drain the kidneys, ureter, and bladder, and can be left indwelling in the prostate and urethra. These stents are now refined to a point where they are comfortable for patients, resistant to incrustation, resistant to infection, and yet provide excellent short- and long-term drainage of the urinary tract without external appliances or tubes.

Urologic Prostheses was compiled to provide a broad view of prosthetic devices used in urologic surgery. In keeping with the recent advances in urologic prosthetic surgery, contributors of recognized authority have been assembled to write expert articles for this book. Each contributing group has been able to bring to their subject significant experience in that area of prosthetic urology to share this experience with the readership and their demonstrated skill in a particular area. Although the reader will note some repetition of subject matter, there will be benefit of this repetition because differences of opinion among various authors in approaching the choice of prosthetic devices and management of specific problems in urologic prosthetic surgery will provide the reader with a complete view of this subspecialty. The clear, concise, and complete discussion of prosthetic urology in this book was made possible by the fine work of the individual contributors, each of whom provided material that is instructional and valuable to all practitioners of urologic prosthetic surgery whether they are at the beginning of their practice or experts in the field of reconstructive and prosthetic surgery. Owing to the wide variety of prosthetic devices available and the recent introduction of some of these technologies, authors have skillfully placed the newer technologies of prosthetic surgery in their proper perspective to assist the reader in assessing their places in urologic surgical practice.

Culley C. Carson III, MD

CONTENTS

Preface v

List of Contributors xi

1 History of Urologic Prostheses 1
Culley C. Carson III

2 Tissue Engineering for the Replacement of Urologic
Organs 9
Anthony Atala

3 Injectable Agents for Urinary Incontinence 29
Edward J. McGuire

4 Injectable Materials for Use in Urology 43
Raul C. Ordorica and Jorge Lockhart

5 Teflon Injection for Incontinence
After Radical Prostatectomy 89
*Choonghee Noh, David Shusterman,
and James L. Mohler*

6 Urethral Stents for Neurogenic Bladder Dysfunction 101
Ian K. Walsh and Anthony R. Stone

7 Urolume Stents in the Management
of Benign Prostatic Hyperplasia 117
*Christopher R. Chapple, J. C. Damian Png,
Jorgen Nordling, and Euan J.G. Milroy*

8 Testicular Prostheses 141
Timothy P. Bukowski

9 Current Status and Future of Penile Prosthesis
Surgery 155
Culley C. Carson III

10 Semirigid, Malleable, and Mechanical Penile Prostheses:
Survey and State of the Art 171
Roy A. Brandell and J. Brantley Thrasher

11 Inflatable Penile Prostheses:
The American Medical Systems' Experience 179
Drogo K. Montague and Kenneth W. Angermeier

12   Experience with the Mentor α-1 191
     Ricardo M. Munarriz and Irwin Goldstein
13   Peyronie's Disease and Penile Implants 201
     Steven K. Wilson and Kevin L. Billips
14   Current Approach to Penile Prosthesis Infection 219
     John J. Mulcahy
15   Reoperation for Penile Prosthesis Implantation 231
     Run Wang and Ronald W. Lewis
16   Corporeal Fibrosis:
     Penile Prosthesis Implantation
     and Corporeal Reconstruction 249
     Kenneth W. Angermeier and Drogo Montague
17   Artificial Urinary Sphincter for Treatment
     of Male Urinary Incontinence 263
     Ananias C. Diokno and Kenneth M. Peters
18   Female Incontinence and the Artificial Urinary
     Sphincter 285
     Irving J. Fishman and F. Brantley Scott

Index 301

CONTRIBUTORS

KENNETH W. ANGERMEIER, MD • *Cleveland Clinic Urological Institute, Cleveland, OH*

ANTHONY ATALA, MD • *Department of Urology, Children's Hospital, Boston, MA*

KEVIN L. BILLIPS, MD • *Private Practice, Edina, MN*

ROY A. BRANDELL, MD • *Section of Urologic Surgery, University of Kansas Medical Center, Kansas City, KS*

TIMOTHY P. BUKOWSKI, MD • *Department of Urologic Surgery, University of North Carolina School of Medicine, Chapel Hill, NC*

CULLEY C. CARSON III, MD • *Department of Urologic Surgery, University of North Carolina School of Medicine, Chapel Hill, NC*

CHRISTOPHER R. CHAPPLE, MD • *Urologic Surgery, Royal Hallamshire Hospital, Sheffield, UK*

ANANIAS C. DIOKNO, MD • *Department of Urology, William Beaumont Hospital, Royal Oak, MI*

IRVING J. FISHMAN, MD • *Department of Urology, Baylor College of Medicine, Houston, TX*

IRWIN GOLDSTEIN, MD • *Department of Urology, Boston University School of Medicine, Boston, MA*

RONALD W. LEWIS, MD • *Section of Urology, Medical College of Georgia, Augusta, GA*

JORGE LOCKHART, MD • *Department of Surgery, University of South Florida College of Medicine, Tampa, FL*

EDWARD J. MCGUIRE, MD • *Department of Surgery, University of Michigan Medical School, Ann Arbor, MI*

EUAN J. G. MILROY, MD • *Urologic Surgery, Royal Hallamshire Hospital, Sheffield, UK*

JAMES L. MOHLER, MD • *Department of Urologic Surgery, University of North Carolina School of Medicine, Chapel Hill, NC*

DROGO K. MONTAGUE, MD • *Cleveland Clinic Urological Institute, Cleveland, OH*

JOHN J. MULCAHY, MD • *Department of Urology, Indiana University School of Medicine, Indianapolis, IN*

RICARDO M. MUNARRIZ, MD • *Department of Urology, Boston University School of Medicine, Boston, MA*

CHOONGHEE NOH, MD • *Department of Urologic Surgery, University of North Carolina School of Medicine, Chapel Hill, NC*

JORGEN NORDLING, MD • *Department of Urology, Herlev Hospital, Copenhagen, Denmark*

RAUL C. ORDORICA, MD • *Department of Surgery, University of South Florida College of Medicine, Tampa, FL*

KENNETH M. PETERS, MD • *Department of Urology, William Beaumont Hospital, Royal Oak, MI*

J. C. DAMIAN PNG, MD • *Urologic Surgery, Royal Hallamshire Hospital, Sheffield, UK*

F. BRANTLEY SCOTT, MD • *Department of Urology, Baylor College of Medicine, Houston, TX*

DAVID SHUSTERMAN, MD • *Department of Urologic Surgery, University of North Carolina School of Medicine, Chapel Hill, NC*

ANTHONY R. STONE, MD • *Department of Urology, University of California-Davis, Sacramento, CA*

J. BRANTLEY THRASHER, MD • *Section of Urologic Surgery, University of Kansas Medical Center, Kansas City, KS*

IAN K. WALSH, MD • *Department of Urology, University of California-Davis, Sacramento, CA*

RUN WANG, MD • *Section of Urology, Medical College of Georgia, Augusta, GA*

STEVEN K. WILSON, MD • *Department of Urology, University of Arkansas, Van Buren, AR*

1 History of Urologic Prostheses

Culley C. Carson, MD

The problem of erectile dysfunction (ED) has been reported since recorded history. Descriptions of erections and ED can be seen in Egyptian tombs, Greek cup paintings, the works of Ovid, the Old Testament, and in the writings of Hypocrites *(1)*. In these early days, cures included prayer, recipes for magic potions and aphrodisiacs, and visits to shamans. Although the placebo effect on ED is clearly important and many of these treatments obviously produced success, agents such as Yohimbine may have had some additional physiologic effect to improve ED. The treatment of ED using prosthetic devices, however, has long been a goal of physicians, urologists, and surgeons.

The first attempt at a penile prosthesis was through the "artificial penis" designed to replace amputated penises from war injuries *(2)*. This concept developed in the 16th century by the French military surgeon, Ambroise Paré, is described in his book "Of the means and manner to repair or supplie the natural or accidental defects or wants of a man's bodie." Paré observed that "those that have their yardes cut off close to their bellies, are greatly troubled in making of urine so that they are constrained to sit downe like women for their ease." Paré created what he termed an "artificial yarde out of firm wood" that served "instead of the yarde in making of water." Although Paré did not discuss the use of his prosthetic penis for sexual intercourse, this early beginning marked the first record of the use of a penile prosthesis *(3)*.

Progress toward a functional penile prosthesis was propelled by the mutilation as a result of war injuries. Penile reconstructive surgery was attempted using tubed pedicle flaps following World War I. The goal of these tubed pedicle flaps was to restore urinary voiding function, as well as coital ability. Although these pedicle tubes were surgically successful, providing rigidity was achieved by placing a segment of rib cartilage in the center of the tube graft. The use of rib cartilage for the purpose of recreating the "os penis" or baculum of lower animals first appeared in literature in 1936 when N.A. Bogoras reported the case of a traumatic penile amputation in (3). He reconstructed the penis by using an abdominal tube pedicle graft in a 4-stage procedure during which a segment of rib cartilage was inserted in the center of the tube graft to provide rigidity. The procedure was successful in restoring sexual function in this patient. Further attempts at penile reconstruction were reported by A.P. Frumkin, a Soviet surgeon whose work is described in (4). Frumkin reconstructed traumatically amputated penises in Russian soldiers injured during World War II. Patients surgically reconstructed presented with partial penile loss to complete loss of the external genitalia. Frumkin modified Bogoras' original description because of the radical nature of injuries that he treated. He used the rib cartilage stent, and when corpus cavernosum was inadequate, secured the stent in the penile remnant using a purse-string procedure. In a procedure, which was to become popular decades later, he improved penile length by sectioning the penile suspensory ligament to provide a more secure base for cartilage implantation. Frumkin reported success with this procedure with patients returning to sexual activity and, in some cases, normal orgasms. Subsequent reports by Bergman and others suggested that creating a new penis over an autografted rib cartilage could be successful (5). Frequently, however, these procedures resulted in stent extrusion, erosion, and often significant and serious penile curvature.

Advancement toward a functional penile implant continued to be an interest in the last half of the 20th century. In the early 1950's, acrylic materials were made available for prosthetic joints, rhinoplasty, and testicular prostheses. Goodwin and Scott, using these acrylic materials, fashioned a stent to provide penile rigidity for penile reconstructions (6). They reported five patients in the 1950's implanted with acrylic stents placed beneath Buck's fascia, but not in the corpora cavernosa. Their initial patients had significant complications of pressure necrosis, draining sinuses, pain, infection, and ultimately implant extrusion. In the 1960's, materials were developed through the space program that were better tolerated in human implantation, were easier to fashion into prosthetic devices and were less associated with infection and extrusion. These materials in the form of silicone rubber elastomer were first implanted in the early 1960's (7). The first silicone prosthesis was implanted in the body in 1959 in the form of a silicone rubber tubing for urethral reconstruction. Following this implantation, silicone breast

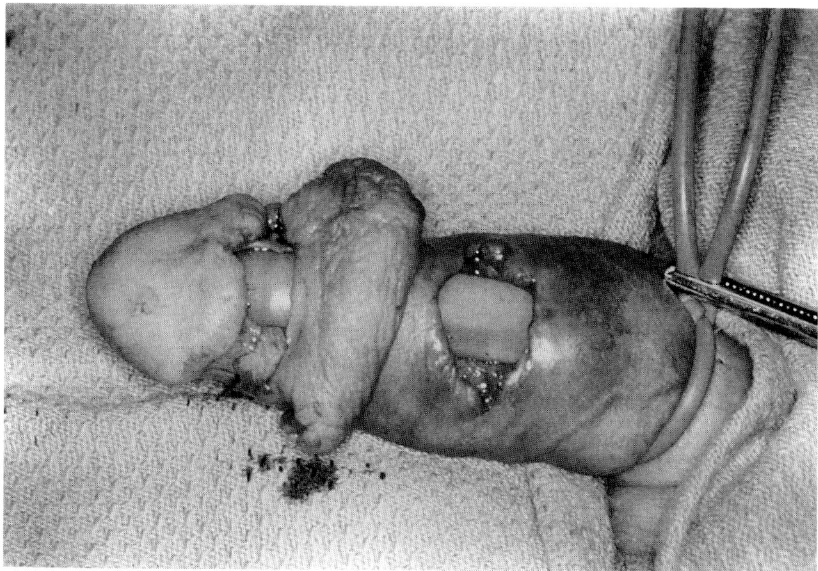

Fig. 1. Pearman penile prosthesis rod surgically placed beneath Buck's fascia.

prostheses were introduced in 1961 and this material was then fashioned into penile prostheses *(8)*. In 1964, Lash, Zimmerman, and Loeffler reported the first penile implants of silicone created from an inlay method used previously in prosthodontics *(9,10)*. Because of its low tissue reactivity, flexibility, rigidity, and durability, silicone rubber became the implant material of choice. Because these early prosthetic devices were placed beneath Buck's fascia in the dorsal midline groove between the corporal bodies, extrusion was frequent. In 1967, Pearman introduced a silicone prosthesis that was trimmable for length and fit beneath Buck's fascia dorsally in hopes of providing fewer complications, more comfort, and better function *(11)* (Fig. 1). Pearman's prosthesis was placed such that the distal portion lay beneath Buck's fascia at the corona and the proximal portion positioned at the suspensory ligament of the penis. Through cadaveric studies, Pearman demonstrated that a plane could be developed at the dorsum of the penis between Buck's fascia and the tunical albuginea from the suspensory ligament to the area just below the corona of the glans penis. He created his prosthesis by making a mold of this space with hot paraffin in cadaveric dissections *(12)*. Because of problems with pain and erosion, however, Pearman redesigned his prosthesis for placement beneath the tunical albuginea to improve stability, comfort, and cosmetic results. Despite these modifications, however, extracavernosal implants continued to be difficult to

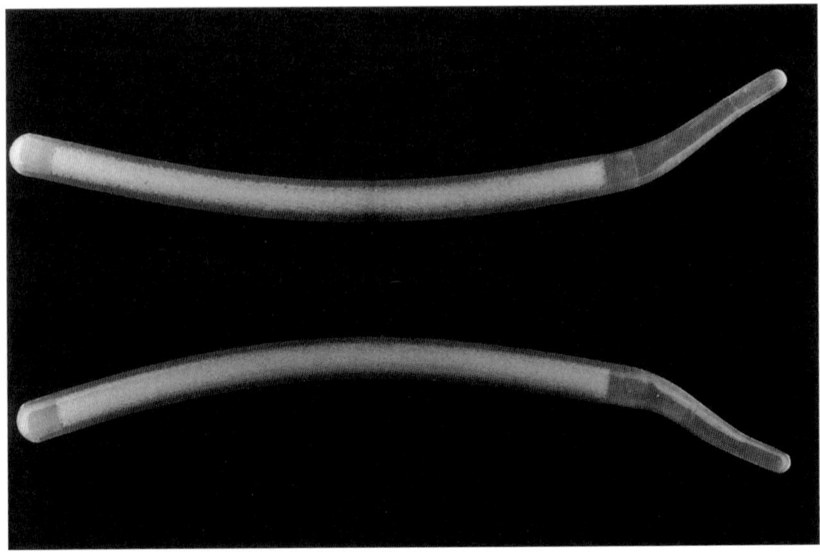

Fig. 2. Small Carrion penile prosthesis.

implant and the results were inconsistent with frequent glans irritation, extrusion, and urethral erosion.

The concept of intracavernosal implants changed the design of penile implants and led to the penile prosthesis implanted in the 21st century. In 1958, G.E. Beheri became frustrated with placement of acrylic stents beneath Buck's fascia and began to implant polyethylene rods in the corpora cavernosa. Beheri reported excellent results in 700 patients in 1966 *(13)*. It was not until 1973, however, when Morales et al. in the United States reported the placement of full-length small-caliber intracavernosal polyethylene rods similar to those used by Beheri in the corpora cavernosa *(14)*. Because these prostheses were stiff, of little flexibility, and quite thin, there was frequent crewel, septal, and distal perforation and erosion. To improve these prostheses and diminish morbidity, experience from the silicone gel breast prostheses was used to create a more flexible, larger prosthesis with a silicone exterior filled with a viscus silicone gel. Because of the vulnerability for leakage of the silicone gel and the short shelf life, these prostheses were implanted in only a few patients *(15)*. The development of the Small Carrion™, prosthesis in 1973 using a silicone rubber exterior with a silicone sponge to provide improved girth, filling of the entire corpus cavernosa, and measurable length set the stage for the modern era in penile prosthesis implantation *(18)* (Fig. 2).

Simultaneously, the inflatable penile prosthesis was being designed by Scott, Bradley, and Timm at the University of Minnesota *(17)*. This prosthesis, consisted of two silicone rubber cylinders placed in the corpora cavernosa and connected to a reservoir, and two pumps to reproduce the natural erectile process and obtain a cosmetically acceptable flaccid state. Small and Carrion in 1973 described the perineal approach for the new type of penile prosthesis implantation, and of 31 patients initially described, only one had less than a satisfactory result *(16)*. In 1977, Finney introduced a flexible prosthesis called the Flexirod prosthesis, which, because of its hinged design, permitted improved concealment *(18)*. A proximal stiff, but multisegmented, end provided trim ability for size adjustment intraoperatively. The issue of concealment continued to be of concern with semirigid penile prostheses and Jonas introduced the Jonas prosthesis in 1980 *(19)*. This prosthesis consisted of a silicone rubber outer sheath with an inner core twisted, braided, or cabled at the end of the prosthesis to a satisfactory position. Changes in surgical approach to include distal penile incisions and local anesthesia have made these prostheses more acceptable surgically for infrequent implanters. These devices continue to be used in selected patients and some patients prefer the reduced mechanical complexity and potential decreased mechanical malfunction.

The development of the inflatable penile prosthesis began with the report in 1973 of Scott et al. who described a prosthesis consisting of two cylindrical cylinders, composed of Dacron™-reinforced silicone rubber, and a reservoir externally controlled by two scrotal pumps. By changing the construction of the cylinders and the high-pressure portion of the system, the Mentor device introduced in the early 1980's changed the construction of the cylinders from silicone rubber to polyurethane *(20)*.

Many other prosthetic devices have been introduced and subsequently eliminated. These include self-contained devices such as the Hydroflex by American Medical Systems, the Flexiflate by Surgitech, the Omniphase by Dacomed *(21)*. In the mid-1980's, a mechanical penile prosthesis termed the omniphase was introduced. Because of mechanical difficulties, however, this was redesigned to the duraphase and subsequently the Dura II by Timm Corporation *(22)*. This prosthesis consists of a central cable and polyethylene cylinder that functions like a "gooseneck lamp" and provides the advantages of a semirigid prosthesis with increased position ability and increased conceal ability.

The concept of a penile prosthesis has intrigued physicians and those suffering from ED for centuries. Anatomic observations of animals in which an os penis or baculum have been described as early as Aristotle.

Prosthetic surgery for ED born from this concept and the war injuries of the 20th century were combined with advances in materials sciences born of the space program to result in the cylinder elastomer prostheses, which have revolutionized medical and surgical treatment. Penile implants, available both in semirigid rod and inflatable design, have been available in their current forms since 1973. Design, material, and surgical changes in these prostheses have resulted in improved reliability, durability, and, ultimately, patient and partner satisfaction. Today, most penile implants placed one of the inflatable variety optimizing function, appearance and concealability with excellent durability *(23)*. Twenty-first century penile prostheses continue to provide excellent erections, excellent flaccidity between erectile events, and superior patient and partner satisfaction rates.

REFERENCES

1. Brendel OJ (1970) The Grecal Roman World. In: *Studies In Erotic Art.* Bowie T, Christenson CV, eds., New York: Basic Books p. 38.
2. Gee WF (1975) A history of surgical treatment of impotence. Urology 5:401.
3. Kim JH, Carson CC (1993) History of urologic prostheses for impotence. Prob Urol 7:283–233.
4. Frumkin AP (1944) Reconstruction of the male genitalia. Am Rev Soviet Med 2:14.
5. Bergman RT, Howard AH, Barnes RW (1948) Plastic reconstruction of the penis. *J Urol* 59:1174.
6. Goodwin WE, Scott WW (1952) Phalloplasty. *J Urol* 68:903.
7. Habal MB (1984) The biologic basis for clinical application of the silicones: a correlate to their biocompatibility. *Arch Surg* 119:843–849.
8. Bretan PN (1989) History of the prosthetic treatment of impotence. *Urol Clin North Am* 16:1–5.
9. Loeffler RA, Sayegh ES, Lash H (1964) The artificial faux penis. *Plast Reconstr Surg* 34:71–73.
10. Lash H, Zimmerman DC, Loeffler RA (1964) Silicone implantation: inlay method. *Plast Reconstr Surg* 34:75–79.
11. Pearman RO (1967) Treatment of organic impotence by implantation of a penile prosthesis. *J Urol* 97:716.
12. Pearman RO (1972) insertion of a silastic penile prosthesis for the treatment of organic sexual impotence. *J Urol* 107:802.
13. Behaeri GE (1996) Surgical treatment of impotence. *Plast Reconstr Surg* 38:92.
14. Morales PA, O'Connor JJ, Hotchkiss RS (1956) Plastic reconstructive surgery after total loss of the penis. *Am J Surg* 92:403.
15. Morales PA, Suarez JB, Delgado J, Whitehead ED (1973) Penile implant for erectile impotence. *J Urol* 109:641.
16. Small MP, Carrion HM, Gordon JA (1975) Small carrion penile prosthesis: new management of impotence. *Urology* 5:479.
17. Scott FB, Bradley WE, Timm GW (1973) Management of erectile impotence: use of implantable inflatable prosthesis. *Urology* 2:80.
18. Finney RP (1984) Finney flexirod prosthesis. *Urology* 23:79–82.

19. Jonas U, Jacobi JH (1980) Silicone cylinder penile prosthesis: description, operative report and results *J Urol* 123:865–868.
20. Wilson SK, Cleves MA, Delk JR (1999) Comparison of mechanical reliability of original and enhanced mentor alpha i penile prosthesis. *J Urol* 162:715–718.
21. Thrasher JB (1993) Self-contained inflatable penile prostheses. *Prob Urol* 7:317–327.
22. Mulcahy JJ (1993) Mechanical penile prostheses. *Prob Urol* 311–3116.
23. Jhaveri FM, Rutledge R, Carson CC (1998) Penile prosthesis implantation surgery: a statewide population based analysis of 2354 patients. *Int J Impot Res* 10:251–254.

2 Tissue Engineering for the Replacement of Urologic Organs

Anthony Atala, MD

Contents

Introduction
Tissue-Engineering Strategies
Cell Delivery Matrices
Tissue Engineering of Urologic Structures
Fetal Tissue Engineering
Gene Therapy and Tissue Engineering
References

INTRODUCTION

Numerous urologic tissue substitutes have been attempted with both synthetic and organic materials *(1)*. The first application of a free-tissue graft for bladder replacement was reported by Neuhoff in 1917, when fascia was used to augment bladders in dogs *(2)*. Since that first report, multiple other free-graft materials have been used experimentally and clinically, including skin, bladder submucosa, omentum, dura, peritoneum, placenta, sero-muscular grafts, and small intestinal submucosa *(3–8)*. Synthetic materials, which have been tried previously in experimental and clinical settings, include polyvinyl sponge, tetrafluoroethylene (Teflon), gelatin sponge, collagen matrices, vicryl matrices, resin-sprayed paper, and silicone *(9–15)*. Some of the aforementioned attempts have not gained clinical acceptance owing to either mechanical, structural, functional, or biocompatibility problems. Permanent synthetic materials have been associated with mechanical failure and calculus formation. Natural

From: *Urologic Prostheses:*
The Complete, Practical Guide to Devices, Their Implantation and Patient Follow Up
Edited by: C. C. Carson © Humana Press Inc., Totowa, NJ

materials usually resorb with time and have been associated with marked graft contracture.

Some of the free grafts utilized for bladder replacement have been able to show a trilayered histologic distribution in terms of a urothelial layer, a midlayer composed of connective tissue, and a muscular layer, all of which have varied in terms of their full development. It has been well established for decades that the bladder is able to regenerate generously over free grafts *(16,17)*. Urothelium is associated with a high replicative capacity. However, the muscle layers are less likely to regenerate in a normal fashion. Both urothelial and muscle ingrowth are believed to be initiated from the edges of the normal bladder toward the region of the free graft *(18)*. Usually, however, contracture or resorption of the graft has been evident. We have hypothesized that the inflammatory response toward the matrix, and the paucity of normal muscle regeneration may contribute to resorption of the free graft when used alone.

TISSUE-ENGINEERING STRATEGIES

The overall failure in the strategies attempted for genitourinary tissue replacement in the past led us to apply the principles of cell transplantation, materials science, and engineering toward the development of a biological substitute that would restore and maintain normal function. Cell transplantation has been proposed for the replacement of a variety of tissues, including skin, pancreas, and liver. However, the concept of urothelial-associated cell transplantation had not been formerly approached in the laboratory setting until earlier this decade because of the inherent difficulties encountered in growing urothelial cells in large quantities. Our laboratory was successful in culturing and greatly expanding urothelial cells from small biopsy specimens. Using our methods of cell culture, we estimate that it would be theoretically possible to expand a urothelial strain from a single specimen that initially covers a surface area of 1 cm^2 to one covering a surface area of more than 4000 m^2 within 8 wk *(19–21)*. This would result in a cell yield that would be sufficient to cover an entire football field. Bladder, ureter, renal pelvis, and corporal cavernosal muscle cells can be equally harvested, cultured, and expanded easily. Based on these observations, we proposed an approach to tissue regeneration by patching isolated cells to support structures that would have a suitable surface chemistry for guiding cell reorganization and growth.

CELL DELIVERY MATRICES

It is known from previous studies that artificial permanent support structures are lithogenic (Teflon, silicone) *(1)*. Investigators have tried permanent homograft or heterograft support structures such as dura, however, these contract with time and are problematic in a clinical setting. Natural permanent support structures, such as denuded bowel, retain their inherent properties and mucosal regrowth invariably occurs with time. A variety of synthetic polymers, both degradable and nondegradable, have been utilized to fabricate tissue engineering matrices *(22)*. Bladder submucosa was proposed as a matrix for tissue regeneration in 1961, and there has been a recent resurgence of interest in this material for bladder replacement *(3,4)*. Intestinal submucosa has also been proposed as a scaffold for the regeneration of urologic tissue *(8)*. All of the materials used until recently in the urinary tract, both synthetic and natural, were applied without the use of cells. A common finding with these materials was usually an adequate histological result, but with a paucity of muscle tissue and subsequent graft contraction and shrinkage *(23,24)*.

Synthetic polymers can be manufactured reproducibly and can be designed to exhibit the necessary mechanical properties *(22)*. Among synthetic materials, resorbable polymers are preferable because permanent polymers carry the risk of infection, calcification, and unfavorable connective tissue response. Polymers of lactic and glycolic acid have been extensively utilized to fabricate tissue engineering matrices *(22)*. These polymers have many desirable features; they are biocompatible, processable, and biodegradable. Degradation occurs by hydrolysis and the time sequence can be varied from weeks to over a year by manipulating the ratio of monomers and by varying the processing conditions. These polymers can be readily formed into a variety of structures, including small diameter fibers and porous films.

The porosity, pore size distribution, and continuity dictate the interaction of the biomaterials and transplanted cells with the host tissue. Fibrovascular tissue will invade a device if the pores are larger than approx 10 µm, and the rate of invasion will increase with the pore size and total porosity of a device *(25,26)*. This process results in the formation of a capillary network in the developing tissue *(26)*. Vascularization of the engineered tissue may be required to meet the metabolic requirements of the tissue and to integrate it with the surrounding host. In urologic applications, it may also be desirable to have a nonporous luminal surface (e.g., to prevent leakage of urine from the tissue).

The direction that we have followed to engineer urologic tissue involves the use of both synthetic (polyglycolic and/or poly-lactic acid and alginate) and natural (bladder submucosa, intestinal submucosa, peritoneum, and reconstituted collagen) biodegradable materials with and without cells.

TISSUE ENGINEERING OF UROLOGIC STRUCTURES

Ureter and Urethra

Urothelial and muscle cells can be expanded in vitro, seeded onto the matrix, and allowed to attach and form sheets of cells. The cell-matrix scaffold can then be implanted in vivo. We have performed a series of in vivo urologic associated cell-matrix experiments. Histologic analysis of human urothelial, bladder muscle, and composite urothelial and bladder muscle-matrix scaffolds, implanted in athymic mice and retrieved at different time-points, indicated that viable cells were evident in all three experimental groups *(27,28)*.

Implanted cells oriented themselves spatially along the matrix surfaces. The cell populations appeared to expand from one layer to several layers of thickness with progressive cell organization with extended implantation times. The matrix alone evoked an angiogenic response by 5 d, which increased with time. Matrix degradation was evident after 20 d. An inflammatory response was also evident at 5 d, and its resolution correlated with the biodegradation sequence. Cell-matrix composite implants of urothelial and muscle cells retrieved at extended times (50 d) showed extensive formation of multilayered sheet-like structures and well-defined muscle layers. Matrices seeded with cells and manipulated into a tubular configuration showed layers of muscle cells lining the multilayered epithelial sheets. Cellular debris appeared reproducibly in the luminal spaces, suggesting that epithelial cells lining the lumina are sloughed into the luminal space. Cell matrices implanted with human bladder muscle cells alone showed almost complete replacement of the polymer with sheets of smooth muscle at 50 d. This experiment demonstrated, for the first time, that composite tissue engineered structures could be created *de novo*. Prior to this study, only single-cell-type tissue engineered structures had been created. The malleability of the synthetic matrix allowed for the creation of cell-matrix implants manipulated into preformed tubular configurations. The combination of both smooth muscle and urothelial cell-matrix scaffolds is able to provide a template wherein a functional ureter or urethra may be created *de novo*.

In the studies performed for tubularized structures, such as ureters and urethras, if an entire segment was replaced, cells were needed in order to prevent contracture. However, if the area replaced was small in at least one of its dimensions, i.e., an onlay graft for urethral replacement, the cells were not essential for adequate healing *(29–31)*. A collagen-based matrix has been used successfully for urethroplasty in patients requiring re-do hypospadias repair (*see* Fig. 1) *(31)*.

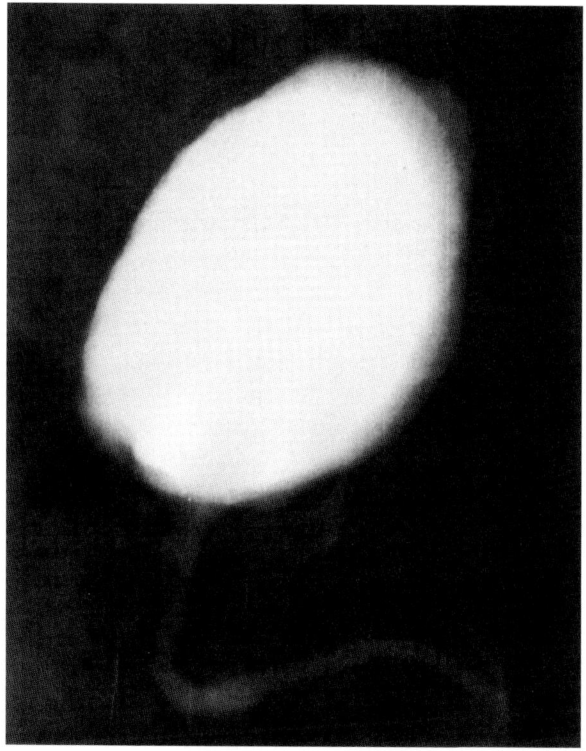

Fig. 1. Radiographic urethrogram of a patient with a reconstructed urethra using a collagen matrix shows maintenance of a wide caliber without any evidence of stricture.

Bladder Engineering

In other sets of experiments, bladder tissue was engineered and used for augmentation using similar techniques as aforementioned *(32)*. Partial cystectomies were performed in beagles. Both urothelial and smooth muscle cells were harvested and expanded separately. Allogenic bladder submucosa obtained from sacrificed animals was seeded with muscle cells on one side and urothelial cells on the opposite side. All beagles underwent cruciate cystotomies on the bladder dome. Augmentation cystoplasty was performed with the allogenic bladder submucosa seeded with cells, and with the allogenic bladder submucosa without cells. Bladders augmented with the allogenic bladder submucosa seeded with cells showed a 99% increase in capacity compared to bladders augmented with the cell-free allogenic bladder submucosa, which showed only a 30% increase in capacity.

In all of the studies performed at our laboratory, whenever entire segments of tissue were replaced, there was a difference evident between matrices used with autologous cells and those used only as a regenerating scaffold. Matrix-cell composites retained most of their implanted diameter, as opposed to matrix only, wherein graft contraction and shrinkage occurred *(33)*.

The results of all our prior studies showed that the creation of artificial bladders may be achieved in vivo, however, much work remained to be done in terms of the functional parameters of these implants. In order to address the functional parameters of tissue-engineered bladders, an animal model was designed that required a subtotal cystectomy with subsequent replacement with a tissue-engineered organ *(34)*.

A total of 18 beagle dogs underwent a trigone-sparing cystectomy. The animals were randomly assigned to one of three groups. Group A (*n*=6) underwent closure of the trigone without a reconstructive procedure. Group B (*n*=6) underwent reconstruction with a cell-free bladder-shaped biodegradable polymer. Group C (*n*=6) underwent reconstruction using a bladder shaped biodegradable polymer that delivered autologous urothelial cells and smooth muscle cells. The cell populations had been separately expanded from a previously harvested autologous bladder biopsy. Preoperative and postoperative urodynamic and radiographic studies were performed serially. Animals were sacrificed at 1, 2, 3, 4, 6, and 11 mo postoperatively. Gross, histological, and immunocytochemical analyses were performed *(34)*.

The cystectomy-only controls and polymer-only grafts maintained average capacities of 24% and 46% of preoperative values, respectively. An average bladder capacity of 95% of the original precystectomy volume was achieved in the tissue-engineered bladder replacements. The subtotal cystectomy reservoirs that were not reconstructed and polymer-only reconstructed bladders showed a marked decrease in bladder compliance (10% and 42%). The compliance of the tissue engineered bladders showed almost no difference from preoperative values that were measured when the native bladder was present (106%). Histologically, the polymer-only bladders presented a pattern of normal urothelial cells with a thickened fibrotic submucosa and a thin layer of muscle fibers. The retrieved tissue-engineered bladders showed a normal cellular organization, consisting of a trilayer of urothelium, submucosa, and muscle (Fig. 2). Immunocytochemical analyses for desmin, α-actin, cytokeratin 7, pancytokeratins AE1/AE3 and uroplakin III confirmed the muscle and urothelial phenotype. S-100 staining indicated the presence of neural structures. The results from this study showed that it is possible to tissue engineer bladders that are anatomically and functionally normal.

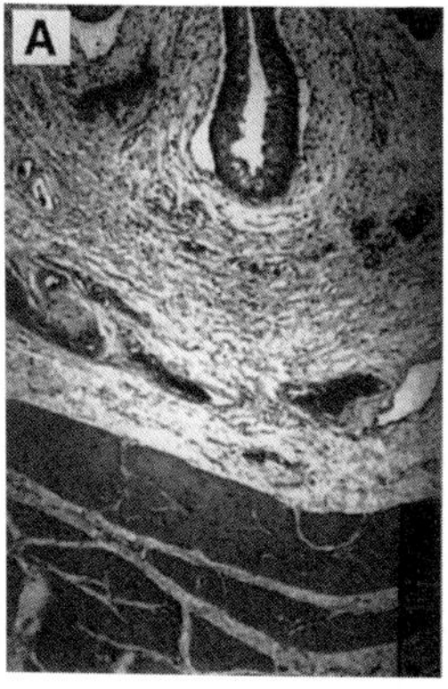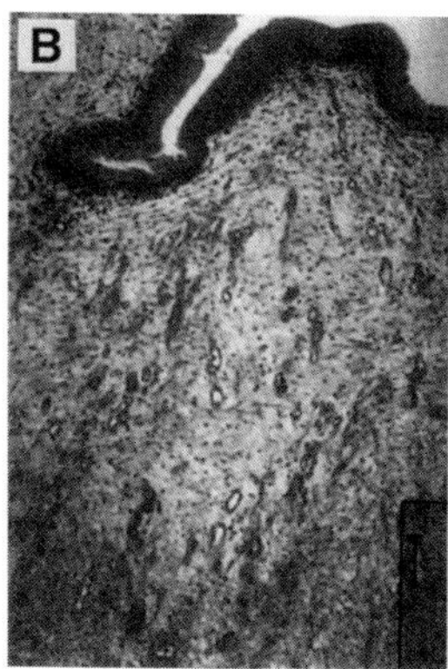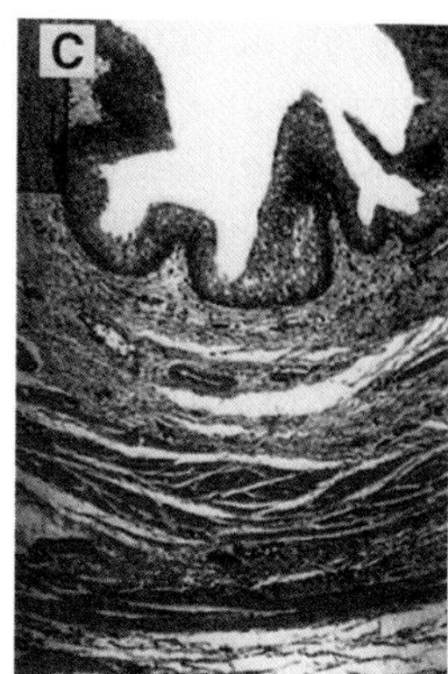

Fig. 2. Histological analysis of canine bladders 6 mo after surgery. Hematoxylin and eosin histological results (orig. magnif. X100) are shown for (**A**) bladder control; (**B**) the bladder dome of the cell-free polymer reconstructed bladder showing extensive fibrosis, and (**C**) the bladder dome of the cell-seeded polymer reconstructed bladder showing a normal architecture.

Genital Tissues

PENILE AND CLITORAL CORPORA CAVERNOSA

A large number of congenital and acquired abnormalities of the genitourinary system, including ambiguous external genitalia, the extrophy-epispadias complex and impotence, would benefit from the availability of transplantable, autologous corpus cavernosum tissue for use in reconstructive procedures. Given the major structural and functional importance of corpora cavernosal tissue, it is clear that the availability of autologous corporal smooth muscle tissue for use in reconstructive procedures would be of great clinical utility, facilitating enhanced cosmetic result, while providing the possibility of *de novo,* functional erectile tissue.

Experiments performed in our laboratory were designed to determine the feasibility of using cultured human corporal smooth muscle cells seeded onto biodegradable matrix scaffolds for the formation of corpus cavernosum muscle in vivo. Primary cultures of human corpus cavernosum smooth muscle cells were derived from operative biopsies obtained during penile prosthesis implantation and vaginal resection. Cells were maintained in continuous multilayered cultures, seeded onto polymers of nonwoven polyglycolic acid, and implanted subcutaneously in athymic mice. Animals were sacrificed at various time-points after surgery and the implants were examined via histology, immunocytochemistry, and Western blot analyses *(35).*

Corporal smooth muscle tissue was identified grossly and histologically at the time of sacrifice. Intact smooth muscle cell multilayers were observed growing along the surface of the polymers throughout all retrieved time-points. There was evidence of early vascular in-growth at the periphery of the implants by 7 d. By 24 d, there was evidence of polymer degradation. Smooth muscle phenotype was confirmed immunocytochemically and by Western blot analyses with antibodies to α-smooth muscle actin.

Further studies were performed wherein corpora cavernosal muscle cells were co-cultured with endothelial cells. The co-cultured cells were seeded on polymers and implanted in vivo. At retrieval, by 42 d, there was tissue organization similar to normal corpora *(36)*. These studies provided the first evidence that cultured human corporal smooth muscle cells could be used in conjunction with biodegradable polymer scaffolds to create corpus cavernosum tissue *de novo*.

In the future, it could be foreseen that corpora cavernosal tissue could be safely and easily obtained under local anesthesia in a percutaneous, office-based procedure. Once harvested, this tissue could be used to establish explant cultures of autologous human corporal smooth muscle cells, fibroblasts, and endothelial cells. These cells, after expansion in vitro, could be seeded onto biodegradable polyglycolic acid polymer scaffolds where they would attach and multiply. Once delivered to the in vivo environment as an autograft in a reconstructive procedure, they might reorganize and resume their highly specialized physiologic function.

PENILE PROSTHESES

Currently, the principal method of reconstructing a phallus when insufficient tissue is present, is to utilize silicone rigid prostheses. Although silicone penile prostheses has been an accepted treatment modality since the 1970s, issues with biocompatibility remain *(37)*. Creation of a natural penile prostheses composed of vascularized autologous tissue may be advantageous. We had previously demonstrated that autologous chondrocytes suspended in biodegradable polymers would form cartilage structures when implanted in vivo *(38,39)*. We recently investigated the possibility of creating a natural phallic prosthesis consisting of autologous chondrocytes, which, if biocompatible and elastic, could be used in patients who require genital reconstruction.

Cartilage was harvested from the articular surface of calf shoulders. Chondrocytes were isolated, grown, and expanded in vitro. The cells were seeded onto preformed cylindrical polyglycolic acid polymer rodsat a concentration of 50×106 chondrocytes/cm^3. Cell-polymer scaffolds were implanted in vivo. Each mouse had two implantation

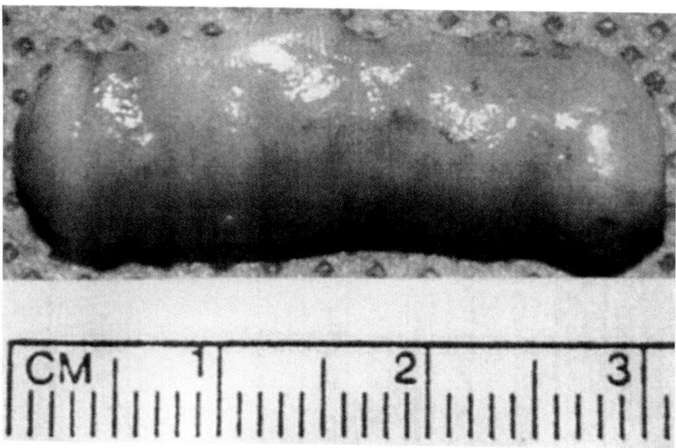

Fig. 3. Penile rod made from autologous cartilage cells.

sites consisting of a polymer scaffold seeded with chondrocytes and a control (polymer alone). The engineered rods were retrieved at 1, 2, 4, and 6 mo after implantation. Stress-relaxation studies to measure biomechanical properties, including compression, tension, and bending, were performed on the retrieved structures. Histological analyses were performed with hematoxylin and eosin, aldehyde fuschin-alcian blue, and toluidine blue staining *(40)*.

Gross examination showed the presence of well-formed milky-white rod-shaped solid cartilage structures which were approximately the same size as the initial implant (*see* Fig. 3). A series of stress-relaxation tests were performed in order to determine whether the engineered cartilage rods possessed the mechanical properties required to maintain penile rigidity. Biomechanical analyses of all specimens demonstrated similar patterns. The compression studies showed that the retrieved cartilage rods were able to withstand high degrees of pressure. A ramp compression speed of 200 μm/s, applied to each cartilage rod up to 2000 μm in distance, resulted in 3.8 kg of resistance. The tension relaxation studies demonstrated that the retrieved cartilage rods were able to withstand stress and were able to return to their initial state while maintaining their biomechanical properties. A ramp-tension speed of 200 μm/s applied to each cartilage rod created a tensile strength of 2.2 kg, which physically lengthened the rods an average of 0.48 cm. Relaxation of tension at the same speed resulted in retraction of the cartilage rods to their initial state. The five cycles of bending studies performed at two different speeds showed that the engineered cartilage rods were durable, malleable, and were able to retain their mechanical properties. None of the rods was ruptured during the biomechanical stress relaxation studies, which showed that the cartilage structures were readily elastic and could withstand high degrees of pressure. Histochemical analyses with hematoxylin and eosin, aldehyde fuschin-alcian blue, and toluidine blue staining demonstrated the presence of mature and well-formed chondrocytes in all the implants. There was no evidence of cartilage formation in the controls.

In a subsequent study, autologous cartilage seeded rods were implanted into rabbit corporas. The scaffolds were able to form cartilage rods in vivo, in the corpora. The engineered penile prostheses were stable, without any evidence of infection or erosion *(41)*.

These preliminary studies indicate that creation of a penile prosthesis composed of chondrocytes can be achieved using biodegradable polymer scaffolds as a cell-delivery vehicle. The engineered tissue forms a cartilaginous structure that resists high pressures. The use of an autologous system would preclude an immunologic reaction. This technology could be useful in the future for the creation of a biocompatible malleable prosthesis for patients undergoing penile reconstruction.

Formation of Renal Structures

End-stage renal failure is a devastating disease that involves multiple organs in affected individuals. Although dialysis can prolong survival for many patients with end-stage renal disease, only renal transplantation can currently restore normal function. Renal transplantation is severely limited by a critical donor shortage. Augmentation of either isolated or total renal function with kidney cell expansion in vitro and subsequent autologous transplantation may be a feasible solution. However, kidney reconstitution using tissue-engineering techniques is a challenging task. The kidney is responsible not only for urine excretion, but for several other important metabolic functions in which critical kidney byproducts, such as renin, erythropoietin, and vitamin D, play a large role. We explored the possibility of harvesting and expanding renal cells in vitro and implanting them in vivo in a three-dimensional organization in order to achieve a functional artificial renal unit wherein urine production could be achieved *(42,43)*. Studies demonstrated that renal cells can be successfully harvested, expanded in culture, and transplanted in vivo where the single suspended cells form and organize into functional renal structures that are able to excrete high levels of uric acid and creatinine through a yellow urine-like fluid. These findings suggest that this system may be able to replace transplantation in patients with end-stage failure.

Other approaches have also been pursued for renal functional replacement. Polysulphone hollow fibers have been prelined with various extracellular matrix (ECM) components and seeded with mammalian renal tubular and endothelial cells *(44)*. Permselective convective fluid transfer and active transport of salt and water were demonstrated. Using this approach, prototypic biohybrid constructs have been developed that are able to replicate the renal excretory functions. In addition, this system is able to facilitate gene and cell therapies by modifying the cells prior to seeding.

Injectable Therapies

URINARY INCONTINENCE AND VESICOURETERAL

Both urinary incontinence and vesicoureteral reflux are common conditions affecting the genitourinary system, wherein injectable bulking agents can be used for treatment. There are definite advantages in treating urinary incontinence and vesicoureteral reflux endoscopically. The method is simple and can be completed in less than 15 min, has a low morbidity, and can be performed in an outpatient basis.

The goal of several investigators has been to find an ideal implant material for the endoscopic treatment of reflux and incontinence. The ideal substance should be injectable, nonantigenic, nonmigratory, volume stable, and safe for human use. Toward this goal, we had previously conducted long-term studies to determine the effect of injectable chondrocytes in vivo *(38)*. We initially determined that alginate, a liquid solution of gluronic and mannuronic acid, embedded with chondrocytes, could serve as a synthetic substrate for the injectable delivery and maintenance of cartilage architecture in vivo. Alginate undergoes hydrolytic biodegradation and its degradation time can be varied depending on the concentration of each of the polysaccharides. The use of autologous cartilage for the treatment of vesicoureteral reflux in humans would satisfy all the requirements for an ideal injectable substance. A biopsy of the ear could be easily and quickly performed, followed by chondrocyte processing, and endoscopic injection of the autologous chondrocyte suspension for the treatment reflux.

Chondrocytes can be readily grown and expanded in culture. Neocartilage formation can be achieved in vitro and in vivo using chondrocytes cultured on synthetic biodegradable polymers *(38)*. In our experiments, the cartilage matrix replaced the alginate as the polysaccharide polymer underwent biodegradation. We then adapted the system for the treatment of vesicoureteral reflux in a porcine model *(39)*.

Six miniswine underwent bilateral creation of reflux. All six were found to have bilateral reflux without evidence of obstruction at 3 mo following the procedure. Chondrocytes were harvested from the left auricular surface of each miniswine and expanded with a final concentration of 50–150 × 10^6 viable cells/animal. The animals then underwent endoscopic repair of reflux with the injectable autologous chondrocyte solution on the right side only.

Cystoscopic and radiographic examinations were performed at 2, 4, and 6 mo after treatment. Cystoscopic examinations showed a smooth bladder wall. Cystograms showed no evidence of reflux on the treated side and persistent reflux in the uncorrected control ureter in all animals. All animals had a successful cure of reflux in the repaired ureter without evidence of hydronephrosis on excretory urography. The harvested ears had evidence of cartilage regrowth within one month of chondrocyte retrieval.

At the time of sacrifice, gross examination of the bladder injection site showed a well-defined rubbery-to-hard cartilage structure in the subureteral region. Histologic examination of these specimens using hematoxylin and eosin stains showed evidence of normal cartilage formation The polymer gels were progressively replaced by cartilage with increasing time. Aldehyde fuschin-alcian blue staining suggested the presence of chondroitin sulfate. Microscopic analyses of the tissues surrounding the injection site showed no inflammation. Tissue sections from the bladder, ureters, lymph nodes, kidneys, lungs, liver, and spleen showed no evidence of chondrocyte or alginate migration, or granuloma formation.

Our studies showed that chondrocytes can be easily harvested and combined with alginate in vitro, the suspension can be easily injected cystoscopically and the elastic cartilage tissue formed is able to correct vesicoureteral reflux without any evidence of obstruction *(39)*.

Using the same line of reasoning as with the chondrocyte technology, our group investigated the possibility of using autologous muscle cells *(45)*. In vivo experiments were conducted in minipigs and reflux was successfully corrected.

The chondrocyte technology is currently being used in FDA-sanctioned studies for in-patients with reflux and incontinence *(see* Fig. 4) *(46)*. In addition to its use for the endoscopic treatment of reflux and urinary incontinence, the system of injectable autologous cells may also be applicable for the treatment of other medical conditions, such as rectal incontinence, dysphonia, plastic reconstruction, and wherever an injectable permanent biocompatible material is needed.

TESTICULAR FUNCTIONAL REPLACEMENT

Leydig cells are the major source of testosterone production in males. Patients with testicular dysfunction require androgen replacement for somatic development. Conventional treatment for testicular dysfunction

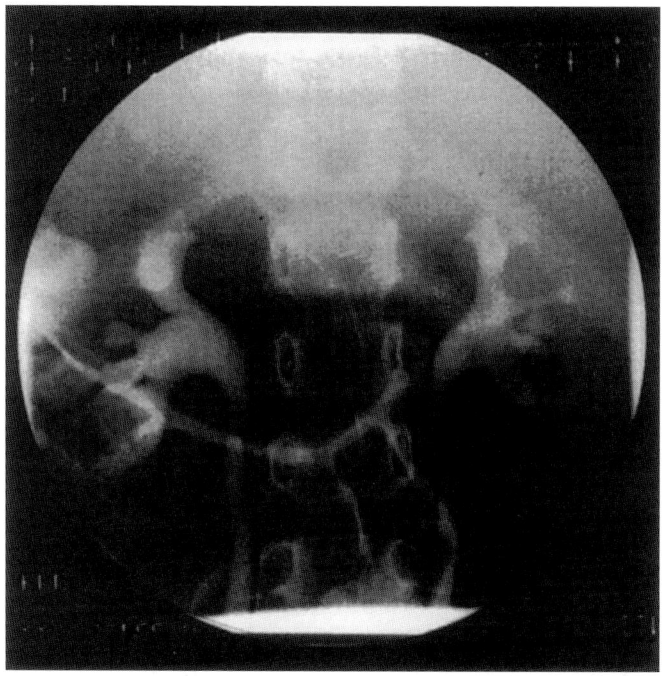

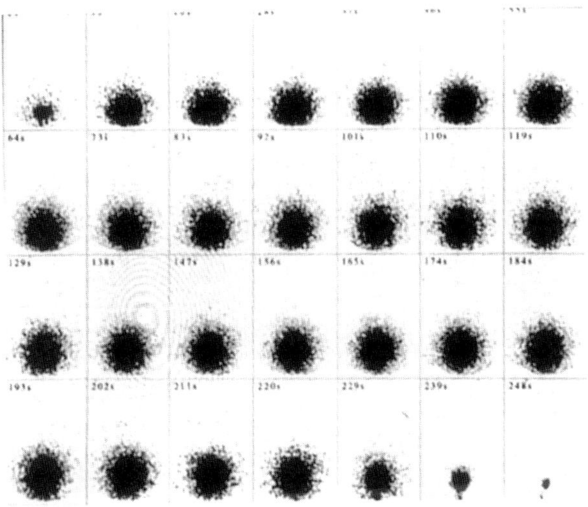

Fig. 4. (Top) Preoperative VCUG in a patient shows bilateral vesicoureteral reflux. (Bottom) Postoperative radionuclide cystogram after endoscopic treatment with autologous engineered chondrocytes shows resolution of reflux bilaterally.

consists of periodic intramuscular (im) injections of chemically modified testosterone, or more recently, of skin patch applications. However, long-term nonpulsatile testosterone therapy is not optimal and can cause multiple problems, including erythropoiesis and bone density changes. The possibility of using leydig cell microencapsulation for controlled testosterone replacement was evaluated *(47)*. Microencapsulated leydig cells may offer several advantages, such as serving as a semipermeable barrier between the transplanted cells and the host's immune system, as well as allowing for the long-term physiological release of testosterone.

Purified leydig cells from rat testes were prepared on a Percoll gradient. Cell viability and identification was performed by Trypan blue and 3b-hydroxysteroid dehydrogenase (3b-HSD), respectively. Leydig cells were suspended in 1.2% sodium alginate solution and extruded through an air-jet nozzle into a 1.5% $CaCl_2$ solution were they gelled, and were further coated with 0.1% poly-L-lysine. The encapsulated cells were pulsed with human chorionic gonadotropin (hCG) every 24 h. The medium was sampled at different time-points after hCG stimulation and analyzed for testosterone production. MTT assay was performed every day to ensure cell viability. Control experiments were performed using nonencapsulated purified leydig cells under the same conditions *(47)*.

More then 90% of the cells recovered from the Percoll gradient stained positively for 3b-HSD. Both Trypan blue exclusion and MTT assays showed that 95% of the cells were viable. Biochemical measurements, which were performed every 4 h, showed that the microencapsulated leydig cells produced testosterone. Testosterone levels in the presence of hCG ranged between 35–60 ng/dL/10*(6)*/24 h. Testosterone levels measured from nonencapsulated leydig cells ranged between 45–50 ng/dL/10*(6)*/24 h.

Microencapsulated leydig cells are viable and are able to produce high levels of testosterone. The microencapsulation system renders the cells nonimmunogenic. These studies suggest that microencapsulated leydig cells may be able to replace or supplement testosterone in situations were anorchia or testicular failure is present.

FETAL TISSUE ENGINEERING

The prenatal diagnosis of patients with bladder disease is now more prevalent. Prenatal ultrasonography allows for a thorough survey of fetal anatomy. The absence of bladder filling, a mass of echogenic tissue on the lower abdominal wall, or a low set umbilicus during prenatal sonographic examination may suggest the diagnosis of bladder exstrophy. These findings and the presence of intraluminal intestinal calcifications suggest the presence of a cloacal malformation.

The natural consequence of the evolution in prenatal diagnosis led to the use of intervention before birth to reverse potentially life-threatening processes. However, the concept of prenatal intervention itself is not limited to this narrow group of indications. A prenatal, rather than a postnatal, diagnosis of exstrophy may be beneficial under certain circumstances. There is now a renewed interest in performing a single-stage reconstruction in some patients with bladder exstrophy. Limiting factors for following a single- or multiple-stage approach may include the findings of a small, fibrotic bladder patch without either elasticity or contractility, or a hypoplastic bladder.

There are several strategies that may be pursued, using today's technological and scientific advances, which may facilitate the future prenatal management of patients with bladder disease. Having a ready supply of urologic-associated tissue for surgical reconstruction at birth may be advantageous. Theoretically, once the diagnosis of bladder exstrophy is confirmed prenatally, a small bladder and skin biopsy could be obtained via ultrasound guidance. These biopsy materials could then be processed and the different cell types expanded in vitro. Using tissue-engineering techniques developed at our center and described previously, reconstituted bladder and skin structures in vitro could then be readily available at the time of birth for a one-stage reconstruction, allowing for an adequate anatomic and functional closure .

Toward this end, we conducted a series of experiments using fetal lambs. *(48,49)*. Bladder exstrophy was created surgically in 10 90–95-d gestation fetal lambs. The lambs were randomly divided into two groups of five. In Group I, a small fetal bladder specimen was harvested via fetoscopy. The bladder specimen was separated and muscle and urothelial cells were harvested and expanded separately under sterile conditions in a humidified 5% CO_2 chamber, as previously described. Seven to ten days prior to delivery, the expanded bladder muscle cells were seeded on one side and the urothelial cells on the opposite side of a 20-cm^2 biodegradable polyglycolic acid polymer scaffold. After delivery, all lambs in Group I had surgical closure of their bladder using the tissue engineered bladder tissue. No fetal bladder harvest was performed in the Group II lambs, and bladder exstrophy closure was performed using only the native bladder. Cystograms were performed 3 and 8 wk after surgery. The engineered bladders were more compliant ($p=0.01$) and had a higher capacity ($p=0.02$) than the native bladder closure group. Histologic analysis of the engineered tissue showed a normal histological pattern, indistinguishable from native bladder at 2 mo *(42)*. Similar prenatal studies were performed in lambs, engineering skin for reconstruction at birth *(49)*.

These studies show that the potential for replicating this technology in humans is possible. Other tissues, such as cartilage, corpora cavernosa, and skeletal muscle can also be harvested and expanded in the same manner. Similar studies addressing these tissues are now in progress in our laboratory.

In addition to being able to manage the bladder exstrophy complex in utero with tissue-engineering techniques, one could also manage patients after birth in a similar manner, whenever a prenatal diagnosis is not assured. In these instances, bladder tissue biopsies could be obtained at the time of the initial surgery. Different tissues could be harvested and stored for future reconstruction, if necessary. A tissue bank for exstrophy complex patients could preserve different cell types indefinitely.

In addition to having an exstrophy complex tissue bank serve as a repository of cells for future tissue reconstitution, it could also serve as a resource to elucidate the cellular, molecular, and genetic mechanisms required for the development and future prevention of these anomalies.

GENE THERAPY AND TISSUE ENGINEERING

Based on the feasibility of tissue-engineering techniques in which cells seeded on biodegradable polymer scaffolds form tissue when implanted in vivo, the possibility was explored of developing a neo-organ system for in vivo gene therapy *(50)*.

In a series of studies conducted in our laboratory, human urothelial cells were harvested, expanded in vitro, and seeded on biodegradable polymer scaffolds. The cell-polymer complex was then transfected with PGL3-luc, pCMV-luc, and pCMVβ-gal promoter-reporter gene constructs. The transfected cell-polymer scaffolds were then implanted in vivo and the engineered tissues were retrieved at different time-points after implantation. Results indicated that successful gene transfer could be achieved using biodegradable polymer scaffolds as a urothelial cell-delivery vehicle. The transfected cell/polymer scaffold formed organ-like structures with functional expression of the transfected genes *(50)*.

This technology is applicable throughout the spectrum of diseases that may be manageable with tissue engineering. For example, one can envision the use of effecting in vivo gene delivery through the ex vivo transfection of tissue engineered cell/polymer scaffolds for the genetic modification of diseased corporal smooth muscle cells harvested from impotent patients. Studies of human corpus cavernosum smooth muscle cells have suggested that cellular overproduction of the cytokine, transforming growth factor-1 (TGF-1) may lead to the synthesis and accumulation of excess collagen in patients with arterial insufficiency resulting in corporal fibrosis. Prostaglandin E1 (PGE1) was shown to suppress this effect in vitro. Theoretically, the in vitro genetic modification of corporal smooth muscle cells harvested from an impotent patient, resulting in either a reduction in the expression of the TGF-1 gene, or the overexpression of genes responsible for PGE1 production, could lead to the resumption of erectile functionality once these cells were used to repopulate the diseased corporal bodies.

REFERENCES

1. Atala A (1997) Tissue engineering in the genitourinary system. In: Atala A, Mooney D, eds, *Synthetic Biodegradable Polymer Scaffolds*. Boston, MA: Birkhauser, pp. 149–164.
2. Neuhof H (1917) Fascial transplantation into visceral defects: An experimental and clinical study. *Surg Gynecol Obstet* 25:383.
3. Tsuji I, Ishida H, Fujieda J (1961) Experimental cystoplasty using preserved bladder graft. *J Urol* 85:42.
4. Probst M, Dahiya R, Carrier S, Tanagho EA (1997) Reproduction of funtional smooth muscle tissue and partial bladder replacement. *Brit J Urol* 79:505.
5. Kelami A, Ludtke-Handjery A, Korb G, Roll J, Schnell J, Danigel KH (1970) Alloplastic replacement of the urinary bladder wall with lyophilized human dura. *Europ Surg Res* 2:195.
6. Jelly O (1970) Segmental cystectomy with peritoneoplasty. *Urol Int* 25:236.
7. Cheng E, Rento R, Grayhack TJ, Oyasu R, McVary KT (1994) Reversed seromuscular flaps in the urinary tract in dogs. *J Urol* 152:2252.
8. Kropp BP, Sawyer BD, Shannon HE, Rippy MK, Badylak SF, Adams MC, et al. (1996) Characterization of small intestinal submucosa regenerated canine detrusor: assessment of reinnervation, in vitro compliance and contractility. *J Urol* 156:599.
9. Gleeson MJ, Griffith DP (1992) The use of alloplastic biomaterials in bladder substitution. *J Urol* 148:1377.
10. Kudish HG (1957) The use of polyvinyl sponge for experimental cystoplasty. *J Urol* 78:232.
11. Bona AV, De Gresti A (1966) Partial substitution of urinary bladder with Teflon prothesis. *Minerva Urol* 18:43.
12. Monsour MJ, Mohammed R, Gorham SD, French DA, Scott R (1987) An assessment of a collagen/vicryl composite memebrane to repair defects of the urinary bladder in rabbits. *Urol Res* 15:235.
13. Tsuji I, Kuroda K, Fujieda J, Shiraishi Y, Kunishima K, Orikasa S (1967) Clinical experience of bladder reconstruction using preserved bladder and gelatin sponge in the case of bladder cancer. *J Urol* 98:91.
14. Fujita K (1978) The use of resin-sprayed thin paper for urinary bladder regeneration. *Invest Urol* 15:355.
15. Rohrmann D, Albrecht D, Hannappel J, Gerlach R, Schwarzkopp G, Lutzeyer W (1996) Alloplastic replacement of the urinary bladder. *J Urol* 156:2094.
16. de Boer WI, Schuller AG, Vermay M, van der Kwast TH (1994) Expression of growth factors and receptors during specific phases in regenerating urothelium after acute injury in vivo. *Am J Path* 145:1199.
17. Baker R, Kelly T, Tehan T, Putman C, Beaugard E (1955) Subtotal cystectomy and total bladder regeneration in treatment of bladder cancer. *J Am Med Assoc* 168:1178.

18. Gorham SD, French DA, Shivas AA, Scott R (1989) Some observations on the regeneration of smooth muscle in the repaired urinary bladder of the rabbit. *Eur Urol* 16:440.

19. Cilento BJ, Freeman MR, Schneck FX, Retik AB, Atala A (1994) Phenotypic and cytogenetic characterization of human bladder urothelia expanded in vitro. *J Urol* 152:665.

20. Tobin MS, Freeman MR, Atala A (1994) Maturational response of normal human urothelial cells in culture is dependent on extracellular matrix and serum additives. *Surgical Forum* 45:786.

21. Freeman MR, Yoo JJ, Raab G, Soker S, Adam RM, Schneck FX, et al. (1997) Heparin-Binding EGF-like growth factor is an autocrine growth factor for human urothelial cells and is synthesized by epithelial and smooth muscle cells in the human bladder. *J Clin Investig* 99:1028.

22. Machluf M, Atala A (1998) Tissue engineering: emerging concepts. *Graft* 1:31.

23. Atala A (1996) Replacement of urologic associated mucosa. *J Urol* 156:338.

24. Atala A (1998) Autologous cell transplantation for urologic reconstruction. *J Urol* 159:2.

25. Wesolowski SA, Fries CC, Karlson KE, et al (1961) Porosity: primary determinant of ultimate fate of synthetic vascular grafts. *Surg* 50:91.

26. Mikos AG, Sarakinos G, Lyman MD, et al. (1993) Prevascularization of porous biodegradable polymers. *Biotechnol Bioeng* 42:716.

27. Atala A, Freeman MR, Vacanti JP, Shepard J, Retik AB (1993) Implantation in vivo and retrieval of artificial structures consisting of rabbit and human urothelium and human bladder muscle. *J Urol* 150:608.

28. Atala A, Vacanti JP, Peters CA, Mandell J, Retik AB, Freeman MR (1992) Formation of urothelial structures in vivo from dissociated cells attached to biodegradable polymer scaffolds in vitro. *J Urol* 148:658.

29. Cliento BG Jr, Atala A (1999) Future frontiers in hypospadias. In: Ehrlich RM, Alter GJ, eds, *Reconstructive and Plastic Surgery of the External Genitalia: Adult and Pediatric.* Philadelphia, PA: W.B. Saunders.

30. Chen F, Yoo J, Atala A (1999) Acellular collagen matrix as a possible "off the shelf" biomaterial for urethral repair. *Urology* 54:1.

31. Atala A, Guzman LF, Retik AB (1999) A novel inert collagen matrix for hypospadias repair. *J Urol* 162:1148–1151.

32. Yoo JJ, Meng J, Oberpenning F, Atala A (1998) Bladder augmentation using allogenic bladder submucosa seeded with cells. *Urology* 51:221.

33. Atala A (1999) Creation of bladder tissue in vitro and in vivo: a system for organ replacement. In: Baskin, Hayward, eds, *Advances in Bladder Research.* New York: Kluwer Academic/Plenum, pp. 31–42.

34. Oberpenning F, Meng J, Yoo JJ, Atala A (1999) Bladder replacement with tissue-engineered neo-organs. *Nature Biotechnology* 17:149.

35. Kershen RT, Yoo JJ, Moreland RB, Krane RJ, Atala A (1998) Novel system for the formation of human corpus cavernosum smooth muscle tissue in vivo. *J Urol* 159:156(suppl).

36. Park HJ, Yoo JJ, Kershen R, Atala A (1999) Reconstitution of corporal tissue using human cavernosal smooth muscle and endothelial cells. *J Urol* 162:1106.

37. Nukui F, Okamoto S, Nagata M, Kurokawa J, Fukui J (1997) Complications and reimplantation of penile implants. *Int J Urol* 4:52.

38. Atala A, Cima LG, Kim W, Paige KT, Vacanti JP, Retik AB, Vacanti CA (1993) Injectable alginate seeded with chondrocytes as a potential treatment for vesicoureteral reflux. *J Urol* 150:745.

39. Atala A, Kim W, Paige KT, Vacanti CA, Retik AB (1994) Endoscopic treatment of vesicoureteral reflux with chondrocyte-alginate suspension. *J Urol* 152:641.

40. Yoo JJ, Lee I, Atala A (1998) Cartilage rods as a potential material for penile reconstruction. *J Urol* 160:1164.

41. Yoo JJ, Park HJ, Lee I, Atala A (1999) Autologous engineered cartilage rods for penile reconstruction. *J Urol* 162:1119–1121.

42. Atala A, Schlussel RN, Retik AB (1995) Renal cell growth in vivo after attachment to biodegradable polymer scaffolds. *J Urol* 153:4(suppl).

43. Yoo J, Ashkar S, Atala A (1996) Creation of fuctional kidney structures with excretion of urine-like fluid in vivo. *Pediatrics* 98S:605.

44. Humes HD, Buffington DA, MacKay SM, Funke AJ, Weitzel WF (1999) Replacement of renal function in uremic animals with a tissue-engineered kidney. *Nature Biotechnol* 17:451.

45. Cilento BG, Atala A (1995) Treatment of reflux and incontinence with autologous chrondrocytes and bladder muscle cells. *Dialog Ped Urol* 18:1.

46. Kershen R, Atala A (1999) New advances in injectable therapies for the treatment of incontinence and vesicoureteral reflux. *Reconstruct Urol* 26:81.

47. Machlouf M, Boorjian S, Caffaratti J, Kershen R, Atala A (1999) Therapeutic delivery of testosterone using microencapsulated leydig cells. *J Urol* 161:311.

48. Fauza DO, Fishman S, Mehegan K, Atala A (1998) Videofetoscopically assisted fetal tissue engineering: bladder augmentation. *J Ped Surg* 33:7.

49. Fauza DO, Fishman S, Mehegan K, Atala A (1998) Videofetoscopically assisted fetal tissue engineering: skin replacement. *J Ped Surg* 33:357.

50. Yoo JJ, Atala A (1997) A novel gene delivery system using urothelial tissue engineered neo-organs. *J Urol* 158:1066.

3

Injectable Agents
for Urinary Incontinence

Edward J. McGuire, MD

CONTENTS

BACKGROUND
INCONTINENCE SUBDIVIDED BY A SPECIFIC TYPE
    OF URETHRAL DYSFUNCTION
COLLAGEN OUTCOME DATA
ANTEGRADE INJECTION
RESULTS IN CHILDREN
OTHER AGENTS
CARBON STEEL PARTICLES
TECHNICAL DETAIL
REFERENCES

BACKGROUND

Injectable materials have been sporadically used for the treatment of urinary incontinence for many years. Solomon Berg, a urologist, reported, at a meeting of the New England Section of the American Urological Association in the late 1970s, that polytetrafluoroethylene paste could be efficacious in the treatment of incontinence when injected into the urethral wall in elderly women *(1)*. The material, polytetrafluoroethylene, had also been used by surgeons for the injection of the vocal cords, when there was paralysis of one cord, to improve phonation as they would later use collagen *(2)*. Kaufman et al. *(3)* and Lewis et al. *(4)* reported rather extensive experience with the use of polytetrafluoroethylene paste in males and in females with incontinence. Patient

From: *Urologic Prostheses:*
The Complete, Practical Guide to Devices, Their Implantation and Patient Follow Up
Edited by: C. C. Carson © Humana Press Inc., Totowa, NJ

selection for the use of this injectable agent was not specifically described, but Politano et al. continued to use the material and to report on efficacy *(5,6)*. Other workers were unable to duplicate precisely the results reported by the Miami group *(7–9)*. In addition, complications related to use of this material began to be reported. Boykin et al. *(10)* described complete urinary obstruction following periurethral polytetrafluoroethylene therapy. Hanau et al. *(11)* described a large Teflon-filled cyst as a complication of periurethral teflon therapy, which had to be evacuated. Dewan and Fraundorfer *(12)* reported migration of periurethral polytetrafluoroethylene into the skin in a patient who had received the material for urinary incontinence. This was associated with an intense itching response. The material was identified in the skin by biopsy. At the Mayo Clinic, Malizia et al. *(13)* reported that polytetrafluoroethylene particles, following periurethral injection in female dogs and male monkeys, migrated to pelvic lymph nodes and the lungs. The material was identified by the Malizia group by X-ray microanalysis. The somewhat unpredictable results, and the description of migration of the particles, lead many workers to abandon polytetrafluoroethylene as a material for bulking the urethra. However, Herschorn and Glazer *(14)* reported a new series with favorable results from teflon injection in women with stress incontinence. Moreover, despite the fact that the material does seem to migrate and to be taken up by regional and distant lymph nodes, there are no reports of adverse effects in humans related to the material, other than that reported by Dewan and Fraundorfer *(12)*.

INCONTINENCE SUBDIVIDED BY A SPECIFIC TYPE OF URETHRAL DYSFUNCTION

Investigation of patients with stress incontinence, using video urodynamics, led to the identification of various subtypes of urethral dysfunction. Type III stress incontinence, probably the most important variant, was characterized by an open nonfunctional vesical outlet on video urodynamic studies when first identified *(see* Fig. 1) *(15)*. The incontinence associated with this abnormality of urethral function is severe. Patients with this kind of incontinence fail standard suspension procedures for stress incontinence *(15–19)*.

Poor or absent function of the proximal urethral sphincter, or Type III stress incontinence, can be diagnosed by video urodynamic studies or leak point pressure testing. In addition to the demonstration that this occurs in some women with stress incontinence *(20,21)*, video urodynamic and other studies show that proximal urethral sphincter dysfunction occurs in males incontinent after radical or nonradical prostatectomy, in most patients with myelodysplasia, in most persons

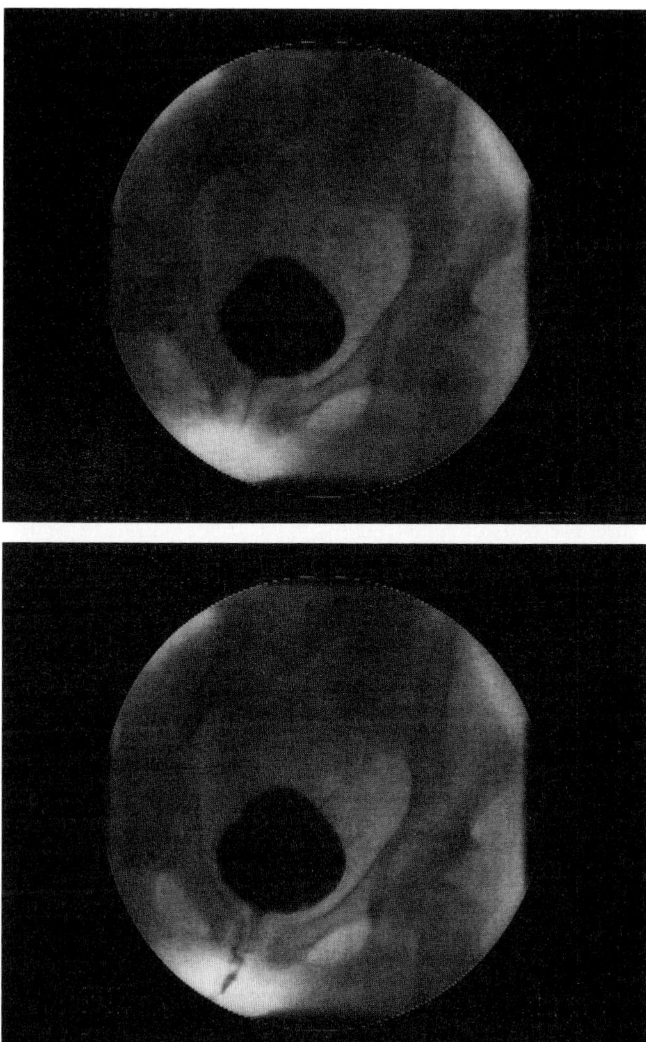

Fig. 1. Upright cystogram in a young woman with congenital absence of proximal sphincter function related to myelodysplasia. Note the leakage that occurred at an abdominal pressure of 16.

with sacral agenesis, and patients with peripheral neuropathy associated with radical pelvic extirpative surgery on the rectum or uterus, and in patients with T12 spinal cord injury *(22–27)*. For these severe kinds of incontinence, only a sling, wrapping the urethra with fascia, an artificial sphincter, or an injectable agent seems to work effectively *(28–29)*. However, a study of a series of young women with myelodysplasia treated with sling procedures for congenital failure of the internal sphincter showed that the local increase in pressure beneath the sling, within the urethral lumen, was actually small. Although the sling did effectively prevent leakage of urine driven by abdominal pressure *(30)*. Parenthetically, children with myelodysplasia treated with the artificial urinary sphincter placed at the bladder neck have a definite propensity to develop upper tract deterioration; something not seen in patients treated by slings *(31)*. Upon investigation, the deterioration in upper tract function turned out to be related to the greater efficacy of closure of the proximal urethra brought about by the artificial sphincter when compared to the sling. The artificial sphincter raised both the detrusor leak point pressure and the abdominal leak point pressure, leading to back pressure effects on the ureter. Although slings are somewhat less efficient overall, in terms of restoration of complete continence, than the artificial sphincter, they are not associated with upper urinary tract deterioration.

Shortliffe et al. *(32)* reported the first successful use of injectable collagen material in women with severe stress incontinence. Although the patients were greatly improved or cured as a result of the injection, the effect of the material injected into the urethra was not discernable by careful, painstaking urethral closing pressure measurements. The concept that incontinence associated with a poorly functional proximal urethra could be treated successfully if the urethra at, or very close to, the bladder neck was simply closed or coapted emerged from this data, and the earlier data in myelodysplastic children. The amount of compressive force required appeared to be relatively low.

COLLAGEN OUTCOME DATA

Despite the rationale for its use, the early clinical trials with collagen resulted in less-than-impressive results. Injection of the material did raise the abdominal leak point pressure, incontinence symptoms often improved, but the effect was unfortunately, usually transient. At first it was not appreciated that multiple injections were required for success, and there was little knowledge about the proper selection of patients for collagen injection therapy. Patients were often "selected" for collagen treatment simply because they failed everything else. With experience, results improved. However, results in women, in virtually any series, are better than those reported for men. Thus Herschorn and Radomski *(33)* reported a 71% dry rate at 1 yr and 46% dry rate at 3 yr without additional collagen therapy. Faerber reported 83% of elderly women with Type I incontinence dry at 10.3 mean mo after the last injection *(34)*.

Richardson et al. *(35)* reported a group of women with intrinsic sphincter dysfunction treated by collagen, with a mean follow-up of

46 mo; 83% of this group were cured, 5% greatly improved, and 17% unchanged or worse. The median number of treatments was 2. The mean increase in the leak point pressure in women who were cured or improved was 65.4 cm/H_2O and in those who did not improve, the increase in leak point pressure was only 14. In the initial experience with collagen, the material was delivered by periurethral injection. Faerber et al. *(36)* showed that for equivalent results, only half the amount of collagen was needed when the material was injected transurethrally. Herschorn et al. *(37)* used on average 12.7 mL of collagen in women and 51.8 mL in men, when the treatment was administered by the periurethral route.

Cespedes et al. *(38)*, in a large series of men with incontinence related to radical prostatectomy, used three or more injections spread over a 4- to 6-mo period and achieved a 70% dry or substantially improved rate. The average amount of collagen used in these male patients was 30 mL. Cross et al. *(39)* used 9 mL of collagen on average and two injections separated by 1 mo to achieve a 74% substantive improvement rate in 139 women, using the transurethral route of injection. Cespedes et al. *(38)* and Cross et al. *(39)* used a dedicated instrument for delivery of collagen with a stable rigid needle. Despite this, the amounts required in men are much higher than that required for women.

ANTEGRADE INJECTION

In an effort to improve results in males, Klutke et al. *(40)* described a technique for antegrade injection of collagen. This necessitated percutaneous access to the bladder and then visualization of the anastomotic ring from above through the bladder. The procedure was associated with good results after one injection in early reports. A later report by Klutke et al. *(41)* noted at a mean follow-up of 28 mo only, 10% of patients were cured and 35% improved. The mean total volume of collagen injected was only 14.5 mL. Although this is a small series, and the results reported are not quite equivalent to those with the transurethral, conventional, injection the amount of collagen used is about 50% of that used in the traditional method.

RESULTS IN CHILDREN

Early results suggested a possible role for collagen in children *(42,43)*, but a lack of durability has led to the gradual abandonment of the agent for treatment of incontinence, even though it is often effective in the short term *(44)*.

OTHER AGENTS

The fact that collagen was efficacious in the short term, but its durability questionable, led to efforts to develop a more stable, longer-lasting material for bulking. Hidar et al. *(45)* reported the results of periurethral injection of silicone microimplants in 25 women with intrinsic sphincter dysfunction. The early success was 80%, but at 3 yr, only 60% were improved. Bugel et al. *(46)* reported that 26% of men with postprostatectomy incontinence related to both radical or nonradical prostatectomy, were improved at 12 mo, but that was a decline from a 40% improvement noted at 1 mo following the injection of the silicone microimplant. Guys et al. *(47)* used Microplastique in children. At 16 mo, mean follow-up 33% of the children were "dry." All of these children had spina bifida. These results are surprisingly close to those outcomes reported for collagen in men, women, and children in many series, including those by Smith et al., Yokoyama et al., Winters et al., O'Connell et al., and Abosief et al. *(48–51)*. That leads to the conclusion that it may be tissue factors that determine outcome here, rather than the material injected.

CARBON STEEL PARTICLES

This is a relatively recent development and consists of small spherical nonreactive carbon steel spheres in a gel vehicle. The injection process is somewhat more difficult than with collagen and a slow injection technique at low pressure is best. Use of the agent takes practice and the agent has not been found very useful in men. Scarring of the urethra in the area of the prostatic anastomosis after radical prostatectomy creates a situation where the material is very difficult to inject. In women, however, reasonable results have been reported and these appear to be relatively durable. The number of published reports on carbon steel particles is still very small.

TECHNICAL DETAIL

Patient Selection for Injectable Material

WOMEN

In general, longer-lasting results will be seen in older women with low Valsalva leak point pressure stress incontinence, and little or no urethral mobility. Reports of short-term success in younger patients with higher leak point pressures and urethral mobility exist, but collagen cannot be considered the most durable or effective method for this kind of incontinence in this age group. Upright video urodynamic studies are the best way to investigate patients and to determine which patient may or may not be acceptable for collagen; however, simple pelvic examination demonstrating a fixed urethra and stress leakage is also a reasonable and accurate method. If this is combined with endoscopy to evaluate the appearance of the bladder outlet and proximal urethra, a good idea of the status of the urethra can be gained.

MEN

Incontinence after radical prostatectomy is associated with rigidity and scarring of the area of the urethral-bladder anastomosis and the short segment of urethra distal to that point, which leads to the external sphincter proper (*see* Fig. 2). Injection into these areas is difficult because the tissue is not very forgiving. Placement of the needle is not as difficult as it is in women because the urethra is rigid and does not move away from the needle (*see* Fig. 3). I like to inject collagen through the anastomotic ring into the tissue just above, if possible. This tissue is softer and takes the collagen better. The volitional sphincter is a pretty definite landmark, and asking the patient to close and open his rectal sphincter shows the operator where the volitional external sphincter is. It is the urethra superior to this point that one needs to inject, but if this area is very short and the anastomosis is close to or virtually on the upper edge of the volitional sphincter, injection is usually futile. In some cases, injection via the external sphincter into the short suprasphincter segment is possible. That means the needle entry point is in the main part of the volitional sphincter. This, however, can be extremely painful. Whether it is or not seems to be somewhat unpredictable. In general, we use two syringes of collagen on each side in men and use the same lateral position for the injection; never at 12:00 or 6:00 because the tissue there is thin. We are prepared to do four to five injections, separated by monthly intervals. If there is no change in symptoms after four injections, and we cannot demonstrate any change in the leak point pressure, we stop the injections.

Complications of injections in males in the office include syncopal episodles, possible allergic reactions, and/or urinary retention, although uncommon. Syncopal episodes may occur following the procedure. This often happens when a patient gets up and walks around. As such, they are difficult to anticipate and we now have the patient stay on the treatment table for 15–20 min following the injection procedure so this simply does not occur. The plane of injection is submucosal, hence, an atrophic on scared urethral lining may prejudice operative results. However, the area of the urethra in which the collagen or other material can be injected for effect is short, beginning at the bladder outlet and ending just above the midurethral high-pressure zone. The latter is the area of the volitional sphincter. Injectable materials cannot be delivered in the area of the volitional sphincter, very efficiently because the operator

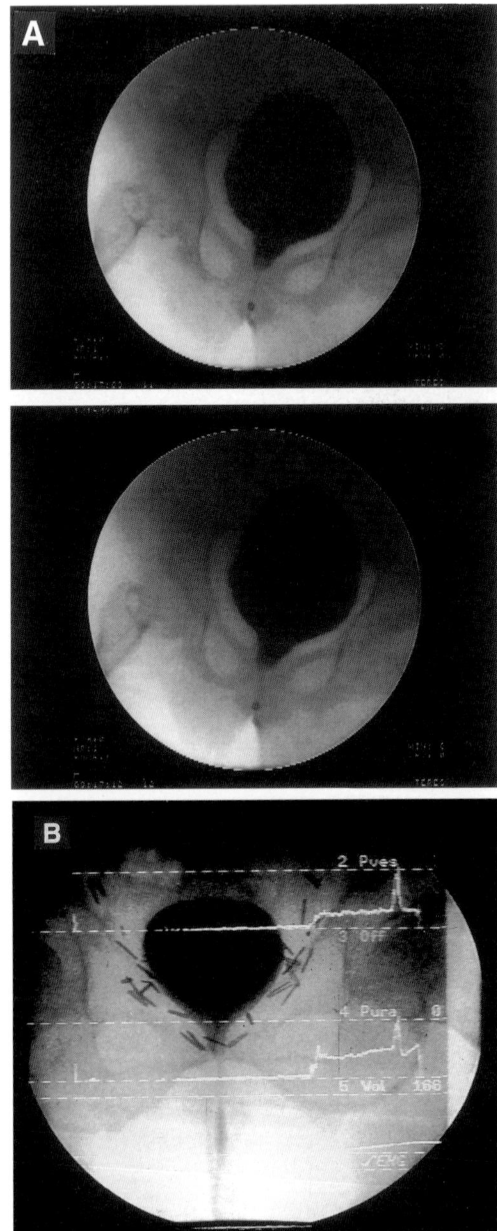

Fig. 2. (A) Typical postprostatecomy incontinence. The radio-opaque maker is located in the external sphincter, which functions normally. The area to be injected is superior to the external sphincter in the area of the anastomosis. Note contrast leaked into the bulbous urethra. **(B)** Leak point pressure testing in a patient with post prostatectomy incontinence. Despite good function of the external sphincter leakage occurs at a pressure of 80 cm. The effect of external sphincter activity is clear: the urethra is *closed* there. but leakage occurs anyway. The injection should be done just at or just distal to the anastomotic ring.

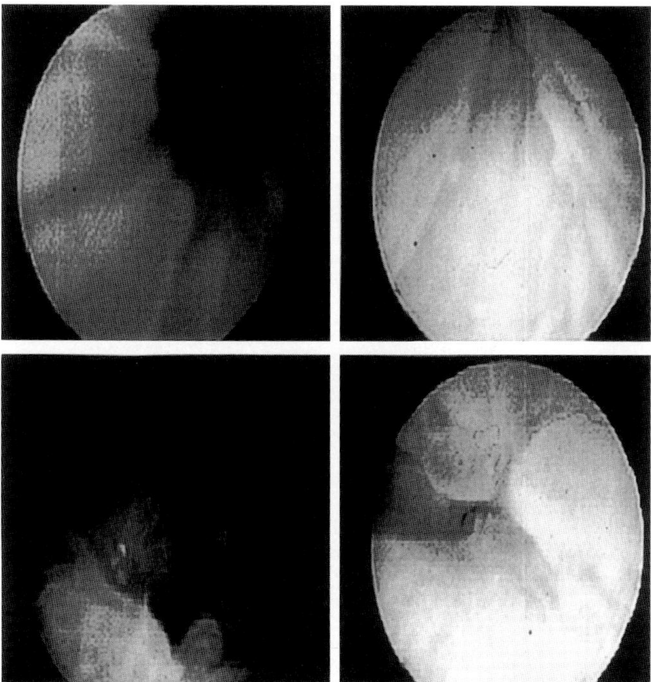

Fig. 3. Injection sequence starting upper left: showing a wide open anastomotic ring. Lower left: detail of edema and poor tissue in the area. Upper right: partial coaptation after 5 mL injection, and reasonable closure after 10 mL injected.

cannot visualize the urethral lumen well, nor can the needle depth be controlled. The urethra superior to this area is the proper site for injection and is relatively easily visualized because it is often wide open. The most effective instrument is a dedicated endoscope for the injection of bulking agents. There are two or three such instruments. A stabilized and rigid needle is best. In addition, the needle should move independently of the instrument, either manually by moving the needle in and out, or by clasping the needle in a working element with a Nesbitt-like feature, so that it can be moved with one finger (*see* Fig. 4). If the needle is not locked to a sliding part of the instrument, two people are required for the injection. This leads to problems as the operator can inadvertently move the endoscope and displace the needle or change the alignment or angle of the needle during the injection process.

Techniques: Collagen

The Wolf instrument is what we use (*see* Fig. 3). It has a 30° lens. The operator locates the bladder neck and moves the endoscope distally, exposing 1.0–1.5 cm of the proximal urethra. The endoscope is then

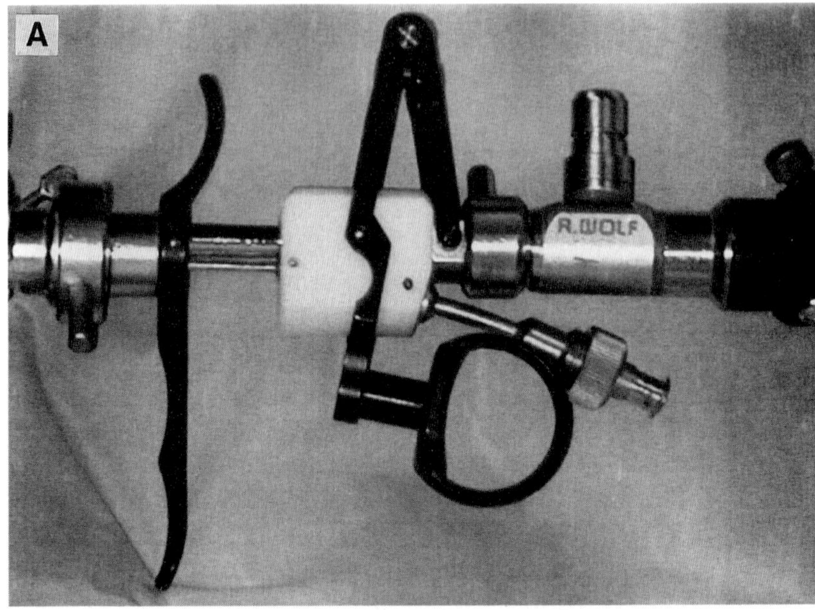

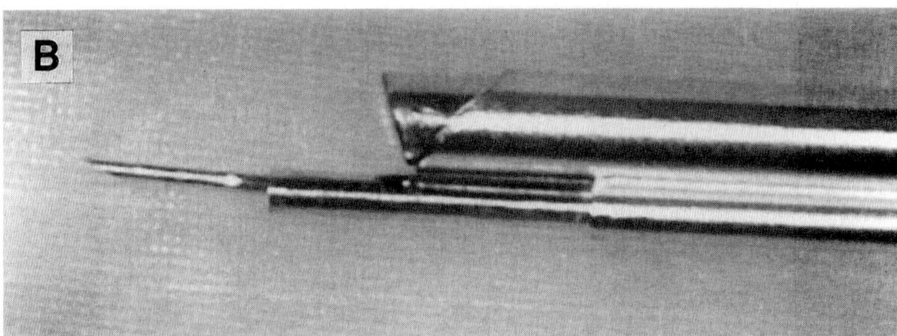

Fig. 4. (A) Detail of the instrument that contains an independent apparatus to move the injection needle. **(B)** Detail of needle at the tip of the instrument.

angled sharply to the left side of the urethra and the needle placed quickly into the mucosa and then the submucosa. Once the mucosa is penetrated, the instrument can be deangulated so that it is again parallel to the long axis of the urethra and the needle advanced along the urethral wall toward the bladder neck. We use for anesthesia 1% Xylocaine, about 0.2 mL is injected with a tuberculin syringe into the submucosal plane. After that, the syringe is changed for a collagen syringe, and the material is injected slowly. Both the local anesthetic and the collagen, when injected, should cause swelling of the urethral mucosa toward the urethral lumen. Usually 2.5 mL of collagen are injected in each side. At

12:00 and 6:00, the urethral tissue is relatively thin and it is hard to get the collagen into the right plane, so injection in this area produces poor coaptation of the lumen at those sites, which is why we tend to use the 3:00 and 9:00 position.

Patients are pretreated with antibiotics and are observed after the procedure to he sure they are able to empty their bladder. Although urinary retention is unusual, when it does occur it is transient. This does not appear to be caused by the collagen itself, but perhaps is a temporary effect of the local anesthetic.

Techniques: Durasphere Injection

The technique is similar, but there is no dedicated instrument, therefore changing syringes requires practice and two people. The injection technique is very different from that of collagen, and local anesthesia because it increases local tissue pressure, seems to interfere with the injection process, creating untoward resistance. Thus, a 10–15 min exposure of the urethra to Xylocaine jelly is preferable to the injection of local anesthetic. The same landmarks are used, but the material must be injected very slowly and very superficially. The needle should be carefully controlled as to the depth that it enters the urethral wall. There are marks on the needle to enable the operator to do so. About 0.5 cm is the maximum that the needle should be advanced. Too much pressure on the device during an injection leads to loss of the gel vehicle, the carbon steel particles line up in the needle and block it, so that one can no longer inject. In our limited experience, durasphere material is more difficult to inject than collagen, but the durability, anecdotally, is better than that of collagen.

REFERENCES

1. Berg, Solomon (1970) Personal comunicators.
2. Ford EN, Staskowski PA, Bless DM (1995) Antolgous collagen vocal cord injection: a preliminary clinical study. *Laryngoscope* 105:944–948.
3. Kaufman M, Lockhart JL, Silverstein NJ, Politano VA (1984) Transurethral polytetrafluoroethylene. Injection for post prostatectomy incontinence. *J Urol* 132:463–464.
4. Lewis RI, Lockhart JL, Politano, VA (1984) Periurethral polytetrafluoroethylene injections in female subjects with neurogenic bladder disease. *J Urol* 131:459–462.
5. Lockhart JL, Walker RD, Vorstman B, Politano VA (1988) Periurethral Polytetra fluoroethylene injections following urethral reconstruction in female patients with urinary incontinence. *J Urol* 140:51–52.
6. Lopez AE, Padron OF, Patsias C, Politano VA (1993) Transurethral polytetrafluoroethylene. Injection in female patients with urinary incontinence. *J Urol* 150:856–858.

7. Kiilholma P, Makinen J (1992) Disappointing effect of endoscopic Teflon injection for female stress incontinence. *Brit J Urol* 69:26–28.

8. Beckingham IJ, Wemyss-Holden C, Lawrence WT (1992) Long term follow up of women treated with periurethral Teflon injections for stress incontinence. *Brit J Urol* 69:580–583.

9. Kabalin JN (1994) Treatment of post prostatectomy stress urinary incontinence. With periurethral polytetrafluoroethylene paste injection. *J Urol* 152:1463–1466.

10. Boykin W, Rodriquez FR, Brizzolara J, Thompson IM, Zeidman EJ (1989) Complete urinary obstruction following periurethral polytetvcfluovoethylene injection for urinary incontinence. *J Urol* 141:1199–1200.

11. Hanau CA, Chancellor MB, Alexander A, et al. (1992) Fine needle aspiration of a periurethral Teflon tilled cyst following radical prostatectomy. *Diagnostic Cystopathol* 8:614–616.

12. Dewan PA, Fraundorfer M (1996) Skin irritation following periurethral polytetrcfiuoroethylene injection for urinary incontinence. *Aust and New Zealand J Surg* 66:57–59.

13. Malizia AA Jr, Reiman HM, Myers RP, Sande JR, et al. (1984) Irritation and granulomataus reaction after periuretheral injection of Polytef (Teflon). *JAMD* 251:3277–3281.

14. Herschorn S, Glazer, AA (2000) Early experience with small volume periuretheral polytetrafluoroethylene for female stress urinary incontinence. *J Urol* 163:1838–1842.

15. McGuire EJ, Lytton B, Pepe V, Kohorn, EI (1976) Stress urinary incontinence. *Obstet Gynecol* 47:255–264.

16. Chancellor MB, Erhard MJ, Kiiholma PS, Karasick S, Rivas DA (1994) Functional urethral closure with pubovaginal sling for destroyed urethra after long term urethral catheterization. *Urology* 43:499–505.

17. Kondo A, Kato A, Gotoh M, Narushima M (1998) Stamey and Gitles procedure long term follow-up in relation to incontinence type and patient age. *J Urol* 160:756–758.

18. Kayigil OS, Iftekhav A (1999) The coexistence of intrinsic sphincter deficiency with type II stress incontinence. *J Urol* 162:1365–1366.

19. Kredar KJ, Austin JC (1996) Treatment of stress urinary incontinence in women with hypermobility and intrinsic sphinter deficiency. *J Urol* 156:1995–1998.

20. English SF, Amundsen C, McGuire EJ (1999) Bladder neck competency at rest in women with incontinence. *J Urol* 161:578–580.

21. McGuire EJ, Cespedes RD (1996) Proper diagnosis: a must before surgery for stress incontinence. *J Endourol* 10:201–205.

22. McGuire EJ, Bloom DA, Ritchey ML (1993) Stress leak point pressure a diagnostic tool for incontinent children. *J Urol* 150:700–702.

23. McGuire EJ, Cespedes RD, O'Connell HE (1996) Leak point pressures. *Urology-Clinics N.A.* 23:253–262.

24. Blaivas JC, Barbalius CA (1983) Characteristics of neural injury after abdomino perineal resection. *J Urol* 129:84–87.

25. McGuire EJ (1988) Myelodysplasia. *Sem Neurourol* 8:145–149.

26. Mundy AR (1982) The anatomical explanation for bladder dysfunction after rectal and uterine surgery. *Brit J Urol* 54:501–503.

27. Woodside JR, McGuire EJ (1979) Urethral hypotonicity after supra sacral spinal cord injury. *J Urol* 121:783–785.

28. Gosalbez R, Castellan M (1998) Defining the role of the bladder neck sling in surgical treatment of urinary incontinence in children *World J Urology* 285–291.

29. Fontaine E, Bendaya S, Desent JF, et al. (1997) Rectus fascia sling and augumentation ileo cystoplasty for neurogenic incontinence in women. *J Urol* 157:109–112.
30. McGuire EI, Wang CC, Usitalo H, et al. (1986) Modified pubovaginal sling in girls with myelodysplasia. *J Urol* 135:94–96.
31. Roth DR, Vyas PR, Kroovand, et al. (1986) Upper urinary tract deterioration in patients with myelodysplasia. *J Urol* 135:528–530.
32. Shortliffe LM, Freiha FS, Kessler R, et al. (1989) Treatment of urinary incontinence by the periurethral implantation of eluturaldehyde cross linked collagen. *J Urol* 141:538–541.
33. Herschorn S, Radomski SB (1997) Collagen injection for stress incontinence patient selection and durability. *International Urology Gynecology J Pelvic Floor Dysfunc* 8:18–24.
34. Faerber G (1996) Endoscopic collagen injection therapy in elderly women with type 1 stress incontinence. *J Urol* 155:512–514.
35. Richardson TD, Kennelly M, Faerber GF (1991) Endoscopic injection of glutaraldehyde cross linked collagen for the treatment of intrinsic sphincter deficiency in women. *J Urol* 46 378–381.
36. Faerber GF, Belville WD, Ohl DA, et al. (1998) Comparsion of transurethral vs periurethral collagen in women with intrinsic sphincter deficiency. *Tech Urol* 4:124–127.
37. Herschorn S, Radomski SB (1992) Early experience with ultraurethral collagen injections for urinary incontinence *J Urol* 148:1797–1800.
38. Cespedes RD, Leng WW, McGuire EJ (1998) Collagen injection therapy for past prostectomy incontinence. *Urology* 54:597–602.
39. Cross C, English SF, Cespedes RD, et al. (1998) A follow-up on transurethral collagen injection therapy for urinary incontinence. *J Urol* 159:106–108.
40. Klutke CL, Nadlen RB, Tieman D, et al. (1999) Early results with antigrade collagen injection for post radical prostatectomy stress urinary incontinence. *J Urol* 156:1703–1706.
41. Klutke JJ, Subir C, Audriale C, et al. (1999) Long term results after anti grade collagen injection for stress incontinence following radical retropubic prostatectomy. *Urology* 53:974–977.
42. Chernoff A, Honowitz M, Comhs A, et al. (1997) Periurethral collagen for the treatment of urinary incontinence in children. *J Urol* 157:2303–2305.
43. Leonard MP, Decter A, Mix LW, et al. (1996) Treatment of urinary incontinence in children by endoscopically directed bladder neck injection of collagen. *J Urol* 156:637–640.
44. Sundaram CP, Reinherg Y, Aliabadi HA (1997) Failure to obtain durable results with collagen implantation in children with urinary incontinence *J Urol* 157:2306–2307.
45. Hidar S, Attyaoui F, deLaval J (2000) Periurethral injection of silicone microparticles in the treatment of sphincter deficiency urinary incontinence. Progress in Urology 10:2 19–23.
46. Bugel H, Pfisterr C, Sibert L, et al. (1999) Intraurethral macroplastic injections in the treatment of urinary incontinence after prostatic surgery. *Prog Urol* 9:1068–1076.
47. Guys IM, Simeoni Alias I, Fakhvu A, et al. (1999) Use of polydimethylsiloxane for endoscopic treatment of urinary incontinence in children. *J Urol* 162:2133–2135.
48. Smith DN, Appell, RA, Rackley RN, et al. (1998) Collagen injection therapy for post prostatectomy incontinence. *J Urol* 160:264–267.

49. Yokoyama E (1995) Contingen Bard Collagen implant: The Japanese experience. *Intl J Urol* 1:11–15.
50. Winters IC, Appell RA (1995) Periurethral injections of collagen in the treatment of intrinsic sphincter deficiency in the female patient *Urol./Clinics NA* 22:673–678.
51. O'Connell HC, McGuire EJ, Abosief S, et al. (1995) Transurethral Collagen Therapy in women. *J Urol* 154:1463–1465.
52. Abosief S, O'Connell HE, Usui A, et al. (1996) Collagen injection for intrinsic sphincter deficiency in men. *J Urol* 155:10–13.

4

Injectable Materials for Use in Urology

Raul C. Ordorica, MD

and Jorge Lockhart, MD

CONTENTS

INTRODUCTION
CONTINENT MECHANISMS IN MEN AND WOMEN
EVALUATION PRIOR TO INJECTION THERAPY FOR ISD
TECHNIQUES OF INJECTION THERAPY FOR CONTINENCE
POSTOPERATIVE CARE FOLLOWING INJECTION THERAPY
    FOR ISD
URETERO–VESICAL JUNCTION PHYSIOLOGY
EVALUATION PRIOR TO INJECTION THERAPY FOR REFLUX
TECHNIQUES OF INJECTION THERAPY FOR REFLUX
POSTOPERATIVE CARE FOLLOWING INJECTION THERAPY
    FOR REFLUX
INJECTION MATERIALS
CONCLUSION
REFERENCES

INTRODUCTION

The injection of bulking agents within urology has primarily confined itself to the urethra and the uretero–vesical junction. Since their inception, the injection of these materials has demonstrated both therapeutic benefit with the advantages of being minimally invasive with reductions in hospital stay, morbitity, and cost *(1)*. From relatively simple beginnings *(2,3)*, there has been a significant increase in available materials, with many more undergoing clinical trial and investigation

From: *Urologic Prostheses:*
The Complete, Practical Guide to Devices, Their Implantation and Patient Follow Up
Edited by: C. C. Carson © Humana Press Inc., Totowa, NJ

(4). Their relative abundance along with the amount of research being performed testifies to the fact that none of these agents are ideal *(5)*. While the search continues, today's urologist has multiple choices regarding the material that best fits their patient's needs. Choosing which bulking agent to use can depend upon the clinical setting, the surgeon's training, and the availability of materials and instruments. This chapter will detail the multiple aspects involved with injection therapy including the pathophysiology of urethral and uretero–vesical junction dysfunction, patient evaluation, injection techniques, and postoperative care. Following is a detailed comparison of injectable materials, including a review of published results along with the ongoing research of newer agents.

CONTINENT MECHANISMS IN MEN AND WOMEN

Continence requires that the urethral transluminal pressure exceeds that of the bladder. Multiple factors are responsible, with significant differences between men and women. The female urethra measures approx 3 cm in length, with its mucosal surface cushioned by the pliant subepithelial tissue formed by the lamina propria and elastic connective tissue. Surrounding this are the bladder neck smooth muscle fibers and slow twitch striated rhabdosphincter, which are present along the proximal two-thirds of the urethra. This complex rests upon the anterior vaginal wall, suspended along the arcus tendinius within the levator musculature. Marked deficiencies in a significant portion of these elements will result in stress incontinence.

The role of the "intrinsic" urethral mechanisms—the seal provided by the mucosal surface bolstered by the underlying connective tissue along with the closure provided by the rhabdosphincter—has gained increasing appreciation in the maintenance of continence. Alterations in this mechanism have been termed Intrinsic Sphincter Deficiency (ISD) *(6)*. Female ISD can develop from multiple causes such as inadequate development, neurologic compromise, vaginal delivery, surgical trauma, estrogen deficiency, or pelvic radiation. Depending on the degree of compromise, the intrinsic sphincter mechanisms can be augmented with the injection of bulking agents beneath the submucosa *(7)*.

The "intrinsic" sphincter mechanisms of the male are anatomically distinct from the female. The continent mechanisms of the male urethra lie within the bladder neck, prostate, and external sphincter. The bladder neck and prostate form an integral mechanism, with circular fibers extending from the detrusor forming the "internal" sphincter. Distal to this lies the external sphincter, which has an internal component with circular slow twitch muscle fibers that surround the anterior two-thirds of the urethra with elastic connective tissue along the posterior aspect.

With two distinct sphincter mechanisms in place, complete dysfunction can be experienced in one with the other maintaining continence. However, if both are affected, incontinence will ensue.

Because of the redundant continent mechanisms of the male, extensive alteration is often required to result in severe enough compromise to cause incontinence. Whereas male ISD can arise from maldevelopment or neurologic compromise, the overwhelming majority of cases are caused by anatomic alteration. These alterations are in the form of transurethral incision or resection, open resection, trauma, or attempts at subsequent repair. Radiation can also affect the tissues, and although it often does not directly result in incontinence, it can have profound effects on attempts to correct the condition.

EVALUATION PRIOR TO INJECTION THERAPY FOR ISD

The evaluation if the lower urinary tract prior to injection therapy requires the establishment of ISD. In addition, overall success with the patient achieving continence is best assured if the storage parameters of the bladder are optimal. This would include bladder capacity as determined by compliance along with detrusor stability. Patient history, voiding diary, urodynamic study, and cystoscopy may be used to assist in determining the bladder's ability to store urine.

History

Patient history should include the type and severity of incontinence, precipitating events, prior therapies, voiding pattern, and any additional factors that may affect outcome. History can be a significant determiner as to whether the patient is suffering from urge or stress incontinence. Increases in abdominal pressure that lead to urine leakage typifies stress incontinence, with urine loss associated with urgency signifying urge incontinence. Confusion may result if increases in abdominal pressure trigger detrusor instability. In addition, patients with stress incontinence may habitually void frequently in order to keep their bladder capacity to a minimum and thus avoid leakage, a pattern more associated with urge incontinence. A voiding diary may be helpful where history is incomplete or to document actual patterns of storage, leaking, and voiding. A patient's voiding pattern may demonstrate their functional bladder capacity and give clues to detrusor function. A patient who historically has had marked urgency, frequency, and nocturia prior to developing stress incontinence may have detrusor instability or decreased compliance, which would make therapy for their ISD suboptimal unless corrected. However, a low functional bladder capacity may also result from severe incontinence with near-continuous urine loss, causing the storage and voiding function of the bladder to remain untested. Therefore, it is often advisable to obtain more objective information of bladder and outlet function beyond history and physical examination, as provided by urodynamic assessment and cystoscopy.

Physical Examination

The physical examination of the incontinent patient can be used to identify stress urinary incontinence (SUI) in both men and women. With a semi-ful bladder, one can demonstrate leakage with maneuvers such as coughing and straining in both the supine and standing position. One should be careful to differentiate the leakage that occurs simultaneous with increases in abdominal pressure from that which occurs immediately thereafter. The latter may be an uninhibited detrusor contraction triggered by the abdominal pressure, and may not resolve with a urethral injection. A possible exception to this is if the inciting event is from urine entering the urethra with such maneuvers. Improved closure of the urethral lumen as afforded by a urethral injection may decrease this trigger. Neuropathology can be suggested by alterations in perineal sensation, loss of anal sphincter tone, and absence of the bulbocavernoses reflex. Vaginal pathology should also be sought, such as bladder neck descensus, cystocele, uterine or vault prolapse, and rectocele.

It has been long held that the ideal candidate for injection therapy is the ISD patient without urethral hypermobility. However, the concept that injection therapy is not of utility in those patients with combined ISD and hypermobility *(8–10)* has been challenged. Herschorn et al. compared outcomes in 187 patients both with and without hypermobility, noting that its presence did not significantly affect success *(11)*. This finding was confirmed by others, also using the injection of Contigen (CR Bard, Murray Hill, NJ) *(12)*, with some finding that patients with hypermobility, in fact, fare better than those with severe ISD *(13–14)*. However, poorer results were found using other injectable agents, including fat *(15)* and silicone microimplants *(16)*. The range of results within the literature may attest to the variable relative contribution of ISD that may be concurrent with hypermobility. Patients with successful injection results may have had more significant ISD or were able to compensate for the isolated hypermobility with augmented intrinsic sphincter function.

Urodynamics

The presence and degree of ISD is best evaluated with the measurement of Valsalva leak pressure *(17)*. The performance of leak pressure measurement has resisted exact standardization, with variations in patient position, catheter size, bladder volume, and method to increase intra-abdominal pressure *(17,18)*. Although there are many techniques used to measure Valsalva leak pressure, it is understood that lower pressure values associated with leakage indicate more severe cases ISD.

Additional urodynamic testing may be performed in evaluating patients prior to injection therapy. Measurement of bladder capacity in the face of extreme ISD may require occlusion of the outlet with a catheter balloon to allow for adequate filling. At best, a low-capacity bladder as a result of altered compliance would result in marked frequency; at worst, an elevation in bladder pressures with "successful" injection would potentiate renal deterioration. The results with detrusor instability are less clear. Intuitively, one would expect that findings of detrusor instability would result in decreased success *(11)*. However, others have found no effect, both in patients with *(19)* and without *(20)* neurogenic disease. A pressure-flow study may demonstrate the presence of both ISD and obstruction, typically in male patients following radical prostatectomy with a fixed narrowed outlet. If the obstruction is not caused by the urodynamic catheter occluding the outlet, then it deserves primary attention. For patients with detrusor acontractility who void by Valsalva, injection therapy may result in greater difficulty in bladder emptying. However, this has not been found in patients with normal voiding *(7,21)*.

Cystoscopy

Cystoscopy can be a useful tool in evaluating the incompetent outlet *(22)*. Whereas it may be inexact in determining the degree of ISD, areas of anatomic deformity can be identified, along with determining the quality of the tissue prior to injection. Marked scarring or atrophy of the outlet may predispose for poor results with little tissue available for injection.

TECHNIQUES OF INJECTION THERAPY FOR CONTINENCE

The primary purpose of injection therapy is to augment urethral coaptation. Adequate increases in urethral resistance can be achieved to overcome elevations in abdominal pressure without significant alteration of urodynamic voiding parameters *(7,23)*. Although an overabundance of injected material can result in urinary retention, this effect is usually transient. Ideal implantation is into the connective tissue layer between the mucosa and the rhabdospincter *(24)*. Injection that is too superficial into the mucosa results in extravasation and loss of the material. Injection that is deep within the rhabdosphinter results in outward expansion without urethral lumen compression. Misdirected injection may also result in rhabdosphincter compromise with a resultant increase in leakage. Preoperative assessment should include the performance of urinalysis to rule out the presence of infection. Both authors use oral flouroquinolone antibiotic prophylaxis that is continued for 1 wk following injection. Injection can be performed under local anesthesia with the placement of 2% lidocaine jelly, either in the office setting or ambulatory surgery suite. Additional anesthetic agent can be placed by local injection and infiltration *(25)*.

Female Urethra

Injection into the female urethral can either be performed using the transurethral (TU) or periurethral (PU) method. The TU method requires placement of the injection needle through the mucosa of the urethra as directed endoscopically (*see* Fig. 1). Flexible endoscopic needles can be passed through routine endoscopes using a catheterizable bridge (Alberrans), with specific working elements available by most manufacturers to enhance control (*see* Fig. 2). The benefits of the TU method include the greater familiarity by most urologists with this technique, with it being easier to place the needle in the desired location under direct vision. The downside is that each injection leaves a mucosal defect for potential material egress. Loss of material can be minimized by not piercing the mucosa directly over the desired site of implantation, but rather allowing the needle to track in the submucosal plane to the area to be injected. Injection should be performed with as few injection passes as possible.

The PU method is performed with use of a 3.5-inch needle outside and parallel to the urethral lumen to the desired location at the proximal one-third of the urethra (*see* Fig. 3). Because the needle length increases the resistance encountered with injection, it precludes injection with more viscous agents such as Teflon or Macroplastique. The perimeatal tissue where the needle will enter at the 3 and 9 o'clock position is initially infiltrated with local anesthetic. Tip location is inferred by needle motion or injection under cystoscopic observation. Attempts at placement under ultrasound guidance without cystoscopic observation have met with less success *(26)*. Once appropriately placed, there is less concern regarding direct extravasation of injected material through the mucosa. However, there is the risk of bladder perforation if the needle is passed too far or for minimal coaptation if the injection is outside of the proper plane. Accurate localization of the needle tip can be assured by initial injection of local anesthetic when one suspects that it is appro-

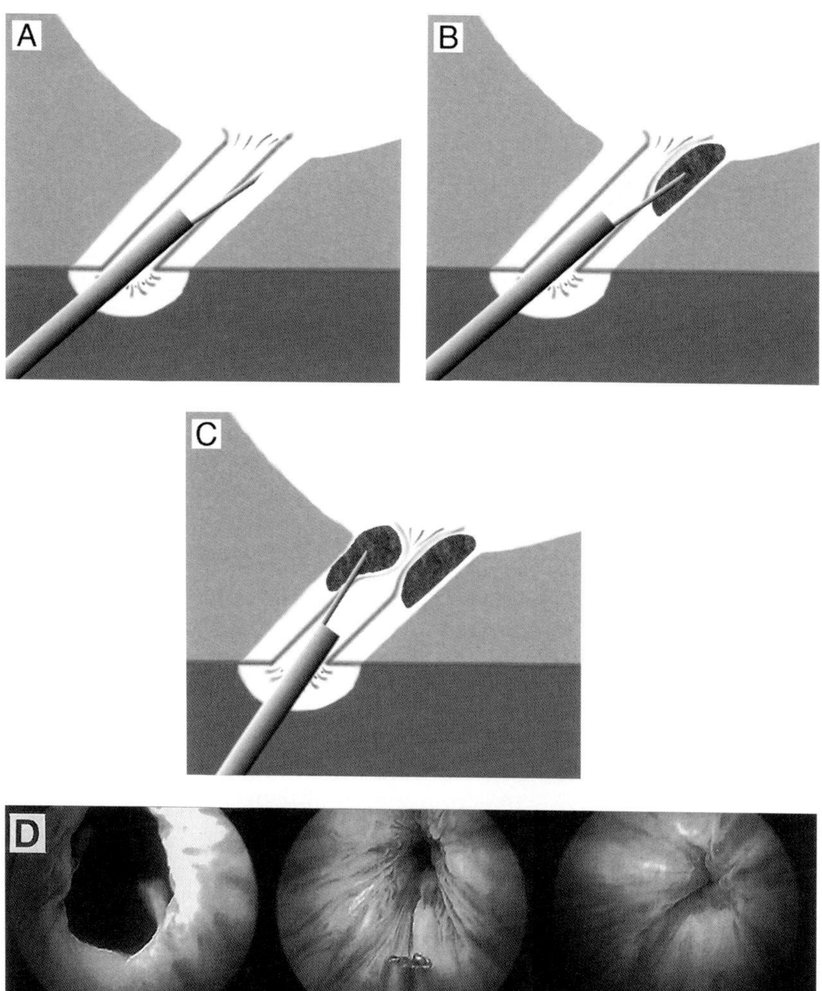

Fig. 1. TU injection of bulking material into the submucosal space. (**A**) Needle placement penetrating submucosa distal injection placement. (**B**) Injection of bulking material with elevation of submucosa. (**C**) Contralateral injection for complete coaptation of proximal urethra. (**D**) Images of TU injection of Durasphere showing coaptation of incompetent bladder neck and proximal urethra (courtesy of Advanced UroScience).

priately placed *(27).* There should be an immediate elevation of the mucosa with minimal volume placed. The use of local anesthetic also provides additional comfort prior to full injection of the bulking agent. The additional use of methylene blue has been described *(28),* although caution should be used with the small risk of allergic response *(29).* Few

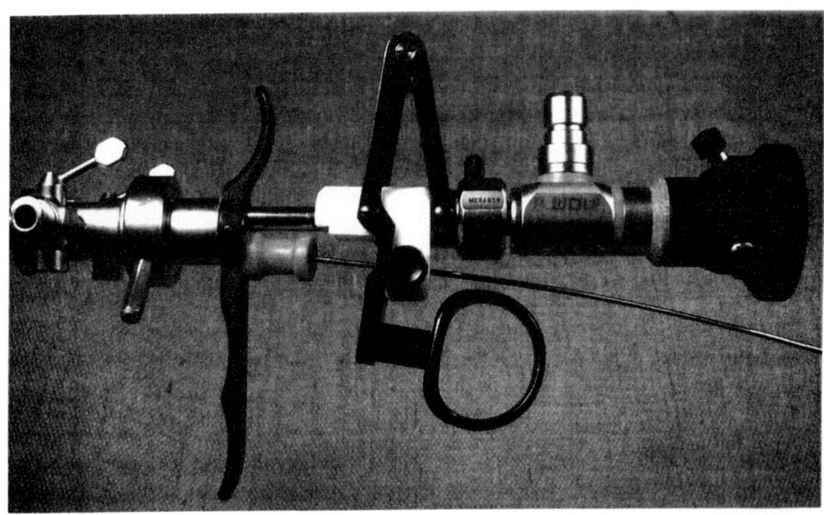

Fig. 2. Endoscopic working element for transurethral injection (courtesy of Wolf).

clinical studies have directly compared the methods of PU and TU injection *(30,31)*, with both looking at injection of bovine glutaraldehyde crosslinked (GAX) collagen. Although there does not appear to be an effect on immediate or long-term results, both groups noted a longer learning curve and higher injection volume with the periurethral method.

Male Urethra

Because of the extensive destruction required for the male to experience stress incontinence, there is often a compromise of the amount of viable epithelium and submucosa into which the bulking agent can be injected. Although the sphincter mechanism of the female is also compromised, there is usually adequate tissue to allow for the injection of material between the rhabdosphincter and the epithelium. For male patients, this results in an increase in the amount of material that must be injected into an area of more compromised tissue with subsequent poorer results *(32)*.

Injection is most typically performed by the TU approach, using the same instrumentation as in female patients. Given the relatively poorer results in comparison to female patients, the transvesical antegrade approach has been developed for the injection of bovine GAX collagen to better access viable tissue at the bladder neck proximal to the external sphincter (*see* Fig. 4). Methods have ranged from using a suprapubic needle, to passing an endoscope through a trocar so as to directly access

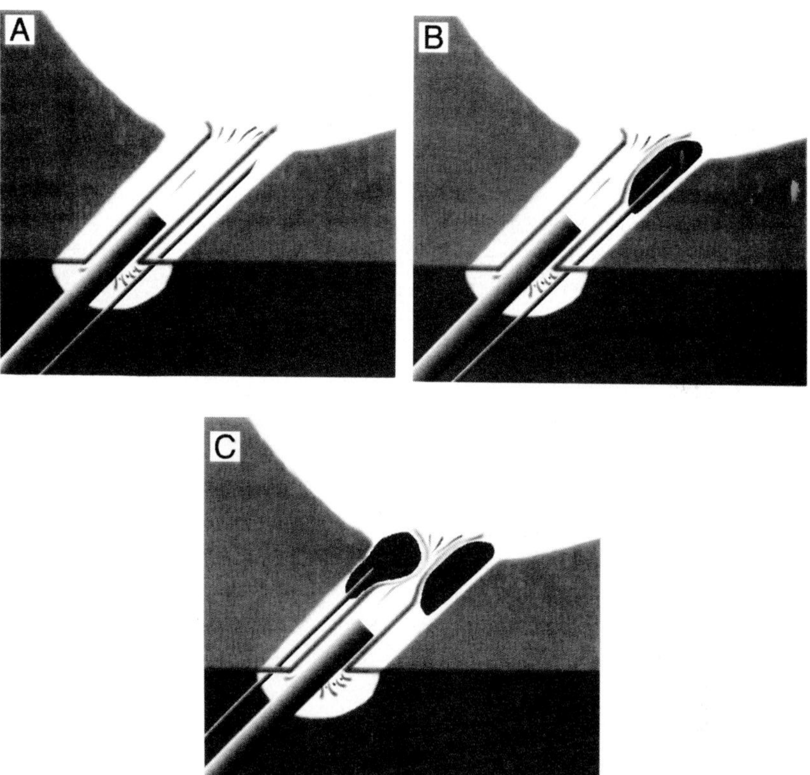

Fig. 3. PU injection of bulking material into the submucosal space. (**A**) Needle is passed parallel to the endoscope to the proximal urethra. (**B**) Injection of bulking material with elevation of submucosa. (**C**) Contralateral injection for complete coaptation of proximal urethra following second needle pass.

the bladder neck *(33–36)*. Although published studies that make direct comparisons are lacking, short-term results by individual authors seem improved using this approach *(37)*. However, subsequent long-term results continue to be disappointing *(38)*.

POSTOPERATIVE CARE FOLLOWING INJECTION THERAPY FOR ISD

The immediate concern following injection is the ability of the patient to void. If unable to void, the patient is conservatively managed with intermittent catheterization with low-caliber catheters to minimize displacement of the bulking agent. In-dwelling catheters are to be avoided because of the potential molding of the implant with resultant poor results. If an in-dwelling catheter is unavoidable because of inability of

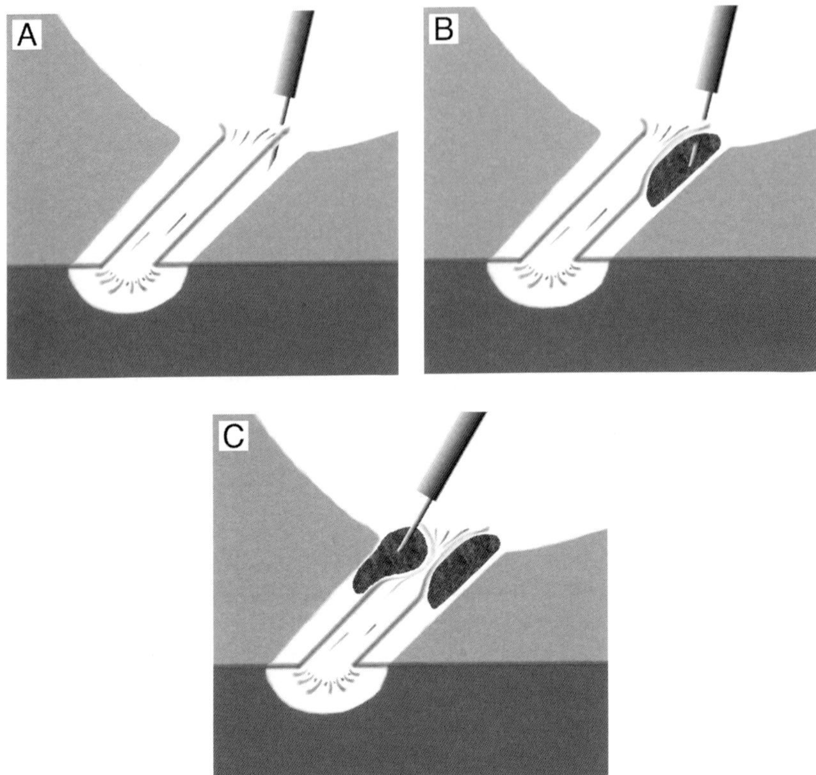

Fig. 4. Antegrade injection of bulking material. (**A**) Needle placement into bladder neck from proximal approach. (**B**) Injection of bulking material with elevation of submucosa. (**C**) Additional injections as required for complete coadaption.

the patient to self-catheterize, than a small lumen in-dwelling catheter can be considered. Urinary retention can be caused by the effects of local anesthesia, edema, and possible overcorrection. Given the temporary nature of these factors, particularly with agents that undergo some resorption of the carrier medium, the retention is usually short lived. Retention may become more problematic as clinicians use newer agents that promise more of a "what you see is what you get" (WYSIWYG) effect with maintenance of initial injection volume. Initial bladder drainage is less problematic in those male patients injected in an antegrade approach using a supra-pubic sheath through which a supra-pubic catheter can be placed. Drainage can be assured until the patient is able to void or for a specified period of time while the bulking agent becomes "set." It is unclear if this method of postoperative management results in better long-term outcome from minimizing tissue motion at the injection site. Once able to void or bladder drainage is assured by whatever means, the patient is discharged until subsequent follow-up.

URETERO–VESICAL JUNCTION PHYSIOLOGY

The uretero–vesical junction allows for the low-pressure peristalsis of urine without reflux. This is created by the anatomic arrangement of the ureter as is passes through the bladder musculature to form the upper trigone. A tunnel is formed through the detrusor fibers that result in the transmission of intravesical pressure against the walls of the ureter causing it to remain closed between ureteric peristaltic boluses. As the bladder distends and the intravesical pressure increases, the actual functional tunnel length increases along with the intraluminal ureteral pressure within the vesical hiatus. This tunnel further elongates during the voiding phase, preventing reflux during elevations in detrusor pressure that characterize bladder emptying.

Chronic increases in bladder pressure, ureteral dilation, or inadequate tunnel length can result in the compromise of the uretero–vesical junction resulting in the reflux of urine. Injection of bulking agents can be used to augment the functional tunnel length and coapt the ureteral lumen. Effective injection requires placement of the material into the submucosa just beneath the ureteral hiatus.

EVALUATION PRIOR TO INJECTION THERAPY
FOR REFLUX

The presence and degree of significant vesicourteral reflux (VUR) is best confirmed with voiding cystourethrography. Intravenous pyelography (IVP) and cystoscopy can be used to identify anatomic relationships and assess for collecting system duplication. Alteration of voiding patterns and findings of bladder wall thickening may suggest increased vesical pressure, which may be the primary cause of the reflux. A history of dysfunctional voiding may provide information regarding the etiology for the reflux. Bladder dysfunction, which results in alterations in storage pressure can result in reflux, as demonstrated by McGuire's sentinal article following patients with myelodysplasia *(39)*. Initial therapy aimed at the bladder dysfunction with improvements in detrusor compliance, capacity, stability, and voiding may result in resolution of the reflux. Finally, if elevated intravesical pressure from whatever cause is not addressed, reflux will recur. Video urodynamic examination can delineate not only alterations in storage and voiding pressure, but also provide information regarding the pressure at which reflux occurs *(40)*.

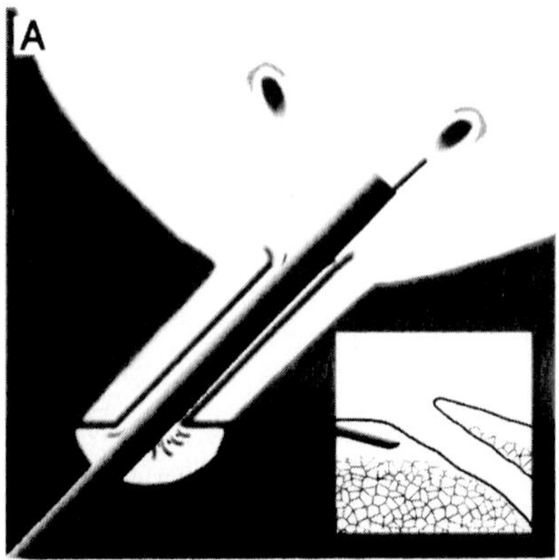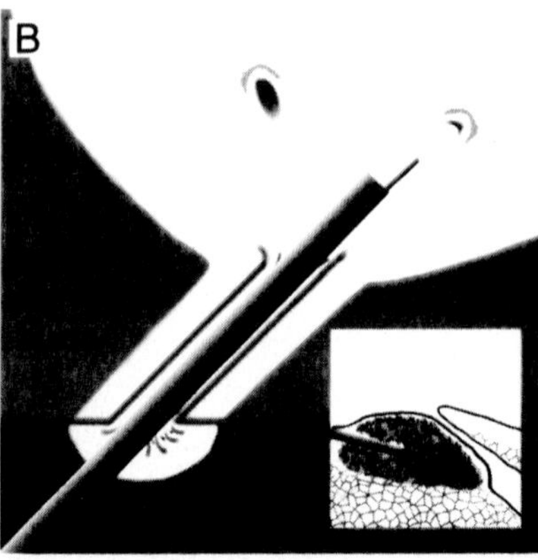

Fig. 5. Subureteral injection of bulking material. (**A**) Needle placement beneath the uretero–vesical junction orifice for injection beneath distal margin of the orifice. (**B**) Bulking material is injected with narrowing of orifice.

Actual bladder capacity may be overestimated if the dilated collecting system(s) hold significant volumes of urine.

TECHNIQUES OF INJECTION THERAPY FOR REFLUX

Given the pediatric population on which this therapy is primarily applied, along with the nature of the injection, procedures are performed under general anesthesia. Injection into the uretero–vesical junction uses the same instrumentation described for TU injection for incontinence. Injection is performed just beneath the ureteral hiatus with swelling of the tissue beneath the ureteral os as described by O'Donnell and Puri *(41)* (*see* Fig. 5). Injection that is placed too deep within the musculature of the bladder diffuses with poorer results *(42)*. As the hiatus is elevated, the configuration of the meatus changes to a small circular opening. Injection therapy has been successfully described in patients with reflux associated with neurogenic bladder *(43,44)*, duplex systems *(45,46)*, posterior urethral valves *(47)*, and endoscopically incised ureteroceles *(48,49)*. Results are better in treating primary vs secondary reflux *(50,51)*.

POSTOPERATIVE CARE FOLLOWING INJECTION THERAPY FOR REFLUX

Performed on an out-patient basis, the patient is discharged following recovery from anesthesia. Antibiotic prophylaxis is continued until resolution from reflux is assured. Unlike incontinence, where recurrence is clinically evident, reflux may recur with little or no symptoms. Therefore, given the potential for recurrence, ongoing surveillance must be performed. Furthermore, because of the potential for ureteral obstruction, initial follow up should include renal ultrasound *(52)*.

INJECTION MATERIALS

What was once only a small field of available materials has increased exponentially into a large array of potential bulking agents. Table 1 lists the injectable agents along with their characteristics, grouped together in rough order of their design. Whereas some of the materials are seeing their first application as a urological bulking agent, many have or are being introduced in plastic surgery or as radiologic embolizing agents. The materials vary in their complexity of production, ease of injection, initial and long-term maintenance of volume, host reaction, and potential for migration. They range from synthetically derived materials to connective tissue matrices to viable autologous tissues with hybrids in between. Some materials function by providing bulk alone, whereas others rely on host fibroblast ingrowth and replacement. Given the multiple clinical settings in which injectable materials are used, there may not be a single agent with all the ideal characteristics. Tables II, III, and IV summarize clinical results of available agents used for female incontinence, male incontinence, and vesicoureteral reflux.

Teflon

Since its initial injection to treat stress incontinence in the early 1970's *(53,54)*, there has been extensive experience with polytetrafluoroethylene paste (Teflon®, DuPont) as an injection material in urology. Currently marketed as Urethrin (Mentor Corp., Santa Barbara, CA), it is available in Europe, but is not FDA approved for urologic use in the United States. It is an inert substance with a particulate size between 4–40 µm that, once injected, is not chemically broken down within the body. The viscosity of the paste requires it to be injected using a large bore needle at substantial pressure, requiring a low-caliber pistol-driven device *(see* Fig. 6). By heating the injection device, the viscosity decreases, which can facilitate injection *(55)*. It has been used for both female and male incontinence, along with reflux. Its use in reflux has been documented since first introduced by Puri and O'Donnell in 1984 *(56)*. These investigators have applied this successfully in children with reflux *(41)*, with published data followed out for 10 years *(47)*. Once injected, there is a persistent inflammatory response to the Teflon particles *(57)*. This response is cause not only for its efficacy, but also for complication, with reports of ureteral obstruction *(58)*, bladder outlet obstruction

Table 1
Injection Materials

Name	Description	Delivery	Advantages	Concerns
Urethrin®	4–40-μm Teflon paste	18-gauge needle high-pressure injection tool	Longest experience	Migration Inflammatory reaction Specialized tool (clinical investigation)
Macroplastique®	200-μm silicone elastomer	18/20-gauge needle high-pressure injection tool	Extensive European experience	Silicone Inflammatory reaction Specialized tool Possible migration (clinical investigation)
Durasphere®	212–500-μm pyrolytic carbon-coated zircinium oxide beads	18-gauge needle special design	FDA-approved Radio opaque Nonmigratory Nonantigenic	Needle clogs
Bioglass	120–355-μm Ceramic beads	16-gauge needle	Nonmigratory	Limited experience Difficult to inject (no further studies)
Urocol	14–400-μm hydroxyapatite tricalcium phosphate	Not reported	Easy to produce	Migration (no further studies)

(continued)

Name	Description	Delivery	Advantages	Concerns
Deflux®	80–120-μm dextranomer microspheres in sodium hyaluronan	23-gauge needle	Easy to produce Ease of injection Nonmigratory	Inflammatory reaction Volume loss over time (clinical investigation)
calcium hydroxylate	75–125-μm particles suspended in a water, glycerin, and sodium carboxy methylcellulose gel	21-gauge needle	Easy to produce Ease of injection Nonmigratory	(clinical investigation)
polyvinyl alcohol	20–500-μm particles	25-gauge needle	Easy to produce Ease of injection	Migration Tomorgenicity (no further studies)
Uryxj	ethylene vinyl alcohol polymer	25-gauge needle	Easy to produce Ease of injection Nonmigratory Forms solid mass upon injection Maintains volume	(clinical investigation)
UroVive®	Detatchable 0.9 cm^3 silicone balloon inflated *in situ*	14-gauge sheath	Nonmigratory Maintains volume Minimal reaction	Silicone large rigid delivery tool (clinical investigation)

(continued)

Table 1 (continued)

Name	Description	Delivery	Advantages	Concerns
silk elastin polymers	Synthetic polymer	Not available	Easy to produce	(clinical investigation) Maintains volume
Hylan B Gel (hylagel-Uro)	> 200-μm Crosslinked hyaluronan Particles	21-gauge needle	Ease of injection Nonmigratory Non-antigenic	Temporary effect with plastic surgery experience (clinical investigation)
Contigen®	GAX bovine collagen	21-gauge needle	Extensive experience Ease of injection Nonmigratory	Pretreatment skin test Volume loss over time Antigenic
small intestine submucosa	Porcine acellular extracellular matrix	20-gauge needle	Tissue ingrowth	Xenograft (clinical investigation)
Urologen	Alllograft acellular dermis (solvent prepared)	21-gauge needle?	Tissue ingrowth Nonantigenic	Cadaveric source Extensive processing (clinical investigation)
Cymetra	100–150-μm Allograft acellular dermis (freeze dried)	23-gauge needle	Tissue ingrowth Nonantigenic	Cadaveric source Extensive processing (clinical investigation)

(continued)

Table 1 (continued)

Name	Description	Delivery	Advantages	Concerns
autologous fat	Liposuction from abdominal wall	18-gauge needle	Abundant supply Nonantigenic	Fat harvesting Large needle Volume loss over time Possible emboli
Chondrogel™	Autologous chondrocytes isolated and cultured for injection	21-gauge needle	Ease of injection Continued growth Nonantigenic Cryopreserved for future injection	Ear biopsy 7-wk culture period Narrow time window for injection (clinical investigation)
Autologous smooth muscle cells	Harvested from bladder	18-gauge needle	Non-antigenic Potential for functional replacement	Bladder biopsy (clinical investigation)

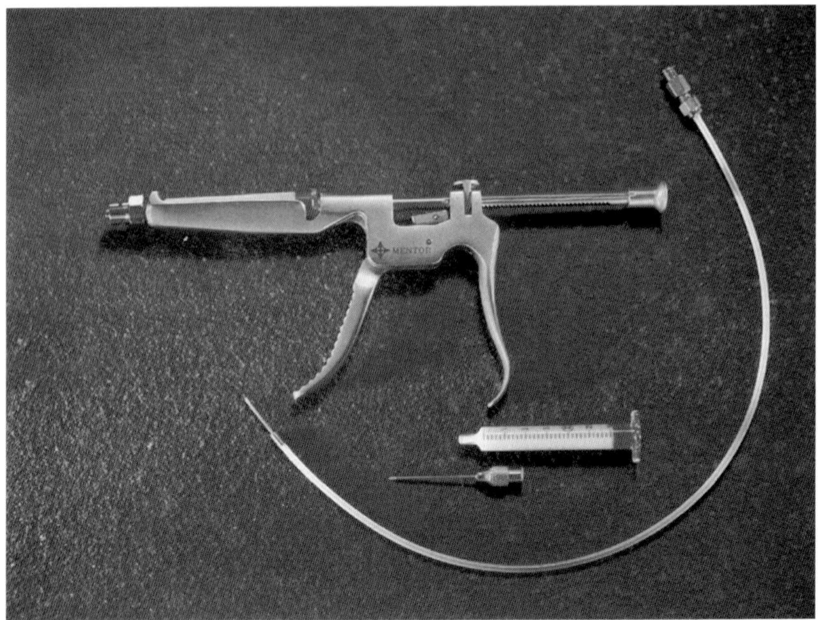

Fig. 6. Teflon injection device with Urethrin syringe and injection needle (courtesy of Mentor).

(59,60), and local granuloma formation *(61–63)*. Despite this reaction, subsequent open surgery does not appear to be hampered in cases of endoscopic failure *(64)*. The major concern associated with the material has been its migratory potential given its relatively small particulate size *(65)*. Migration has primarily been reported to lung parenchyma in human subjects *(66,67)*, although more distant migration has been reported *(68)*. Initial animal studies have demonstrated migration to pelvic nodes, lung, spleen, kidneys, and brain *(69)*. Miyakita demonstrated in a dog model that it required actual intra-arterial injection to result in brain emboli, without emboli resulting from low-volume periurethral injection *(70)*. Low volumes are typically used for reflux, with this concept further extended by Herschorn in treating 46 female patients with ISD using low-volume periurethral Teflon injections *(71)*. Larger volumes are used for male incontinence, with the largest series by Politano with favorable results *(72)*.

Silicone Elastomer

Macroplastique (Uroplasty, Minneapolis, MN) consists of silicone elastomer with a mean diameter of 200 µm suspended in a polyvinylpyrrolidone hydrogel. The elastomer size is designed to prevent the migra-

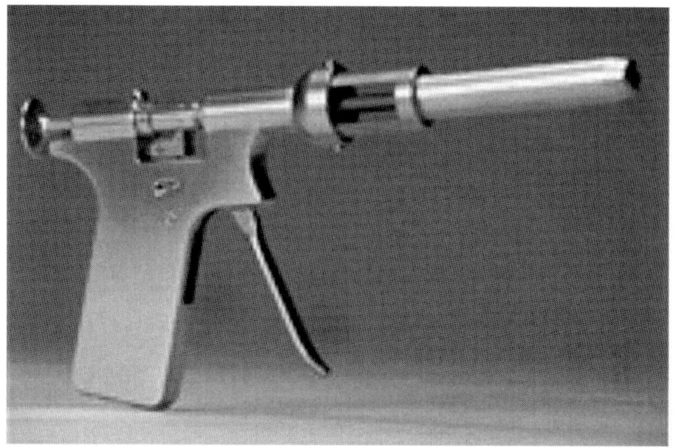

Fig. 7. Macroplastique injection device (courtesy of Uroplasty).

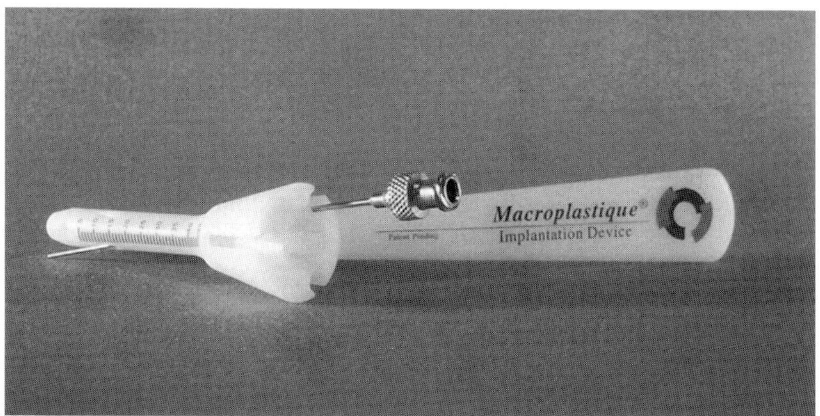

Fig. 8. Macroplastique injection guide (courtesy of Uroplasty).

tion that can occur with smaller particles *(73,65)*. The injection of the viscous material requires substantial pressure, and although it can be injected through an 18-gage needle for adults and a 20-gauge needle for children, it requires an injection device (*see* Fig. 7). Most commonly, the material is injected in a TU fashion, although it has also been performed periurethally *(74)*. The manufacturer also supplies an injection device to allow for TU injection in female patients without the use of an endoscope (*see* Fig. 8), although the benefits of this method for a urologist familiar with endoscopy is unclear. Once injected, the PVP hydrogel is absorbed and the elastomers are engulfed in an acute and then chronic low-grade inflammatory response with subsequent collagen deposition. It has been applied to female, male, and pediatric ISD, along with vesico-ureteral reflux (VUR) (*see* Tables 2, 3, and 4). Its benefit in each of these categories does not vary from other published data of available agents. Although the material, along with the resultant host reaction appear to persist, the benefits of the injection tends to wane over time *(74–77)*. Unlike adverse events involving large volume silicone gel implants, there has been no reports directly related to the injection of silicone elastomer as formulated in Macroplastique. The material is available in Europe, but not yet approved in the United States.

Durasphere

Made of pyrolytic carbon-coated zirconium oxide beads, Durasphere[®] (Advanced UroScience, Inc., St. Paul, MN) was FDA approved for injection for ISD in September 1999. Pyrolytic carbon is biocompatible and does not require skin testing, being nonantigenic with a record of artificial heart valve use for more than 30 yr. The material does not require refrigeration with a shelf life of 6 mo. The suspension is implanted transurethrally, requiring a specialized 18-gauge needle with an internally tapered hub to minimize clogging. The gel component of the preparation results in decreased material leakage from the injection site. The particle size is 212–500 μm, which prevents migration. Once injected, there is a persistent mild chronic inflammatory response with minimal granuloma formation. Over 6 mo, this is replaced with collagen deposition. The material is radio-opaque and can be seen on plain radiograph (*see* Fig. 1D). The multicenter study performed for approval compared the Durasphere to GAX bovine collagen (Contigen) *(78)*. Twelve-month data included 235 patients with ISD, of whom 115 received the Durasphere. Of these patients, 43% received a single treatment, 40% received two treatments, and 13% received three treatments. Of the patients injected with Duraphere, 66.1% had an improvement of incontinence grade of 1 or more at 12 mo, identical to the Contigen group. Although there was also significant improvement in pad weight, incontinence episodes, and quality of life, there was no significant difference in these parameters between the Durasphere and Contigen. Durasphere did have less material injected (4.83 mL vs 6.23 mL; $p<0.001$), with a higher acute urgency and retention rate (24.7%, 16.9%) than in the Contigen group (11.9%, 3.4%) ($p=0.002$, $p<0.001$). This was postulated by the FDA panel to be caused by the initial inflammatory reaction to the material. Other adverse events were minimal and equivalent. There was no evidence of material loss or migration as observed by KUB at 12 mo (*see* Fig. 10). Postmarket approval studies are underway to evaluate 5-yr data, along with its applicability for male incontinence.

Bioglass

Ceramic beads measuring 120–355 µm have been suspended in hyaluronan for injection. Initial studies using New Zealand white rabbits with the material injected into the dome of the bladder were followed from 2 to 12 wk at 2-wk intervals *(79)*. Tissue specimens from sacrificed animals showed no evidence of particle migration. Subsequent work using Yucatan minipigs with injection of the material into the bladder neck showed an elevation in the urethral pressure profile without evidence of migration. Suspensions of smaller particles have also been investigated. Urocol (Genesis Medical Ltd., London UK) was formed by a ceramic suspension of 60% hydroxyapatite and 40% tricalcium phosphate. With a mean particle size of 14 µm, the material was readily phagocytized by macrophages and monocytes in a rat model *(65)*.

Dextranomers

Dextran is a polysaccharide that can be crosslinked to form microspheres. Dextranomer microspheres suspended in sodium hyaluronan (Deflux, Questor AB, Uppsala, Sweden) have been used as a bulking agent in animals and human clinical studies. Initially applied for VUR *(80)*, it has since been clinically studied for ISD in female patients *(81)*. The material is easily produced and injected, with a particle size of 80–120 µm that resists migration *(82)*. Initial human studies have demonstrated its safety with relative ease of injection *(81)*. There was a 20% retention rate upon injection that may attest to the maintenance of initial volume. Upon injection, the implant is infiltrated with fibroblasts, inflammatory cells, and foreign body giant cells *(83)*. Following the initial reaction, there is an increase in extracellular matrix with blood vessel ingrowth. Animal studies have demonstrated a 23% decrease in volume over 12 mo. Limited human studies have demonstrated short-term benefit with the need for longer term follow-up.

Calcium Hydroxylate

Calcium hydroxylate can be manufactured into particles that range between 75–125 µm in size. Suspended in a gel carrier of water, glycerin, and sodium carboxy methylcellulose, the material can be injected using a 21-gauge needle. Following injection, the carrier is biodegraded and the calcium hydroxylate particles have fibroblast infiltration with connective tissue ingrowth. The particles are not encapsulated, and there is no bone deposition. The material is currently manufactured by Bioform, Inc. (Milwaukee, WI). Having been studied in an animal model, it has undergone pilot investigation in the United States in patients with ISD.

Table 2
Injection Therapy for Incontinence: Female

Author	Material	Method	# Patients	Types	Follow-up	Success
Teflon®	Lockhart (19)	TU	20	urethral reconstruction		60%
	Lotenfoe (133)	TU	21	Type III	11 mo	56%
	Herschorn (134)	PU	46	ISD	24 mo	60%
	Lopez (135)	TU	128	74 SUI	31 mo	76%
				22 Neurogenic		73%
				11 Congenital		91%
				8 Trauma		62%
				13 Other		46%
	Kiilholma (136)	TU	22		60 mo	18%
	Politano (137)	PU		54	6 mo–16 yr	71%
Macroplastique®	Henella (138)	TU	40	ISD	3 mo	74%
	Guys (139)	TU	25	ISD	23 mo	44%
	Sheriff (140)	TU	34	ISD	24 mo	48%
	Harriss 97 (141)	PU	40	genuine	36 mo	58%
Durasphere®	FDA study (142)	TU	115	ISD	12 mo	66%
UroVive®	Diamond (143)	PU	3	ISD	6 mo	66%
	Pycha (144)	PU	20	10 Type III	35.5 mo	100%
				6 Type I/III		88%
				4 Type II/III		25%

Deflux®	Stenberg (145)	TU	20	genuine	6 mo	85%
Contigen®	Ang (146)	PU	105	ISD	12 mo	82%
	Cross (147)	PU	139	ISD	18 mo	93%
	Herschorn (148)	PU	187	54 Type I	22 mo	72%
				70 Type II		77%
				63 Type III		75%
	Corcos (149)	PU	40	8 Type I	50 mo	88%
				20 Type II		65%
				12 Type III		67%
	Gorton (150)	PU	53	genuine	60 mo	26%
fat	Haab (151)	PU	45	ISD	7 mo	13%
	Garibay (152)	PU	15	ISD	12 mo	23%
	Palma (153)	PU	30	ISD	12 mo	31–64%
	Su (154)	PU	26	ISD	12 mo	65%
	Santarosa (155)	PU	12	ISD	18 mo	78%
			3	hypermobility		0%
Chondrogel™	Lloyd (156)	TU	32	ISD	12 mo	84%

Table 3
Injection Therapy for Incontinence: Male

Author	Material	Method	# Patients	Dignoses	Follow-up	Success
Teflon®	Politano (157)	TU	720	RRP		67%
				TURP	12 mo	88%
				simple		74%
	Stanisic (158)	TU	20	RRP	17 mo	
				simple		
	Kabalin (159)	TU	13	8 RRP	11–36 mo	25%
				5 TURP		20%
Macroplastique®	Duffy (28)	TU	12	epispadius	11 mo	75%
	Bugel (160)	TU	15	9 RRP	12 mo	26%
				4 TURP		
				2 simple		
	Guys (161)	TU	19	neurogenic	23 mo	21%
UroVive®	Diamond (90)	TU	5	neurogenic	6 mo	63%
Contigen®	Aboseif (162)	TU	88	47 RRP	10 mo	66%
				7 RRP & XRT		57%
				7 TURP		43%
				24 Other		21%
				3 Neurogenic		100%

	Cummings (163)	TU	19	RRP	10 mo	58%
	Elsergany (164)	TU	35	31 RRP	18 mo	51%
				4 TURP		
	Faerber (165)	TU	68	47 RRP	38 mo	15%
				8 XRT		25%
				4 Cryo		25%
				4 Salvage		0%
				5 TURP		80%
	Kuznetsov (166)	TU	41	RRP	19 mo	20%
	Sanchez-Ortiz (167)	TU	31	RRP	15 mo	35%
	Martins (168)	TU	46	RRP	26 mo	24%
	Smith (169)	TU	62	54 RRP	29 mo	36%
				8 TURP		62%
	Appell (170)	Antegrade	24	RRP	12 mo	38%
	Klutke (171)	Antegrade	20	RRP	28 mo	45%
Fat	Garibay (172)	TU	5	TURP	12 mo	0%
	Santarosa (155)	TU	6	3 RRP	18 mo	0%
				3 TURP		33%

Table 4
Injection Therapy for VUR

Material	Author	# units	Follow-up	Success
Teflon[®]	Sauvage *(173)*	201	3 mo	92%
	Geiss *(174)*	1290	12 mo	82%
	Blake *(175)*	115	3–36 mo	79%
	Puri *(176)*	143	24–66 mo	88%
Macroplastique[®]	Dodat *(177)*	253	12 mo	84%
UroVive[®]	Palma *(178)*	2	3 mo	100%
Deflux[®]	Stenberg *(179)*	101	3 mo	68%
Contigen[®]	Reunanen *(180)*	159	48 mo	21–82%
	Leonard *(181)*	92	12 mo	65%
	Haferkamp *(182)*	58	37 mo	9%
	Frey *(183)*	204	33 mo	63%
Fat	Chancellor *(184)*	12	6 mo	29%
Chondrogel[®]	Diamond *(185)*	46	3 mo	83%

Polyvinyl Alcohol

Polyvinyl alcohol has been widely applied as an embolizing agent *(84–86)*. Although this inert biocompatible material is easy to handle and inject, its particle size range between 20–500 µm has led to some concern regarding its migratory potential *(87)*. Once injected, it results in a fibrotic reaction that persists over time. Whereas investigation in urology demonstrated its persistence within the bladder wall of New Zealand white rabbits at 3 mo *(88)*, its tumorgenic potential has been raised based on additional animal models *(89)*.

Ethylene Vinyl Alcohol

Ethylene vinyl alcohol is a biocompatible polymer that, once in contact with the body tissue or fluids, precipitates into a coherent solid mass to serve as a bulking agent. Developed as an embolizing agent (EMBOLYX, Micro Therapeutics, Inc., Irvine, CA) for vascular application, URYXJ is being investigated in urology as a bulking material by a subsidiary company (Genyx Medical, Inc., Irvine, CA). The ethylene vinyl alcohol is dissolved in dimethyl sulfoxide (DMSO), which acts as a carrier for injection. Once the dissolved material contacts the body tissue or fluids, the DMSO rapidly dissipates from the polymer. At room temperature, the material is a nonviscous liquid, easily passing through a 25-gauge needle. Upon warming to body temperature, the material rapidly solidifies

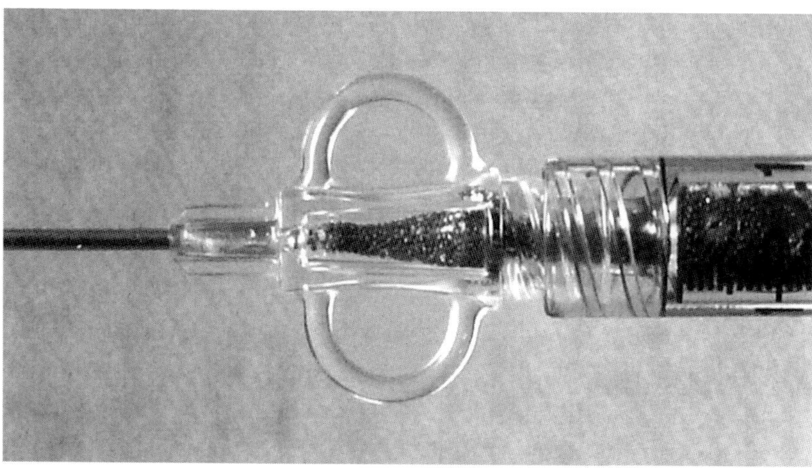

Fig. 9. Durasphere injection needle demonstrating tapered hub to facilitate flow and minimize jamming of material (courtesy of Advanced UroScience).

to an inert pliant solid. This rapid formation into a coherent mass would preclude its migration that may occur with smaller particles. Its ease of manufacture and introduction would make it readily available as an implant material and is currently undergoing clinical investigation.

Microballoon System

UroVive (American Medical Systems, Minnetonka, MN) is a self-contained Microballoon System, as previously investigated by Uro Surge (Iowa City, IA). The balloon is made of silicone that is inflated with up to 0.9 cm^3 of an inert liquid (polyvinylpyrrolidone hydrogel) (*see* Fig. 11). The benefits of this system are that it would be nonmigratory and retain its volume. Histologic examinations of the implant in an animal model at 3 mo demonstrated minimal reaction *(90)*. It appears to be better suited for patients without hypermobility, as noted by Pycha who followed 10 patients with pure ISD for a mean of 36 mo with all having continued benefit (paper abstract). This is in contrast to 4/ 10 patients with hypermobility that had recurrence of their incontinence. The few erosions noted occurred with urethral laceration or superficial injection.

The noninflated system is implanted using endoscopic guidance much like other injectable agents, however, requiring the use of a 14-gauge sheath. This system has been applied for both male and female patients with incontinence *(91)*, along with patients with VUR (Palma, aua abstract, Atlanta, 2000). In female patients, the procedure may be best performed periurethrally to maintain mucosal integrity. The distortion created by passing the 14-gage sheath and trocar in the periurethral space can be minimized by stabilizing the urethra by grasping the meatus with an Allis clamp. Following balloon inflation, the system detaches with removal of the sheath, remaining filled with its integral check valve. This device is undergoing further investigation.

Silk-Elastin Polymer

Synthetically manufactured (Protein Polymer Technologies, Inc., San Diego, CA) and injectable through a 25-gauge needle, the material transforms from a polymer solution to a firm, pliant hydrogel. Preclinical studies have reportedly shown the product to be biocompatible, nonimmunogenic, resistant to migration, and durable. Preservation of volume following injection results in the ability to accurately implant the material without the need to overinject to obtain the desired results. The material is undergoing clinical investigation.

Hylan B Gel

Hylanuronan is a major component of connective tissue, formed by repeating dimers of glucuronic acid and N-acetyl glucosamine. This large polysaccharide helps form the elastoviscous fluid matrix in which collagen and elastic fibers are embedded. Its chemical structure is the same throughout nature, and thus is extremely biocompatible. In its native form, hyaluronan turns over quickly with a half-life of 1–2 d. Hylan B gel (Hylaform®, Biomatrix Corp., Ridgefield, NJ) is a derivative of hyaluronan for dermatologic use, with the formation of sulfonyl-*bis*-ethyl crosslinks to resist degradation. It is derived from rooster combs *(92)*, and has not demonstrated any cellular or humoral reaction in both animal *(93)* and human investigations *(92)*. It is easily injected using a 30-gauge needle, and has been compared favorably to bovine GAX collagen for wrinkles and scars *(94)*. In a series of 177 patients who were followed for a minimum of 1 yr, the mean duration of effectiveness was 21 wk. It is currently being investigated as an injectable agent for urinary incontinence under the name Hylagel-Uro®.

Contigen

Contigen is GAX bovine collagen FDA approved for urologic application since 1993. The crosslinking is to stabilize the collagen and prevent degredation. It is also enzymatically treated to remove its antigenic telemeres and minimize host reaction. Although initially reported in 1989 for urologic use *(95)*, it has been long available to plastic surgery for dermal injection (Zyderm, CR Bard). It is primarily made up of type I collagen *(95%)* with a small amount of type III collagen (5%), suspended in an aqueous medium at a concentration of 35 mg/mL.

Allergic response can occur, with possible sensitization from bovine products with approx 28% of the patients treated having demonstrated specific antibodies against bovine type I collagen *(96)*. The allergic response is primarily IgG, IgA, and IgM mediated, and most typically results in an irritation and erythema at the injection site. This is more relevant in plastic surgical applications where the potential for a local reaction is cosmetically undesirable. Whereas IgE-mediated anaphylactic responses have not been reported, systemic side effects such as arthralgia have occurred *(97)*. To preclude against any reaction, a skin test is performed with a 1-cm^3 noncrosslinked aliquote placed subcutaneously to test for allergic response. The skin test requires a 4-wk waiting period with a reaction rate of 3%. Even following a negative skin test, 0.9% of patients will demonstrate an allergic response following subsequent urethral injection *(98)*. Some authors have called for the performance of two sequential skin tests to decrease the potential of injection into a sensitized individual *(99)*.

The urethral application is relatively simple to inject with the ability to infuse it through a 21-gauge needle, either transurethrally or periurethrally. Upon injection, there is some immediate absorption of the aqueous portion with a reduction in the infused volume. This is being addressed by investigation of a higher concentration formulation of GAX collagen at 65 mg/mL (GAX 65) that has greater retention of the infused volume *(100)*. Although the connective tissue makeup would seem to invite capillary ingrowth and further native collagen deposition *(105)*, the material is relatively inert with subsequent resorption requiring additional injection or alternative therapy. For those female patients treated for ISD. Ang noted that the mean time to relapse was 13.3 mo *(102)*, Herschorn demonstrated that the probability of remaining dry was 71%, 58%, and 46% and 1, 2, and 3 yr following successful injection *(11)*.

Smooth Intestine Submucosa

Smooth intestine submucosa (SIS) is an acellular extracellular matrix derived from porcine small intestine. The material retains its three-dimensional architecture and contains collagen, proteoglycans, glycosaminoglycans, and functional growth factors. The material acts as a scaffold for ingrowth of host fibroblasts and muscle cells. Volume maintenance of this material relies on this host tissue ingrowth, and thus differs from GAX bovine collagen that appears to persist because of its inate bulk alone. Injection of the material can be performed using a 20-gauge needle. It has been applied both within *(103)* and cross species

(104) with injection into the bladder. When used as a xenograft, reports indicate that there is more of an inflammatory reaction, with tissue ingrowth still occurring. The material can be irradiated, which appears to result in its persistence over nonirradiated SIS. It is postulated that this may result in partial crosslinking of the collagen, which results in its persistence until tissue ingrowth can occur *(104)*. This material has also been investigated as a scaffold seeded with smooth muscle cells forming a composite graft for bladder augmentation *(105)*.

Allogenic Collagen

The use of collagen has appeal in providing a natural substance as a bulking agent. However, the lack of long-term efficacy and antigenicity of bovine GAX collagen has led to further investigation of allogenic sources. The use of autologous or allogenic tissue eliminates the need to enzymatically treat the collagen to remove the telopeptides that are the antigenic component. Because the telopeptides are also essential to the architecture of the collagen fibers, the preserved morphology may result in improved host tissue ingrowth and preservation of bulk. Autologous collagen derived from dermis injected into the bladders of New Zealand white rabbits demonstrated preservation of the implant with neovascularization and minimal tissue reaction at 50 d *(106)*.

Subsequent work by Cozzolino et al. using the same animal model, compared it to bovine GAX collagen at 3 mo *(111)*. The authors demonstrated the intact arrangement of the autologous collagen with greater fibroblastic and vascular infiltration without a marked inflammatory response in comparison to the bovine collagen implant. The mechanical and enzymatic dispersion techniques used in these investigations has been further applied to human dermis. Urologen® (Collagenesis, Inc., Beverly, MA) is a cadaveric human tissue matrix, primarily composed of collagen fibrils, elastic network, and glycosaminoglycans. Pilot data looking at 18 female patients with ISD showed equivalent results in comparison to bovine GAX collagen. Preliminary data from on-going IDE feasibility clinical studies confirm this, whereas noting that average total treatment volume appears to be less with Urologen in comparison to bovine GAX collagen. The manufacturer has similar products (Dermalogen®, Autologen®) *(108–111)* for dermatologic and plastic surgical use. Results appear to be promising, with a single complication of a foreign body reaction noted in the literature *(112)*. Using an alternative technique of chemical processing with subsequent freeze drying, Alloderm® (Lifecell, Branchburg, NJ) has also been developed as an allogenic acellular tissue matrix. Currently used in the plastic surgery arena, it is available in sheets or micronized into an injectable form (Cymetra®). Both forms have been compared favorably within plastic surgery to GAX bovine collagen, with greater tissue ingrowth, reduced inflammatory response, and persistence in volume *(113)*. Urologic clinical studies are being sponsored as part of a joint venture by Boston Scientific Corp. (Natick, MA). The potential for disease transmission using cadaveric sources should be prevented by donor screening and tissue preparation into acellular preparations.

Fat

At a urological historical point when there was increased interest in agents other than Teflon, attention increasingly turned to fat for injection. The abundance of available material and its pliant nature would potentially make it an ideal candidate for autologous injection. Harvested from the abdominal wall using liposuction techniques, the material can then be immediately injected into the urethra. Relatively large bore needles are used to minimize adipocyte injury *(114)*. There is a range of results from the literature regarding efficacy. Recent initial interest was raised by Santiago Gonzalez de Garibay reporting on both men and women with ISD, along with patients with reflux *(115)*. Santarosa and Blaivas generated interest in the United States in the use of fat with good results using repeat injections in women with ISD without hypermobility *(15)*. The lack of benefit shown in women with hypermobility was not confirmed in Su's larger study *(116)*. Palma demonstrated that results are improved if patients are given repeat injections *(117)*, supporting techniques of small-volume repeat injections rather than a large-volume single injection. In one study comparing fat to bovine GAX collagen in female patients with ISD, the 7-mo success rate using fat showed a 31% cure or improved, significantly less than collagen at 71% *(118)*. Results using fat for male incontinence are uniformly poor, other than anecdotal reports. Its use for treating reflux has been limited and without encouraging results *(119)*. Success depends in large part on implant viability with volume maintenance from 0–50%. Investigation in the plastic surgery arena has demonstrated similar discouraging results with injected material *(120,121)*. Using an animal model, Matthews demonstrated greater viability if the fat was harvested from a perivesical source rather than from the abdominal wall *(122)*. Work outside of urology has demonstrated possible improved results with better tissue handling, culture techniques, and the addition of growth factors *(123–128)*. Fat emboli have occurred, with one death being attributed to this *(129)*.

Chondrogel

Cell culture techniques are being applied within urology to allow for the injection of chondrocytes as a bulking agent. Chondrogel (Curis, Cambridge, MA) is formed by autologous chondrocytes that are suspended in alginate. The chondrocytes are isolated from a biopsy of the posterior aspect of the outer ear through a 2-cm incision performed under local anesthesia (*see* Fig. 12). Two 4-mm^2 pieces of cartilage are harvested and shipped in a vial containing cell culture medium. The isolation and culturing of the chondrocytes requires 7 wk preparation, with the ability to cryopreserve the cells for subsequent injection. Although they can be stored in their frozen state, once shipped for implant, the preparation must be injected within a 24–48-hr time frame. The injection of the material is relatively straightforward with the ability to pass it through a standard 21-gauge needle. There is an initial loss in volume secondary to absorption of the alginate that is offset by subsequent chondrocyte growth. The tissue growth that occurs may augment urethral function 3–6 mo following initial injection Future injections are possible from cryopreserved material, requiring 4-wk time frame to thaw and prepare. This material has been applied to both urinary incontinence from ISD and VUR *(130)*. It is currently undergoing further clinical trial in the United States.

Smooth Muscle

The ultimate form in the replacement of urethral tissue has been in the harvesting and implantation of bladder smooth muscle into the urethra *(131)*. Using an animal model, cultured myoblasts were transduced with adenovirus to allow identification following injection. Following implantation, viable myoblasts were identified with myotubule formation. Whereas this approach may provide for the regeneration of specific urethral tissue, rather than merely the placement of nonphysiologic bulk, actual function would need to be demonstrated. Other investigators have injected fetal bladder tissue for implantation in a refluxing lamb model, precluding the need for bladder biopsy *(132)*.

CONCLUSION

Submucosal injection of bulking materials can be used to treat intrinsic sphincter deficiency and the incompetent uretero–vesical junction. Careful evaluation of bladder function can best assure success and long-term benefit. Injections are minimally invasive, with at most requiring brief anesthesia performed in an ambulatory setting. Experience in female incontinence has been better than in male patients, even with

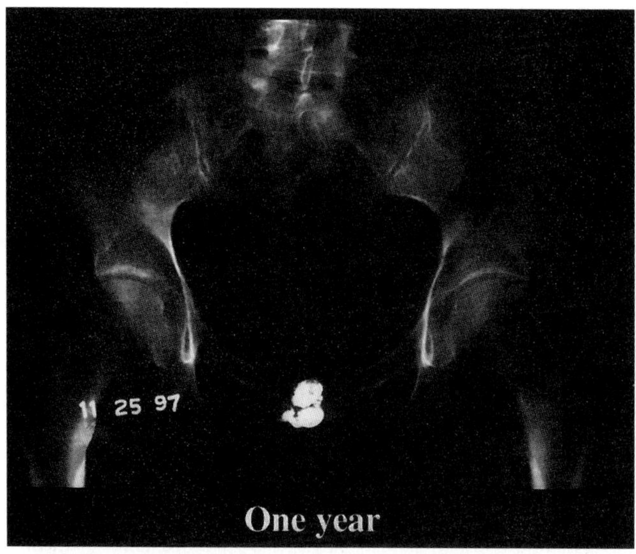

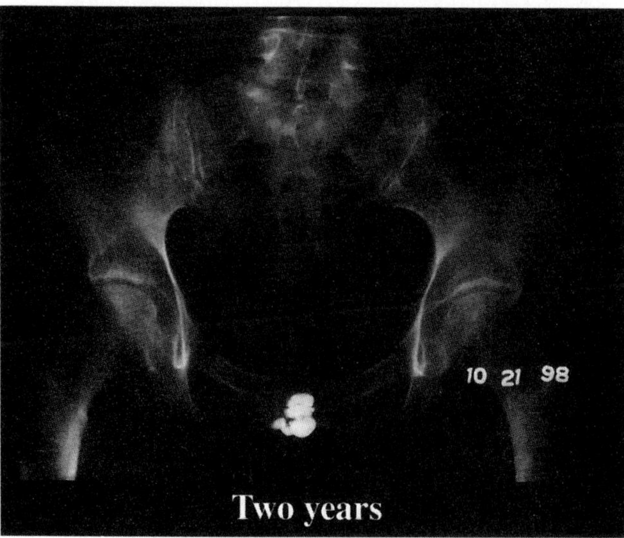

Fig. 10. KUB of Durasphere implant at 1 and 2 yr (courtesy of Advanced UroScience).

antegrade techniques to better access viable tissue. Even with successful injection for reflux, patients must have continued surveillance to monitor for recurrence. The few agents that are currently FDA approved for use in urology are offset by a large assortment being investigated. Materials range from inert synthetic bulking agents to connective tissue

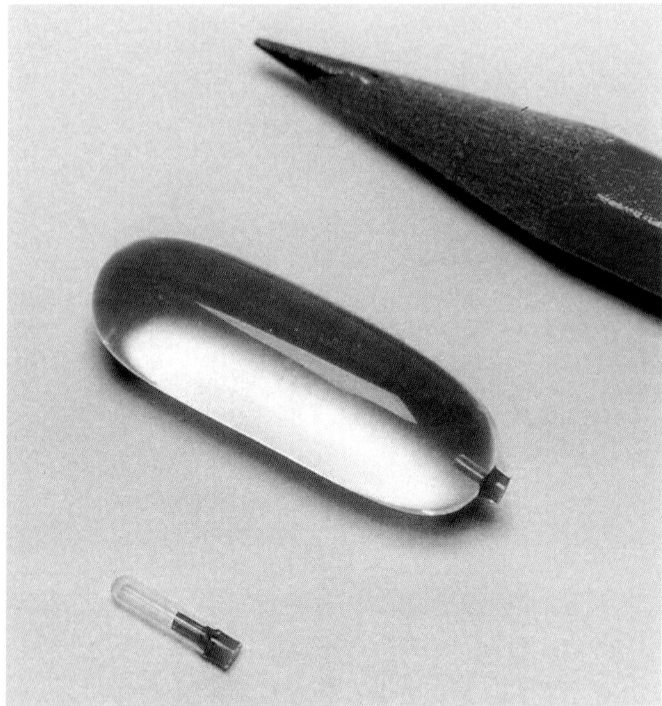

Fig. 11. UroVive implant prior to and following inflation compared to pencil tip (courtesy of AMS).

matrices to viable tissue graft implants. Although the ideal agent remains to be elucidated, patients will continue to be benefited using available techniques and materials. As we increase our understanding of implant technology and lower urinary tract physiology, the injection of bulking agents will play an increasing role in urology.

REFERENCES

1. Leonard MP, Decter A, Mix LW, Johnson HW, Coleman GU (1996) Endoscopic treatment of vesicoureteral reflux with collagen: preliminary report and cost analysis. *J Urol* 155:1716.
2. Schultheiss D, Hofner K, Oelke M, Grunewald V, Jonas U (2000) Historical aspects of the treatment of urinary incontinence. *Eur Urol* 38:352.
3. Benshushan A, Brzezinski A, Shoshani O, Rojansky N (1998) Periurethral injection for the treatment of urinary incontinence. *Ob stet Gynecol Surv* 53:383.
4. Joyner BD, Atala A (1997) Endoscopic substances for the treatment of vesicoureteral reflux. *Urology* 50:489.
5. Su TH, Hsu CY, Chen JC (1999) Injection therapy for stress incontinence in women. *Int Urogynecol J Pelvic Floor Dysfunct* 10:200.

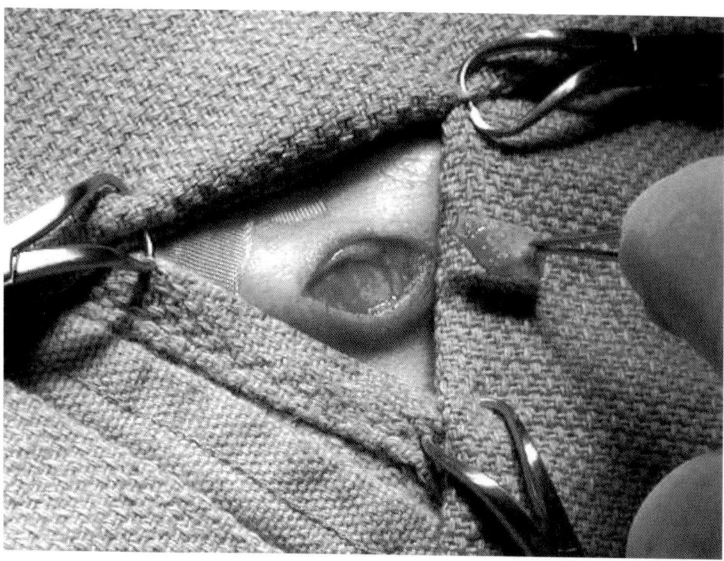

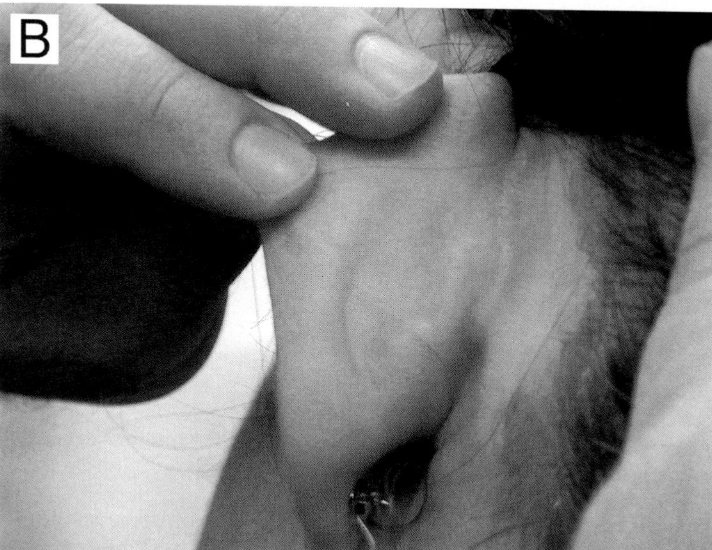

Fig. 12. Ear incision for cartilage harvesting (courtesy of Curis). (**A**) Harvesting of cartilage from posterior aspect of outer ear for subsequent tissue culture and expansion. (**B**) Healed incision site at 4 mo.

6. McGuire EJ (1995) Diagnosis and treatment of intrinsic sphincter deficiency. *Int J Urol* 2 Suppl 1:7.
7. Monga AK, Stanton SL (1997) Urodynamics: prediction, outcome and analysis of mechanism for cure of stress incontinence by periurethral collagen. *Br J Obstet Gynaecol* 104:158.

8. Appell RA (1994) Collagen injection therapy for urinary incontinence. *Urol Clin North Am* 21:177.

9. Kreder KJ, Austin JC (1996) Treatment of stress urinary incontinence in women with urethral hypermobility and intrinsic sphincter deficiency [see comments]. *J Urol* 156:1995.

10. Stricker PD (1995) Proper patient selection for Contigen Bard Collagen implant. *Int J Urol* 2.

11. Herschorn S, Steele DJ, Radomski SB (1996) Followup of intraurethral collagen for female stress urinary incontinence. *J Urol* 156:1305.

12. Steele AC, Kohli N, Karram MM (1900) Periurethral collagen injection for stress incontinence with and without urethral hypermobility [see comments]. *Obstet Gynecol* 95:327.

13. Homma Y, Kawabe K, Kageyama S, Koiso K, Akaza H, Kakizoe T, Koshiba K, Yokoyama E, Aso Y (1996) Injection of glutaraldehyde cross-linked collagen for urinary incontinence: two-year efficacy by self-assessment. *Int J Urol* 3:124.

14. Gorton E, Stanton S, Monga A, Wiskind AK, Lentz GM, Bland DR (2000) Periurethral collagen injection: a long-term follow-up study. *Br J Urol Int* 84:966.

15. Santarosa RP, Blaivas JG (1994) Periurethral injection of autologous fat for the treatment of sphincteric incontinence [see comments]. *J Urol* 151:607.

16. Barranger E, Fritel X, Kadoch O, Liou Y, Pigne A (2000) Results of transurethral injection of silicone micro-implants for females with intrinsic sphincter deficiency [In Process Citation]. *J Urol* 164:1619.

17. McGuire EJ (1995) Urodynamic evaluation of stress incontinence. *Urol Clin North Am* 22:551.

18. Badlani G, Ravalli R, Moskowitz MO (1993) A tool for the objective assessment of passive incontinence. *Contemp Urol* 5:29.

19. Lockhart JL, Walker RD, Vorstman B, Politano VA (1988) Periurethral polytetrafluoroethylene injection following urethral reconstruction in female patients with urinary incontinence. *J Urol* 140:51.

20. Kim YH, Kattan MW, Boone TB (1997) Correlation of urodynamic results and urethral coaptation with success after transurethral collagen injection. *Urology* 50:941.

21. Stanton SL, Monga AK (1997) Incontinence in elderly women: is periurethral collagen an advance? *Br J Obstet Gynaecol* 104:154.

22. Cundiff GW, Bent AE (1997) The contribution of urethrocystoscopy to evaluation of lower urinary tract dysfunction in women. *Int Urogynecol J Pelvic Floor Dysfunct* 7:307.

23. Vesey SG, Rivett A, O'Boyle PJ (1988) Teflon injection in female stress incontinence. Effect on urethral pressure profile and flow rate. *Br J Urol* 62:39.

24. Rivas DA, Chancellor MB, J-B L, Hanau C, Bagley DH, Goldberg B (1996) Endoluminal ultrasonographic and histologic evaluation of periurethral collagen injection. *J Endourol* 10:61.

25. Andersen R (2000) Urethral anesthesia for periurethral bulking procedures in women. Obstet Gynecol, 95:.

26. Gottfried HW, Maier S, Gschwend J, Brandle E, Hautmann RE (1996) [Minimally invasive treatment of stress urinary incontinence by collagen administration. Comparison between endosonography controlled and transurethral submucous collagen injection]. *Urologe A* 35:6.

27. Ordorica R (1997) Collagen injection techniques. *UroTrends* 2:1.

28. Neal DE Jr, Lahaye ME, Lowe DC (1995) Improved needle placement technique in periurethral collagen injection. *Urology* 45:865.
29. Gousse AE, Safir MH, Madjar S, Ziadlourad F, Raz S (2000) Life-threatening anaphylactoid reaction associated with indigo carmine intravenous injection. *Urology* 56:508.
30. Faerber GJ, Belville WD, Ohl DA, Plata A (1998) Comparison of transurethral versus periurethral collagen injection in women with intrinsic sphincter deficiency. *Tech Urol* 4:124.
31. Von Heland M, Mantovani F, Zanetti G, Ceresoli A, Ginepri A, Frascaro E, et al. (1998) [Urethral implantation of collagen in the treatment of urinary incontinence. Comparison of transurethral and periurethral approach]. *Minerva Urol Nefrol* 50:213.
32. McGuire EJ, English SF (1997) Periurethral collagen injection for male and female sphincteric incontinence: indications, techniques, and result. *World J Urol* 15:306.
33. Klutke CG, Nadler RB, Andriole GL (1995) Surgeon's workshop: antegrade collagen injection: new technique for postprostatectomy stress incontinence. *J Endourol* 9:513.
34. Appell RA, Vasavada SP, Rackley RR, Winters JC (1996) Percutaneous antegrade collagen injection therapy for urinary incontinence following radical prostatectomy. *Urology* 48:769.
35. Edelstein RA, Razdan S, Joseph RG, Babayan RK (1998) Surgeon's workshop: a simple method of antegrade collagen placement for postprostatectomy incontinence. *J Endourol* 12:389.
36. Loughlin KR, Comiter CV (1999) New technique for antegrade collagen injection for post-radical prostatectomy stress urinary incontinence. *Urology* 53:410.
37. Klutke CG, Tiemann DD, Nadler RB, Andriole GL (1996) Antegrade collagen injection for stress incontinence after radical prostatectomy: technique and early results. *J Endourol* 10:279.
38. Klutke JJ, Subir C, Andriole G, Klutke CG (1999) Long-term results after antegrade collagen injection for stress urinary incontinence following radical retropubic prostatectomy. *Urology* 53:974.
39. Flood HD, Ritchey ML, Bloom DA, Huang C, McGuire EJ (1994) Outcome of reflux in children with myelodysplasia managed by bladder pressure monitoring. *J Urol* 152:1574.
40. Willemsen J, Nijman RJ (2000) Vesicoureteral reflux and videourodynamic studies: results of a prospective study. *Urology* 55:939.
41. O'Donnell B, Puri P (1984) Treatment of vesicoureteric reflux by endoscopic injection of Teflon. *Br Med J (Clin Res Ed)* 289:7.
42. Brown S, Stewart RJ, O'Hara MD, Hill CM (1991) Histological changes following submucosal Teflon injection in the bladder. *J Pediatr Surg* 26:546.
43. Kaplan WE, Dalton DP, Firlit CF (1987) The endoscopic correction of reflux by polytetrafluoroethylene injection. *J Urol* 138:953.
44. Sugiyama T, Hashimoto K, Kiwamoto H, Ohnishi N, Esa A, Park YC, Kurita T, Kohri K (1996) Endoscopic correction of vesicoureteral reflux in patients with neurogenic bladder dysfunction. *Int Urol Nephrol* 27:527.
45. Farkas A, Moriel EZ, Lupa S (1990) Endoscopic correction of vesicoureteral reflux: our experience with 115 ureters. *J Urol* 144:534.
46. Dewan PA, O'Donnell B (1991) Polytef paste injection of refluxing duplex ureters. *Eur Urol* 19:35.

47. Puri P, Kumar R (1996) Endoscopic correction of vesicoureteral reflux secondary to posterior urethral valves. *J Urol* 156:680.

48. Diamond T, Boston VE (1987) Reflux following endoscopic treatment of ureteroceles. A new approach using endoscopic subureteric Teflon injection. *Br J Urol* 60:279.

49. Viville C (1990) Endoscopic treatment of ureterocele and antireflux injection with Teflon paste. *Eur Urol* 17:321.

50. Simsek F, Dillioglugil O, Ilker Y, Akdas A (1995) Correction of primary and secondary vesicoureteral reflux by subureteric Teflon injection. *Int Urol Nephrol* 27:51.

51. Angulo JM, Arteaga R, Rodriguez Alarcon J, Fernandez T, Arnet R (1996) [Our experience in endoscopic teflon treatment in vesicoureteral reflux in children]. *Cir Pediatr* 8:161.

52. Mann CI, Jequier S, Patriquin H, LaBerge I, Homsy YL (1988) Intramural Teflon injection of the ureter for treatment of vesicoureteral reflux: sonographic appearance. *AJR Am J Roentgenol* 151:543.

53. Politano VA, Small MP, Harper JM, Lynne CM (1974) Periurethral teflon injection for urinary incontinence. *J Urol* 111:180.

54. Berg S (1973) Polytef augmentation urethroplasty. Correction of surgically incurable urinary incontinence by injection technique. *Arch Surg* 107:379.

55. Lotenfoe R, O'Kelly JK, Helal M, Lockhart JL (1993) Periurethral polytetrafluoroethylene paste injection in incontinent female subjects: surgical indications and improved surgical technique [see comments]. *J Urol* 149:279.

56. Puri P, O'Donnell B (1984) Correction of experimentally produced vesicoureteric reflux in the piglet by intravesical injection of Teflon. *Br Med J (Clin Res Ed)* 289:5.

57. Kossovsky N, Millett D, Juma S, Little N, Briggs PC, Raz S, Berg E (1992) In vivo characterization of the inflammatory properties of poly(tetrafluoroethylene) particulates [published erratum appears in *J Biomed Mater Res* (1992) 26(2):269]. *J Biomed Mater Res* 25:1287.

58. Martinez-Pineiro L, Leon J Jd, Cozar JM, Navarro J, E CB, Martinez-Pineiro JA (1989) [Obstructive uropathy secondary to the periurethral injection of teflon paste]. *Arch Esp Urol* 42:571.

59. McKinney CD, Gaffey MJ, Gillenwater JY (1994) Bladder outlet obstruction after multiple periurethral polytetrafluoroethylene injections. *J Urol* 153:149.

60. Boykin W, Rodriguez FR, Brizzolara JP, Thompson IM, Zeidman EJ (1989) Complete urinary obstruction following periurethral polytetrafluoroethylene injection for urinary incontinence. *J Urol* 141:1199.

61. Kiilholma PJ, Chancellor MB, Makinen J, Hirsch IH, Klemi PJ (1994) Complications of Teflon injection for stress urinary incontinence. *Neurourol Urodyn* 12:131.

62. Ferro MA, Smith JH, Smith PJ (1988) Periurethral granuloma: unusual complication of Teflon periurethral injection. *Urology* 31:422.

63. Aragona F, D'Urso L, Scremin E, Salmaso R, Glazel GP (1997) Polytetrafluoroethylene giant granuloma and adenopathy: long-term complications following subureteral polytetrafluoroethylene injection for the treatment of vesicoureteral reflux in children. *J Urol* 158:1539.

64. Lacombe A (1990) Ureterovesical reimplantation after failure of endoscopic treatment of reflux by submucosal injection of polytef paste. *Eur Urol* 17:318.

65. Solomon LZ, Birch BR, Cooper AJ, Davies CL, Holmes SA (2000) Nonhomologous bioinjectable materials in urology: 'size matters'? *Br J Urol Int* 85:641.

66. Leth PM (1994) [Spread of teflon particles from periurethrally injected teflon paste to pulmonary tissue]. *Ugeskr Laeger* 156:981.

67. Claes H, Stroobants D, Van Meevbeek J, Verbeken E, Knockaert D, Baert L (1989) Pulmonary migration following periurethral polytetrafluoroethylene injection for urinary incontinence [see comments]. *J Urol* 142:821.

68. Dewan PA, Fraundorfer M (1996) Skin migration following periurethral polytetrafluoroethylene injection for urinary incontinence. *Aust N Z J Surg* 66:57.

69. Malizia AA Jr, Reiman HM, Myers RP, Sande JR, Barham SS, Jr BR, Dewanjee MK, Utz WJ (1984) Migration and granulomatous reaction after periurethral injection of polytef (Teflon). *JAMA* 251:3277.

70. Miyakita H, Puri P (1994) Particles found in lung and brain following subureteral injection of polytetrafluoroethylene paste are not teflon particles. *J Urol* 152:636.

71. Herschorn S, Glazer AA (2000) Early experience with small volume periurethral polytetrafluoroethylene for female stress urinary incontinence [see comments]. *J Urol* 163:1838.

72. Politano VA (1992) Transurethral polytef injection for post-prostatectomy urinary incontinence. *Br J Urol* 69:26.

73. Henly DR, Barrett DM, Weiland TL, O'Connor MK, Malizia AA, Wein AJ (1995) Particulate silicone for use in periurethral injections: local tissue effects and search for migration. *J Urol* 153:2039.

74. Harriss DR, Iacovou JW, Lemberger RJ (1997) Peri-urethral silicone microimplants (Macroplastique) for the treatment of genuine stress incontinence [see comments]. *Br J Urol* 78:722.

75. Hidar S, Attyaoui F, de Leval J (2000) [Periurethral injection of silicone microparticles in the treatment of sphincter deficiency urinary incontinence]. *Prog Urol* 10:219.

76. Koelbl H, Saz V, Doerfler D, Haeusler G, Sam C, Hanzal E (1998) Transurethral injection of silicone microimplants for intrinsic urethral sphincter deficiency. *Obstet Gynecol* 92:332.

77. Sheriff MK, Foley S, Mcfarlane J, Nauth-Misir R, Shah PJ (1997) Endoscopic correction of intractable stress incontinence with silicone micro-implants. *Eur Urol* 32:284.

78. Inc AU (1999) Summary of safety and effectiveness data: Durasphere injectable bulking agent.

79. Walker RD, Wilson J, Clark AE (1992) Injectable bioglass as a potential substitute for injectable polytetrafluoroethylene. *J Urol* 148:645.

80. Stenberg A, Lackgren G (1995) A new bioimplant for the endoscopic treatment of vesicoureteral reflux: experimental and short-term clinical results. *J Urol* 154:800.

81. Stenberg A, Larsson G, Johnson P, Heimer G, Ulmsten U (1999) DiHA Dextran Copolymer, a new biocompatible material for endoscopic treatment of stress incontinent women. Short term results. *Acta Obstet Gynecol Scand* 78:436.

82. Stenberg AM, Sundin A, Larsson BS, Lackgren G, Stenberg A (1997) Lack of distant migration after injection of a 125iodine labeled dextranomer based implant into the rabbit bladder. *J Urol* 158:1937.

83. Stenberg A, Larsson E, Lindholm A, Ronneus B, Stenberg A, Lackgren G (2000) Injectable dextranomer-based implant: histopathology, volume changes and DNA-analysis. *Scand J Urol Nephrol* 33:355.

84. Kunstlinger F, Brunelle F, Chaumont P, Doyon D (1981) Vascular occlusive agents. *AJR Am J Roentgenol* 136:151.

85. Barry JW, Bookstein JJ (1981) Transcatheter hemostasis in the genitourinary tract. *Urol Radiol* 2:211.

86. Belis JA, Horton JA (1982) Renal artery embolization with polyvinyl alcohol foam particles. *Urology* 19:224.

87. Jack CR Jr, Forbes G, Dewanjee MK, Brown ML, Earnest F IV (1985) Polyvinyl alcohol sponge for embolotherapy: particle size and morphology. *AJNR Am J Neuroradiol* 6:595.

88. Merguerian PA, McLorie GA, Khoury AE, Thorner P, Churchill BM (1990) Submucosal injection of polyvinyl alcohol foam in rabbit bladder. *J Urol* 144:531.

89. Canning D (1991) New implants for endoscopic correction in the nineties and beyond. *Dialog Pediatr Urol* 14:6.

90. Yoo JJ, Magliochetti M, Atala A (1997) Detachable self-sealing membrane system for the endoscopic treatment of incontinence. *J Urol* 158:1045.

91. Diamond DA, Bauer SB, Retik AB, Atala A (2000) Initial experience with the transurethral self-detachable balloon system for urinary incontinence in pediatric patients. *J Urol* 164:942.

92. Manna F, Dentini M, Desideri P, De Pita O, Mortilla E, Maras B (2000) Comparative chemical evaluation of two commercially available derivatives of hyaluronic acid (hylaform from rooster combs and restylane from streptococcus) used for soft tissue augmentation. *J Eur Acad Dermatol Venereol* 13:183.

93. Larsen NE, Pollak CT, Reiner K, Leshchiner E, Balazs EA (1994) Hylan gel biomaterial: dermal and immunologic compatibility. *J Biomed Mater Res* 27:1129.

94. Piacquadio D, Larsen N, Denlinger J, Balazs E (1998) Hylan B Gel (Hylaform) as a Soft Tissue Augmentation Material. *Tissue Augmentation in Clinical Practice: Procedures and Techniques*, (Klein, A. W., ed.) Marcel-Dekker, Inc., New York, NY.

95. Shortliffe LM, Freiha FS, Kessler R, Stamey TA, Constantinou CE (1989) Treatment of urinary incontinence by the periurethral implantation of glutaraldehyde cross-linked collagen. *J Urol* 141:538.

96. McClelland M, Delustro F (1996) Evaluation of antibody class in response to bovine collagen treatment in patients with urinary incontinence [see comments]. *J Urol* 155:2068.

97. Stothers L, Goldenberg SL (1998) Delayed hypersensitivity and systemic arthralgia following transurethral collagen injection for stress urinary incontinence [see comments]. *J Urol* 159:1507.

98. Stothers L, Goldenberg SL, Leone EF (1998) Complications of periurethral collagen injection for stress urinary incontinence. *J Urol* 159:806.

99. Elson ML (1999) Re: Delayed hypersensitivity and systemic arthralgia following transurethral collagen injection for stress urinary incontinence [letter; comment]. *J Urol* 161:610.

100. Frey P, Mangold S (1995) Physical and histological behavior of a new injectable collagen (GAX 65) implanted into the submucosal space of the mini-pig bladder. *J Urol* 154:812.

101. Frey P, Lutz N, Berger D, Herzog B (1994) Histological behavior of glutaraldehyde cross-linked bovine collagen injected into the human bladder for the treatment of vesicoureteral reflux. *J Urol* 152:632.

102. Ang LP, Tay KP, Lim PH, Chng HC (1997) Endoscopic injection of collagen for the treatment of female urinary stress incontinence. *Int J Urol* 4:254.
103. Knapp PM, Lingeman JE, Siegel YI, Badylak SF, Demeter RJ (1994) Biocompatibility of small-intestinal submucosa in urinary tract as augmentation cystoplasty graft and injectable suspension. *J Endourol* 8:125.
104. Furness PD III, Kolligian ME, Lang SJ, Kaplan WE, Kropp BP, Cheng EY (2000) Injectable small intestinal submucosa: preliminary evaluation for use in endoscopic urological surgery [In Process Citation]. *J Urol* 164:1680.
105. Zhang Y, Kropp BP, Moore P, Cowan R, Furness PD III, Kolligian ME, et al. (2000) Coculture of bladder urothelial and smooth muscle cells on small intestinal submucosa: potential applications for tissue engineering technology. *J Urol* 164:928.
106. Cendron M, DeVore DP, Connolly R, Sant GR, Ucci A, Calahan R, Klauber GT (1995) The biological behavior of autologous collagen injected into the rabbit bladder. *J Urol* 154:808.
107. Cozzolino DJ, Cendron M, DeVore DP, Hoopes PJ (1999) The biological behavior of autologous collagen-based extracellular matrix injected into the rabbit bladder wall. *Neurourol Urodyn* 18:487.
108. Fagien S (2000) Facial soft-tissue augmentation with injectable autologous and allogeneic human tissue collagen matrix (autologen and dermalogen). *Plast Reconstr Surg* 105:362.
109. Apesos J, Muntzing MG II (2000) Autologen [In Process Citation]. *Clin Plast Surg* 27:507.
110. Goode RL (2000) Current status of "soft" implant materials for the face. *Arch Facial Plast Surg* 1:60.
111. Sclafani AP, Romo T III, Parker A, McCormick SA, Cocker R, Jacono A (2000) Autologous collagen dispersion (Autologen) as a dermal filler: clinical observations and histologic findings [In Process Citation]. *Arch Facial Plast Surg* 2:48.
112. Moody BR, Sengelmann RD (2000) Self-limited adverse reaction to human-derived collagen injectable product [In Process Citation]. *Dermatol Surg* 26:936.
113. Sclafani AP, Romo T III, Jacono AA, McCormick S, Cocker R, Parker A (2000) Evaluation of acellular dermal graft in sheet (AlloDerm) and injectable (micronized AlloDerm) forms for soft tissue augmentation. Clinical observations and histological analysis. *Arch Facial Plast Surg* 2:130.
114. Lewis CM (1993) The current status of autologous fat grafting. *Aesthet Plast Surg* 17:109.
115. Santiago Gonzalez, de GA, Castro Morrondo J, Castillo Jimeno JM, Sanchez Robles I, Sebastian Borruel JL (1989) [Endoscopic injection of autologous adipose tissue in the treatment of female incontinence]. *Arch Esp Urol* 42:143.
116. Su TH, Wang KG, Hsu CY, Wei HJ, Yen HJ, Shien FC (1998) Periurethral fat injection in the treatment of recurrent genuine stress incontinence. *J Urol* 159:411.
117. Palma PC, Riccetto CL, Herrmann V, Netto NR Jr (1997) Repeated lipoinjections for stress urinary incontinence. *J Endourol* 11:67.
118. Haab F, Zimmern PE, Leach GE (1997) Urinary stress incontinence due to intrinsic sphincteric deficiency: experience with fat and collagen periurethral injections [see comments] [published erratum appears in *J Urol* (1997) 158(1):188]. *J Urol* 157:1283.
119. Chancellor MB, Rivas DA, Liberman SN, Moore J Jr, Staas WE Jr (1994) Cystoscopic autogenous fat injection treatment of vesicoureteral reflux in spinal cord injury. *J Am Paraplegia Soc* 17:50.

120. Billings E Jr, May JW Jr (1989) Historical review and present status of free fat graft autotransplantation in plastic and reconstructive surgery [see comments]. *Plast Reconstr Surg* 83:368.

121. Ersek RA (1991) Transplantation of purified autologous fat: a 3-year follow-up is disappointing [see comments]. *Plast Reconstr Surg* 87:219.

122. Matthews RD, Christensen JP, Canning DA (1994) Persistence of autologous free fat transplant in bladder submucosa of rats. *J Urol* 152:819.

123. Eppley BL, Sadove AM (1991) A physicochemical approach to improving free fat graft survival: preliminary observations. *Aesthet Plast Surg* 15:215.

124. Fagrell D, Enestrom S, Berggren A, Kniola B (1996) Fat cylinder transplantation: an experimental comparative study of three different kinds of fat transplants. *Plast Reconstr Surg* 98:90.

125. Ullmann Y, Hyams M, Ramon Y, Beach D, Peled IJ, Lindenbaum ES (1998) Enhancing the survival of aspirated human fat injected into nude mice. *Plast Reconstr Surg* 101:1940.

126. Yuksel E, Weinfeld AB, Cleek R, Wamsley S, Jensen J, Boutros S, et al (2000) Increased free fat-graft survival with the long-term, local delivery of insulin, insulin-like growth factor-I, and basic fibroblast growth factor by PLGA/PEG microspheres. *Plast Reconstr Surg* 105:1712.

127. Nishimura T, Hashimoto H, Nakanishi I, Furukawa M (2000) Microvascular angiogenesis and apoptosis in the survival of free fat grafts. *Laryngoscope* 110:1333.

128. Har-Shai Y, Lindenbaum ES, Gamliel-Lazarovich A, Beach D, Hirshowitz B (2000) An integrated approach for increasing the survival of autologous fat grafts in the treatment of contour defects. *Plast Reconstr Surg* 104:945.

129. Currie I, Drutz HP, Deck J, Oxorn D (1998) Adipose tissue and lipid droplet embolism following periurethral injection of autologous fat: case report and review of the literature. *Int Urogynecol J Pelvic Floor Dysfunct* 8:377.

130. Diamond DA, Caldamone AA (1999) Endoscopic correction of vesicoureteral reflux in children using autologous chondrocytes: preliminary results. *J Urol* 162:1185.

131. Chancellor MB, Yokoyama T, Tirney S, Mattes CE, Ozawa H, Yoshimura N, et al. (2000) Preliminary results of myoblast injection into the urethra and bladder wall: a possible method for the treatment of stress urinary incontinence and impaired detrusor contractility. *Neurourol Urodyn* 19:279.

132. Zhang Y., Bailey R.R. (1998) Treatment of vesicoureteric reflux in sheep model using subureteric injection of cultured fetal bladder tissue. *Pediatr Surg Int* 13:32–36.

133. Lotenfoe R, O'Kelly JK, Helal M, Lockhart JL (1993) Periurethral polytetrafluoroethylene paste injection in incontinent female subjects: surgical indications and improved surgical technique [see comments]. *J Urol* 149:279.

134. Herschorn S, Glazer AA (2000) Early experience with small volume periurethral polytetrafluoroethylene for female stress urinary incontinence [see comments]. *J Urol* 163:1838.

135. Lopez AE, Padron OF, Patsias G, Politano VA (1993) Transurethral polytetrafluoroethylene injection in female patients with urinary continence. *J Urol* 150:856.

136. Kiilholma P, Makinen J (1992) Disappointing effect of endoscopic Teflon injection for female stress incontinence. *Eur Urol* 20:197.

137. Politano VA (1982) Periurethral polytetrafluoroethylene injection for urinary incontinence. *J Urol* 127:439.

138. Henalla SM, Hall V, Duckett JR, Link C, Usman F, Tromans PM, van Veggel L (2000) A multicentre evaluation of a new surgical technique for urethral bulking in the treatment of genuine stress incontinence. *Br J Obstet Gynecol* 107:1035.
139. Guys JM, Simeoni-Alias J, Fakhro A, Delarue A (2000) Use of polydimethyl-siloxane for endoscopic treatment of neurogenic urinary incontinence in children [see comments]. *J Urol* 162:2133.
140. Sheriff MK, Foley S, Mcfarlane J, Nauth-Misir R, Shah PJ (1997) Endoscopic correction of intractable stress incontinence with silicone micro-implants. *Eur Urol* 32:284.
141. Harriss DR, Iacovou JW, Lemberger RJ (1997) Peri-urethral silicone microimplants (Macroplastique) for the treatment of genuine stress incontinence [see comments]. *Br J Urol* 78:722.
142. Inc AU (1999) Summary of safety and effectiveness data: Durasphere injectable bulking agent.
143. Diamond DA, Bauer SB, Retik AB, Atala A (2000) Initial experience with the transurethral self-detachable balloon system for urinary incontinence in pediatric patients. *J Urol* 164:942.
144. Pycha A, Klingler CH, Haitel A, Heinz-Peer G, Marberger M (1998) Implantable microballoons: an attractive alternative in the management of intrinsic sphincter deficiency. *Eur Urol* 33:469.
145. Stenberg A, Larsson G, Johnson P, Heimer G, Ulmsten U (1999) DiHA Dextran Copolymer, a new biocompatible material for endoscopic treatment of stress incontinent women. Short term results. *Acta Obstet Gynecol Scand* 78:436.
146. Ang LP, Tay KP, Lim PH, Chng HC (1997) Endoscopic injection of collagen for the treatment of female urinary stress incontinence. *Int J Urol* 4:254.
147. Cross CA, English SF, Cespedes RD, McGuire EJ (1997) A followup on transurethral collagen injection therapy for urinary incontinence. *J Urol* 159:106.
148. Herschorn S, Steele DJ, Radomski SB (1996) Followup of intraurethral collagen for female stress urinary incontinence. *J Urol* 156:1305.
149. Corcos J, Fournier C (1999) Periurethral collagen injection for the treatment of female stress urinary incontinence: 4-year follow-up results. *Urology* 54:815.
150. Gorton E, Stanton S, Monga A, Wiskind AK, Lentz GM, Bland DR (2000) Periurethral collagen injection: a long-term follow-up study. *Br J Urol Int* 84:966.
151. Haab F, Zimmern PE, Leach GE (1997) Urinary stress incontinence due to intrinsic sphincteric deficiency: experience with fat and collagen periurethral injections [see comments] [published erratum appears in *J Urol* (1997) 158(1):188]. *J Urol* 157:1283.
152. Santiago Gonzalez, de GA, Castro Morrondo J, Castillo Jimeno JM, Sanchez Robles I, Sebastian Borruel JL (1989) [Endoscopic injection of autologous adipose tissue in the treatment of female incontinence]. *Arch Esp Urol* 42:143.
153. Palma PC, Riccetto CL, Herrmann V, Netto NR Jr (1997) Repeated lipoinjections for stress urinary incontinence. *J Endourol* 11:67.
154. Su TH, Wang KG, Hsu CY, Wei HJ, Yen HJ, Shien FC (1998) Periurethral fat injection in the treatment of recurrent genuine stress incontinence. *J Urol* 159:411.
155. Santarosa RP, Blaivas JG (1994) Periurethral injection of autologous fat for the treatment of sphincteric incontinence [see comments]. *J Urol* 151:607.
156. Lloyd L, Bent R, Tutrone G, Badlani G, Kennelly M (2000) Treatment of intrinsic sphincter deficiency using autologous ear cartilage as a bulking agent. *Am Urolog Assoc 95th Ann Meet* 332.

157. Politano VA (1992) Transurethral polytef injection for post-prostatectomy urinary incontinence. *Br J Urol* 69:26.
158. Stanisic TH, Jennings CE, Miller JI (1991) Polytetrafluoroethylene injection for post-prostatectomy incontinence: experience with 20 patients during 3 years. *J Urol* 146:1575.
159. Kabalin JN (1994) Treatment of post-prostatectomy stress urinary incontinence with periurethral polytetrafluoroethylene paste injection. *J Urol* 152:1463.
160. Duffy PG, Ransley PG (1998) Endoscopic treatment of urinary incontinence in children with primary epispadias. *Br J Urol* 81:309.
161. Bugel H, Pfister C, Sibert L, Cappele O, Khalaf A, Grise P (1999) [Intraurethral Macroplastic injections in the treatment of urinary incontinence after prostatic surgery]. *Prog Urol* 9:1068.
162. Aboseif SR, O'Connell HE, Usui A, McGuire EJ (1996) Collagen injection for intrinsic sphincteric deficiency in men [see comments]. *J Urol* 155:10.
163. Cummings JM, Boullier JA, Parra RO (1996) Transurethral collagen injections in the therapy of post-radical prostatectomy stress incontinence. *J Urol* 155:1011.
164. Elsergany R, Ghoniem GM (1998) Collagen injection for intrinsic sphincteric deficiency in men: a reasonable option in selected patients [see comments]. *J Urol* 159:1504.
165. Faerber GJ, Richardson TD (1997) Long-term results of transurethral collagen injection in men with intrinsic sphincter deficiency. *J Endourol* 11:273.
166. Kuznetsov DD, Kim HL, Patel RV, Steinberg GD, Bales GT (2000) Comparison of artificial urinary sphincter and collagen for the treatment of postprostatectomy incontinence [In Process Citation]. *Urology* 56:600.
167. Sanchez-Ortiz RF, Broderick GA, Chaikin DC, Malkowicz SB, Van Arsdalen K, Blander DS, Wein AJ (1997) Collagen injection therapy for post-radical retropubic prostatectomy incontinence: role of Valsalva leak point pressure. *J Urol* 158:2132.
168. Martins FE, Bennett CJ, Dunn M, Filho D, Keller T, Lieskovsky G (1997) Adverse prognostic features of collagen injection therapy for urinary incontinence following radical retropubic prostatectomy [see comments]. *J Urol* 158:1745.
169. Smith DN, Appell RA, Rackley RR, Winters JC (1998) Collagen injection therapy for post-prostatectomy incontinence. *J Urol* 160:364.
170. Appell RA, Vasavada SP, Rackley RR, Winters JC (1996) Percutaneous antegrade collagen injection therapy for urinary incontinence following radical prostatectomy. *Urology* 48:769.
171. Klutke JJ, Subir C, Andriole G, Klutke CG (1999) Long-term results after antegrade collagen injection for stress urinary incontinence following radical retropubic prostatectomy. *Urology* 53:974.
172. AS., G.d., Castillo Jimeno JM, Villanueva Perez I, Figuerido Garmendia E, Vigata Lopez MJ, Sebastian Borruel JL (1992) [Treatment of urinary stress incontinence using paraurethral injection of autologous fat]. *Arch Esp Urol* 44:595.
173. Sauvage P, Geiss S, Saussine C, Laustriat S, Becmeur F, Bientz J, et al. (1990) Analysis and perspectives of endoscopic treatment of vesicoureteral reflux in children with a 20-month follow-up. *Eur Urol* 17:310.
174. Geiss S, Alessandrini P, Allouch G, Aubert D, Bayard M, Bondonny JM, et al. (1990) Multicenter survey of endoscopic treatment of vesicoureteral reflux in children. *Eur Urol* 17:328.

175. Blake NS, O'Connell E (1989) Endoscopic correction of vesico-ureteric reflux by subureteric Teflon injection: follow-up ultrasound and voiding cystography. *Br J Radiol* 62:443.
176. Puri P (1990) Endoscopic correction of primary vesicoureteric reflux by subureteric injection of polytetrafluoroethylene [see comments]. *Lancet* 335:1320.
177. Dodat H, Valmalle AF, Weidmann JD, Collet F, Pelizzo G, Dubois R (1999) [Endoscopic treatment of vesicorenal reflux in children. Five-year assessment of the use of Macroplastique]. *Prog Urol* 8:1001.
178. Palma P, Almeida M, Nardi A, Ricetto L (2000) Self-detachable balloon system (UroVive) for complex vesicoureteral reflux (VUR). *Am Urolog Assoc 95th Ann Meet*.
179. Stenberg A, Lackgren G (1995) A new bioimplant for the endoscopic treatment of vesicoureteral reflux: experimental and short-term clinical results. *J Urol* 154:800.
180. Reunanen M (1996) Correction of vesicoureteral reflux in children by endoscopic collagen injection: a prospective study. *J Urol* 154:2156.
181. Leonard MP, Canning DA, Peters CA, Gearhart JP, Jeffs RD (1991) Endoscopic injection of glutaraldehyde cross-linked bovine dermal collagen for correction of vesicoureteral reflux [see comments]. *J Urol* 145:115.
182. Haferkamp A, Contractor H, Mohring K, Staehler G, Dorsam J (2000) Failure of subureteral bovine collagen injection for the endoscopic treatment of primary vesicoureteral reflux in long-term follow-up. *Urology* 55:759.
13. Frey P, Lutz N, Jenny P, Herzog B (1995) Endoscopic subureteral collagen injection for the treatment of vesicoureteral reflux in infants and children. *J Urol* 154:804.
184. Chancellor MB, Rivas DA, Liberman SN, Moore J Jr, Staas WE Jr (1994) Cystoscopic autogenous fat injection treatment of vesicoureteral reflux in spinal cord injury. *J Am Paraplegia Soc* 17:50.
185. Diamond DA, Caldamone AA (1999) Endoscopic correction of vesicoureteral reflux in children using autologous chondrocytes: preliminary results. *J Urol* 162:1185.

5 Teflon Injection for Incontinence After Radical Prostatectomy

Choonghee Noh, MD, David Shusterman, MD and James L. Mohler, MD

CONTENTS

ANATOMY
HISTORY OF TEFLON INJECTION
SELECTION OF CANDIDATES FOR TEFLON INJECTION
OPERATIVE TECHNIQUE OF TEFLON INJECTION
RESULTS OF TEFLON INJECTIONS AT UNC
OTHER TREATMENT OPTIONS FOR POSTPROSTATECTOMY
    INCONTINENCE
CONCLUSION
REFERENCES

Urinary incontinence is a frequent complication after radical prostatectomy; rates vary widely depending on the skill and experience of the surgeon, patient age, and criteria used for reporting incontinence. A study of a large group of Medicare beneficiaries who underwent radical prostatectomy showed that almost half of the survey respondents reported daily urinary leakage, 32% required protection or used a penile clamp, and 6% required surgical intervention for treatment of urinary incontinence *(1)*. Postradical prostatectomy incontinence impairs quality of life and results in significant patient expense.

From: *Urologic Prostheses:*
The Complete, Practical Guide to Devices, Their Implantation and Patient Follow Up
Edited by: C. C. Carson © Humana Press Inc., Totowa, NJ

ANATOMY

In males, two separate continence zones are recognized: 1) the proximal urethral sphincter (PUS) that includes the bladder neck, prostate gland, and prostatic urethra to the veru montanum and 2) the distal urethral sphincter (DUS) that extends from the veru montanum to the bulbar urethra. The DUS has three principal components: 1) the intrinsic rhabdosphincter that contains slow-twitch fibers capable of sustaining the tone of the urethral lumen over prolonged periods; 2) the periurethral extrinsic skeletal muscle layer composed primarily of fast-twitch fibers that supplement the activity of the rhabdosphincter under stress conditions; and 3) the intrinsic smooth muscle layer, a continuation of the superficial layer of the detrusor muscle lining the posterior prostatic urethra *(2)*. After radical prostatectomy, the PUS and proximal portion of the DUS, including the veru montanum and the prostatic apex, are removed. Therefore, postoperative continence depends exclusively on the distal sphincteric mechanism.

In addition to an intact distal urethral sphincter, normal bladder function (normal bladder capacity and compliance without detrusor instability) is required to preserve continence after radical prostatectomy. Any bladder dysfunction resulting in an intravesical pressure that exceeds the distal urethral sphincter resistance will result in urinary incontinence *(3)*.

HISTORY OF TEFLON INJECTION

Teflon paste, Polytef,® is a 50% suspension of polytetrafluoroethylene particles in the carrying vehicle, glycerin. Glycerin is quickly absorbed after injection. Teflon is an inert particulate substance that causes a foreign body reaction with histiocyte infiltration and encapsulation by fibrous tissue *(4)*. Although Teflon induces chronic inflammation, it has not been associated with secondary malignancy *(5)*.

Murless *(6)* first used a sclerosing agent for treatment of urinary incontinence in 1938 when he injected sodium morrhuate in the anterior vaginal wall. The resulting scarring compressed the urethra and produced temporary continence. Arnold reported the use of Teflon injection for vocal cord augmentation in 1962 *(7)*. Beginning in 1964, Politano et al. pioneered the use of Teflon for the endoscopic treatment of urinary incontinence *(8)*. From 1964 to 1978, Teflon injections were made transperineally. Since 1978, injections were performed transurethrally; the technique was simpler and improved results *(8–10)*.

Politano reported on more than 1000 injections performed on 720 patients (average 1.4 injections per patient and 18 mL Teflon per injection). The results of the injection were graded as excellent (when patients were completely continent and used no protective pads or tissues), good (when patients improved and required minimal protection), or failed. Teflon injection was successful in 88% of patients who had incontinence after transurethral resection of the prostate (TURP), 74% of patients incontinent after open prostatectomy, and 67% of patients incontinent after radical prostatectomy *(8)*. Postoperative complications were minimal and consisted primarily of several days of irritative symptoms. A few patients had prolonged perineal pain that responded well to antiinflammatory drugs. He identified three patterns of response to Teflon injections. The first group improved immediately and remained dry. The second group resolved their incontinence slowly over a period of 3–7 mo. The third group was dry immediately postoperatively but began to leak 1–3 wk later. These patients became dry in approximately 3–7 mo. He recommended waiting at least 6 mo before considering reinjection *(8)*.

Teflon particles have an irregular surface and diameter of 5–100 μm; more than 90% of particles are less than 40 μm in diameter. Particles less than 60 μm in size may be injected directly into capillaries, embolize and give rise to distant granulomas *(11)*. In addition, Teflon particles are phagocytized into the reticuloendothelial system and may migrate to regional lymph nodes and beyond *(12)*. This phenomenon was first reported in 1983 when a 76-yr-old man treated for urinary incontinence with periurethral Teflon was found to have pulmonary Teflon granulomas at autopsy 4 yr following therapy *(13)*. Animal studies with dogs and monkeys injected with periurethral Teflon had Teflon particle migration and resultant granuloma formation in the pelvic lymph nodes, lungs, brain, kidneys, and spleen *(11)*. A large granulomatous reaction may occur at the initial injection site that may persist and enlarge for several years. Politano has not found any evidence of complications from Teflon particle migration in 720 cases treated since 1964 *(8)*. Teflon has been used medically for more than three decades in vascular grafts, heart valves, aortic implants, cerebral shunts and shunts for hemodialysis and for vocal cord augmentation. In spite of the long and safe use of Teflon, concerns regarding the possibility of particulate migration and embolization with granuloma formation have curtailed use of Teflon injections for treatment of urinary incontinence.

SELECTION OF CANDIDATES FOR TEFLON INJECTION

Patients who have postradical prostatectomy incontinence in spite of treatment with Kegel exercises, bladder relaxants, biofeedback, and mechanical aids may be considered for Teflon injection. Urinary tract infection is excluded and chance of prostate cancer cure estimated. Cystoscopy should be performed to exclude anastomotic and urethral strictures and visualize the distal urethral sphincter.

Urodynamic evaluation should be performed to exclude detrusor instability and neurogenic bladder. The need for urodynamic evaluation in patients with postprostatectomy incontinence was reviewed recently *(14)*. In our referral practice experience, 3 of 21 patients considered for Teflon injection were found to have contraindications for the procedure. One had unrecognized detrusor failure and his overflow incontinence was managed with intermittent clean catheterization, and two had detrusor instability as the primary cause of urinary incontinence that responded to imipramine whereas anticholinergics had failed.

Patients are counseled that the chance of resolution of urinary incontinence depends upon the degree of incontinence and post-radical prostatectomy treatments. Overall, 50% of patients will benefit—total urinary incontinence resolves rarely, whereas mild stress urinary incontinence resolves usually. Salvage radiotherapy probably prevents Teflon injection success. Resolution of urinary incontinence may require as many as three treatments. The risks of Teflon injection appear low.

OPERATIVE TECHNIQUE OF TEFLON INJECTION

The patient is placed in the dorsal lithotomy position under intravenous sedation and a broad-spectrum antibiotic administered. General or spinal anesthesia cannot be used as they prevent participation of the patient in the procedure that is essential for identification of the distal urethral sphincter. A 22-French cystoscopic sheath with a 12-degree lens is used to identify the distal urethral sphincter (*see* Fig. 1). The patient may perform a Valsalva maneuver to assist with identification of the distal urinary sphincter. Once the sphincter is identified, sedation is deepened.

Irrigation fluid is warmed and tubes of Teflon are kept in hot water at all times. Teflon paste becomes too dense at room or body temperature to pass through injection needles. A standard injection needle (17 gage) has been altered by placing a black ring 0.75 in (19 mm) from its tip (Lancet needle, Cook Company). The needle is passed through the scope and inserted just distal to the distal urethral sphincter and advanced 0.75 in so that the needle tip lies within the external urinary sphincter. Teflon paste is injected at 12 o'clock (*see* Fig. 2), 3 o'clock (*see* Fig. 3) and 9 o'clock. The floor is elevated last with a 6 o'clock injection (*see* Fig. 4). Most patients require 3–4 cm^3 at each site in order to achieve the goal

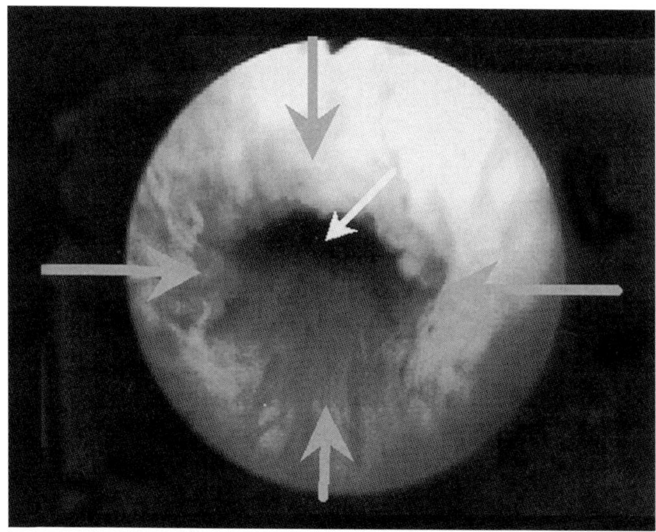

Fig. 1. Distal urethral sphincter. (Small, white arrow—urethra lumen; large, gray arrows—sphincter).

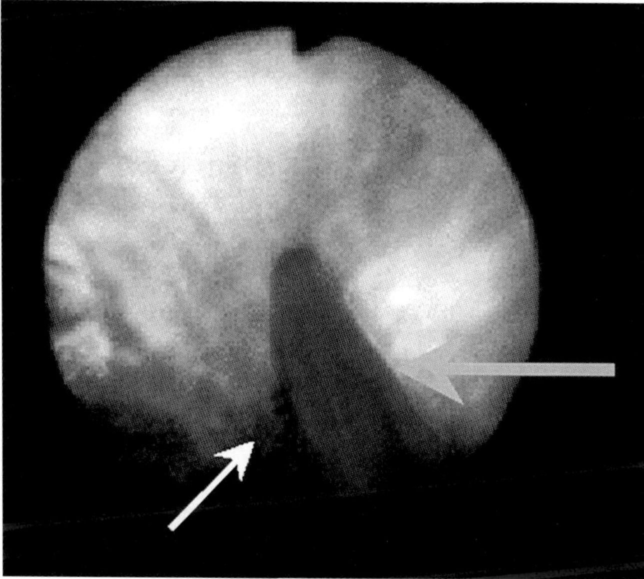

Fig. 2. Teflon injection at 12 o'clock. (Small, white arrow—urethral lumen; large, gray arrow—needle).

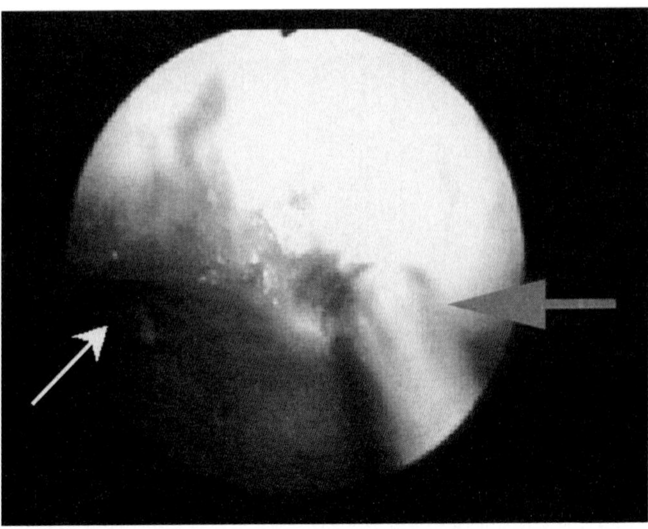

Fig. 3. Teflon injection at 3 o'clock. (Small, white arrow—urethral lumen; large, gray arrow—needle).

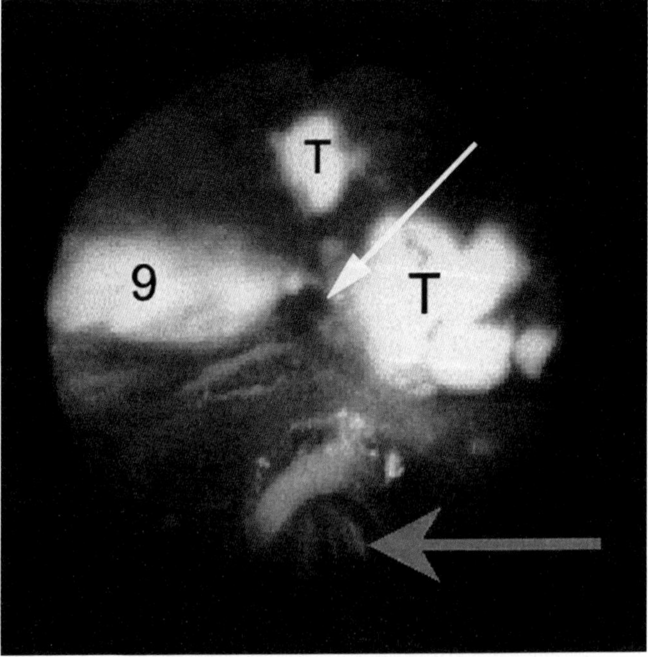

Fig. 4. Teflon injection at 6 o'clock. Teflon bolster is visible at 9 o'clock *(9)*. Teflon is floating freely in urethral lumen (T). (Small, white arrow—urethral lumen; large, gray arrow—needle).

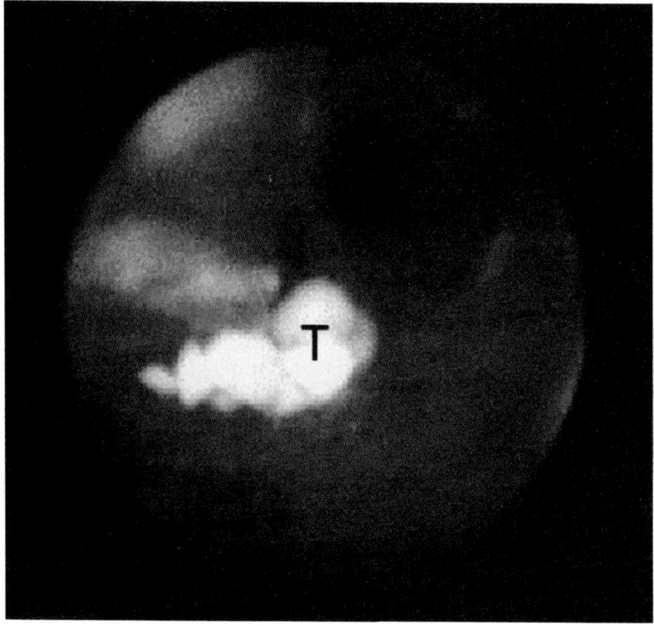

Fig. 5. Apposition of distal urethral sphincter at completion of Teflon injection. Teflon is floating freely in urethral lumen (T).

of complete apposition of the distal urethral sphincter (*see* Fig. 5). The injections must be performed quickly so that passage of the cystoscope into the bladder for drainage is not required since loss or compression of the Teflon bolsters would be risked.

With the bladder full at the end of the case and needle and the cystoscope removed, leakage should not occur, but abdominal compression usually produces a good urinary stream. Patients are discharged to home when sedation has worn off and they have voided successfully. Approximately 20% of patients will suffer postinjection urinary retention and a 12-French coude Foley catheter is placed carefully; the patient returns for a voiding trial 2–3 d later. Broad-spectrum antibiotics are continued for 10 d and ibuprofen is prescribed for pelvic discomfort that occurs in approx 20% of patients. Patients will frequently have immediate continence that worsens over several days as the acute inflammation from the injections subside and the Teflon bulk is reduced as a result of loss of the glycerine vehicle. The granulomatous response to Teflon injection restores Teflon bulk over several months. Therefore, patients return to clinic in 3 mo to report on continence status. Reinjection is considered 6 mo postoperatively. Up to three sessions of Teflon injections are performed before other options may be considered.

RESULTS OF TEFLON INJECTIONS AT UNC

Eighteen men incontinent after radical prostatectomy have received a total of 28 Teflon injections since 1993 (*see* Table 1). Patients ranged in age from 51–81 yr. Radical prostatectomy was complicated by bladder neck strictures in five men and urethral stricture, periurethral fibrosis, and rectal injury in one patient each. Three patients received salvage radiation therapy. Teflon injection was performed 14 mo to 140 mo and average 30 mo after radical prostatectomy. Urodynamic study was performed in 15 patients. Average residual urine was 20 cm^3 and average bladder capacity was 264 cm^3. Detrusor instability was found in 8 patients (53%) and distal urethral sphincter deficiency was demonstrated in 12 patients (80%).

Nine patients were injected once, eight patients twice and one patient three times. Each session of injections used an average of 15 cm^3 of Teflon: the average amount of Teflon used for first, second, and third injections were 16, 15, and 8 cm^3, respectively. Urinary retention occurred after 5 of 28 (18%) Teflon injections. There have been no other complications.

All patients used three pads or more daily to control urinary leakage prior to Teflon injection; seven patients were totally incontinent. Five patients are not evaluable because of recent treatment and one patient failed to return after injection and is lost to follow-up; two irradiated patients have failed; among 10 nonirradiated patients, two failed, three are cured, two use a security pad, and four use one or two pads daily.

OTHER TREATMENT OPTIONS FOR POSTPROSTATECTOMY INCONTINENCE

Collagen Injection

Collagen is available as a highly purified bovine collagen that is 3% cross-linked with glutaraldehyde (Contigen®); crosslinking stabilizes the molecules and reduces the rate of reabsorption. Bovine collagen is a foreign protein that may elicit cellular and humeral responses; skin testing is required 30 d before treatment although anaphylactic reactions have occurred even after negative skin tests *(16)*. Collagen elicits little local tissue reaction and granulomas do not occur nor have any reports described migration of the injected material *(17)*.

Collagen begins to degrade 12 wk after injection and degrades completely after 9–19 mo. Repeat injections are therefore required in the majority of patients. Of 257 incontinent postprostatectomy patients treated with transurethral injection and followed for a mean of 28 mo

Table 1
Results of Teflon Injections

Age	Time from RP (yr)	DI	SD	Post-RP incontinence	Inj	Amount (cc)	Time since last inj (mo)	Results
70	1.3	yes	yes	4 pads/d	2	12, 10.5	81	cured
72	1.3	yes	yes	total	3	28, 22, 8	54	cured
74	3.5	yes	yes	4–6 pads/d	1	13	16	cured
65	1.3	no	yes	4–5 pads/d	1	16.5	4	security pad
74	2	no	yes	total	1	18	4	security pad
61	2	no	no	4–6 pads/d	2	20, 16	58	1 pad
78	1.5	yes	no	3 pads/d	1	14.5	3	1 pad
68	2	—	—	2–4 pads/d	1	13.5	4	2 pads
77	2	yes	yes	4 pads/d	2	18, 16	16	2 pads
64	1.5	yes	yes	5–6 pads/d	2	16, 12	3	failed, awaiting AUS
51	4	no	yes	total	1	5	84	unknown
63	2	no	yes	8 pads/d	1	13	3	failed, awaiting reinjection
64	1.3	yes	yes	4 pads/d	1	18	13	failed, awaiting reinjection
81	12	no	yes	total	2	13, 15	3	failed, awaiting reinjection
54	2	yes	no	total	2	16.5, 16	1	pending
61	3	—	—	total*	2	17, 16	15	failed, AUS
83	2	—	—	total*	2	16, 11.5	21	failed, AUS
68	3	no	yes	3–5 pads/d*	1	15.5	1	pending

DI =detrusor instability; SD = sphincteric deficiency; INJ = Teflon injections; AUS = artificial urinary sphincter; * patients had salvage radiation therapy.

97

(range 12–48 mo), 20% of patients were dry and 39% were significantly improved. Patients required an average of 4.4 injections (range 1 to 11) and required an average total of 36.6 cm^3 of collagen *(18)*.

Two other injectables offer potential benefits compared to both collagen and Teflon. Autologous fat injection has the advantages of ready availability, biocompatibility, and lower expense. However, autologous fat injection has been used in only six men with postprostatectomy incontinence and may not produce durable results *(19)*. Silicone rubber *(20)*, bioglass *(21)* and, more recently, carbon particles have been suggested for use as injectables for treatment of urinary incontinence.

Artificial Urinary Sphincter (AUS) Implantation

The artificial urinary sphincter (AUS) may restore continence even in men with severe or continuous urinary leakage. Revisions (32% of 2606 patients) *(22)* are frequently necessary due to erosion, infection, and mechanical problems. Manual dexterity is required to operate the device, physiological voiding is not attained, and the device and its placement are expensive. Moreover, many men will require 1 to 2 pads daily after placement of a single cuff and choose implantation of a second cuff *(23,24)*. Artificial sphincter implantation cured incontinence in 76% (range, 20% to 96%) and cured or improved incontinence in 89% (range, 84% to 96%) of 286 men when results described in five studies were combined *(24)*.

The Male Bulbourethral Sling Procedure

Sling procedures have been used for many years to treat women with intrinsic sphincter deficiency. A similar procedure has been devised for use in men with urinary incontinence after radical prostatectomy. Among 64 patients who underwent the bulbourethral sling procedure for severe postprostatectomy incontinence, 36 *(56%)* became dry and 5 (8%) improved significantly. In 17 patients, 23 retightening procedures were performed that increased the success rate to 75%. The revision, erosion, and infection rates were 27, 6, and 3%, respectively. Many patients experienced perineal discomfort that may last 3 mo or more and some patients experienced long-term numbness or pain *(25)*.

Chronic Urinary Catheterization

Chronic indwelling catheters are associated with a high rate of complications, especially urinary tract infections, and should be used only when other management options have failed *(26)*. Condom catheters cause abrasions, dermatitis, penile ischemia or necrosis, and maceration, but the frequency of these complications is unknown. Use of a condom catheter brings an increased risk of urinary tract infection; 24-h/d users have a higher frequency of infection than nonusers and nighttime-only users have an intermediate risk of infection *(27)*.

CONCLUSION

Teflon injection of the distal urethral sphincter for urinary incontinence was pioneered by Politano. In a limited experience, we have achieved good results with Teflon injection for postradical prostatectomy incontinence. Teflon injection can be performed as an out-patient procedure under sedation and cures some men who suffer even total urinary incontinence after radical prostatectomy. Teflon injection offers more durable results than collagen but may migrate or embolize to cause granulomas in regional lymph nodes or distant organs. Although Teflon injection appears safe over four decades of use, newer and more biocompatible materials may prove better. Teflon injection may be offered to men who suffer post-radical prostatectomy urinary incontinence prior to resorting to implantation of artificial urinary sphincters or performance of male bulbourethral sling procedures.

REFERENCES

1. Fowler FJ, Barry MJ, Lu-Yao G, et al. (1995) Effect of radical prostatectomy for prostate cancer on patient quality of life: results from a Medicare survey. *Urology* 45:1007.
2. Turner-Warwick R (1983) The sphincter mechanisms: Their relation to prostatic enlargement and its treatment. In: *Benign Prostatic Hypertrophy*. Hinman F, Jr., ed., New York: Springer-Verlag, pp. 809–828.
3. Leach GE, Chi-Ming Y, Donovan BJ (1987) Post prostatectomy incontinence: the influence of bladder dysfunction. *J Urol* 138:574.
4. O'Donnell B, Puri P (1986) Endoscopic correction of primary vesico-ureteral reflux. *Br J Urol* 58:601.
5. Dewan PA (1992) Is injected polytetrafluoroethylene (Polytef) carcinogenic? *Br J Urol* 69:29.
6. Murless BC (1938) The injection treatment of stress incontinence. *J Obs Gynaecol Br Emp* 45:67.
7. Arnold GE (1962) Vocal rehabilitation of paralytic dysphonia. IX. Technique of intracordal injection. *Arch Otolaryngol* 76:358.
8. Politano VA (1992) Transurethral polytef injection for post-prostatectomy urinary incontinence. *Br J Urol* 69:26.
9. Politano VA, Small MP, Harper JM, et al. (1974) Periurethral teflon injection for urinary incontinence. *J Urol* 111:180.
10. Kaufman, M, Lockhart JL, Silverstein MJ, et al. (1984) Transurethral polytetrafluoroethylene injection for post-prostatectomy urinary incontinence. *J Urol* 132:463.
11. Malizia, A.A., Reiman HM, Myers RP, et al. (1984) Migration and granulomatous reaction after periurethral injection of Polytef (Teflon). *JAMA* 251:3277.

12. Aaronson IA (1995) Current status of the 'STING': an American perspective. *Br J Urol* 75:121.
13. Mittleman RE, Marraccini JV (1983) Pulmonary Teflon granulomas-following periurethral Teflon injection for urinary incontinence. *Arch Path Lab Med* 107:611.
14. Haab F, Yamaguchi R, Leach GE (1996) Postprostatectomy incontinence. *Urol Clin North Am* 23:447.
15. Lipsky H, Wuernschimmel E (1993) Endoscopic treatment of vesicoureteric reflux with collagen. Five years' experience. *Br J Urol* 72:965.
16. Vandenbossche M, Delhove O, Dumortier P, et al. (1993) Endoscopic treatment of reflux: experimental study and review of Teflon and collagen. *Eur Urol* 23:386.
17. Gorton E, Stanton S, Monga A, et al. (1999) Periurethral collagen injection: a long-term follow-up study. *Br J Urol* 84:966.
18. Cespedes RD, Leng WW, McGuire EJ (1999) Collagen injection therapy for postprostatectomy incontinence. *Urology* 54:597.
19. Santarosa RP, Blaivas JG (1994) Periurethral injection of autologous fat for the treatment of sphincteric incontinence. *J Urol* 151:607.
20. Chaliha C, Williams G (1995) Periurethral injection therapy for the treatment of urinary incontinence. *Br J Urol* 76:151.
21. Walker RD, Wilson J, Clark AE (1992) Injectable bioglass as a potential substitute for injectable polytetrafluoroethylene. *J Urol* 148:645.
22. Hajivassilioiu CA (1999) A review of the complications and results of implantation of the AMS artificial urinary sphincter. *Eur Urol* 35:36.
23. Brito CG, Mulcahy JJ, Mitchell ME, et al. (1993) Use of a double cuff AMS 800 urinary sphincter for severe stress incontinence. *J Urol* 149:283.
24. Montague DK, Angermeier KW (2000) Postprostatectomy urinary incontinence: the case for artificial urinary sphincter implantation. *Urology* 55:2.
25. Schaeffer AJ, Clemens JQ, Ferrari M, et al. (1998) The male bulbourethral sling procedure for post-radical prostatectomy incontinence. *J Urol* 159:1510.
26. Warren JW (1997) Catheter-associated urinary tract infections. *Infect Dis Clin North Am* 11:609.
27. Ouslander JG, Greengold B, Chen S (1987) External catheter use and urinary tract infections among incontinent male nursing home patients. *J Am Geriatr Soc* 35:1063.

6 Urethral Stents for Neurogenic Bladder Dysfunction

Ian K. Walsh, MD, FRCSUROL
and Anthony R. Stone, MD, FRCSED

CONTENTS

INTRODUCTION
TYPES OF URETHRAL STENTS
CONCLUSION
REFERENCES

INTRODUCTION

In the United States alone, more than 10,000 traumatic spinal cord injuries occur each year, predominantly affecting males in the 20–40-yr-old age group *(1,2)*. Spinal cord injury may also result from myelopathy, myelitis, arachnoiditis, vascular disease, or arteriovenous malformations. Traumatic lesions are most commonly sited at the thoracolumbar vertebral level, corresponding to the suprasacral spinal cord. In patients with suprasacral, subpontine lesions, the typical neurogenic bladder behavior pattern emerges as one of involuntary external sphincter contraction occurring simultaneously with hyperreflexic detrusor contractions. This detrusor-sphincter dyssynergia (DSD) results in dangerously high intravesical pressures, which pose significant risks for the upper tracts, with complications such as vesicoureteral reflux, hydronephrosis, calculus formation, sepsis, and renal decompensation occurring in more than 50% of patients if left untreated *(3)*. Current management of DSD is directed toward reducing intravesical pressures with antimuscarinic

From: *Urologic Prostheses:*
The Complete, Practical Guide to Devices, Their Implantation and Patient Follow Up
Edited by: C. C. Carson © Humana Press Inc., Totowa, NJ

medication and minimizing intravesical volumes via intermittent catheterization. Most paraplegics, however, lack the level of manual dexterity required to self-catheterize effectively and must rely upon intermittent catheterization by their care taker. Some paraplegics may also find self-catheterization either difficult to perform or they may cooperate poorly with their catheterization regimen. In such cases, drainage may be ensured by the use of an in-dwelling urethral catheter, but this is limited by the almost inevitable development of urethral erosion, chronic infection, and calculus formation. Suprapubic catheterization circumvents some of these problems, but long-term use is still associated with considerable morbidity in the form of chronic urinary tract infection, squamous metaplasia, and calculus development.

The results of medical management of DSD are consistently disappointing. Centrally acting muscle relaxants are ineffective and peripherally acting agents are associated with significant toxicity *(4,5)*. Administering the skeletal muscle relaxant baclofen intrathecally may, however, effectively reduce DSD in up to 40% of patients *(6)*.

External sphincterotomy was first introduced by Watkins in 1936 as a method for ablating outlet resistance and is purported to provide low-pressure drainage *(7)*. Despite initial enthusiasm, sphincterotomy has been shown to be hampered by a failure to fully eliminate residual urine, the potential for significant hemorrhage and the need to repeat the procedure in up to one-quarter of patients *(8,9)*. Patients are also reliant upon condom catheter drainage. Less than 50% of patients continue with this drainage method in the long term *(10)*. An alternative method to surgical external sphincterotomy is sphincter ablation by direct injection of Botulinum toxin. Although less invasive than surgical incision, this method provides only temporary relief, repeat injections are necessary every couple of months *(11)*. Balloon dilatation is another alternative, but this is restricted by recurrent obstruction and excessive bleeding *(12)*.

In view of the difficulties encountered in establishing low-pressure bladder emptying in these patients, therapeutic innovations continue to be introduced. Intraurethral stent placement was first introduced by Fabian in 1980 as an alternative to long-term in-dwelling urethral catheterization *(13)*. Intraurethral stents have thus become recognized as a minimally invasive, effective treatment option for urethral strictures and prostatic obstruction *(14,15)*. The attractive features of an in-dwelling stent include potential reversibility and provision of a wide lumen, which facilitates both urinary drainage and instrumentation. The disadvantages include biocompatibility concerns, hyperplastic reactions, encrustation, infection, and calculus formation *(16)*. The application of intraurethral stent placement to the management of DSD has been investigated in several studies in the last decade and these will be discussed in this chapter.

TYPES OF URETHRAL STENTS

Lower urinary tract stents are broadly categorized as being permanent or temporary. Whereas temporary stents (Urospiral, Prostacoil, Prostacath) have become popular in managing prostatic obstruction and urethral strictures, clinical experience in managing DSD with these devices is limited. To date, the most extensive clinical experience reported in this area has been with the Urolome™ permanent stent (known as the Medinvent Wallstent in Europe). Temporary stents include the include the Memokath and Memotherm prostheses.

Permanent Stents

The Urolume prosthesis (American Medical Systems; Minnetonka, MN; Medinvent SA, Lausanne, Switzerland) was originally developed as a self-expanding endoprosthesis to maintain patency of stenotic arteries following balloon angioplasty. The device exerts a strong, continuous, outward radial force and has also found clinical application in the non-surgical treatment of biliary strictures *(17,18)*. Its utility in managing bulbar urethral strictures was first described by Milroy in 1988 *(19)*. The stent is composed of a braided, pliable, self-expanding cylindrical mesh of corrosion-resistant, nonmagnetic super-alloy wire (*see* Fig. 1). The radial mesh design exerts an outward force against the urethral lumen to maintain patency of up to 42-Ch.

Stent placement is performed endoscopically. The stent is packaged preloaded on a 24-Ch cystourethroscopic insertion tool. Although several stent lengths are available commercially, a 3-cm stent appears to be the most effective for optimum external sphincter bridging *(12)*. The insertion tool is introduced into the urethra and advanced to the verumontanum under direct vision via a 0° cystoscopy lens. Landmarks for correct placement are from the distal half of the verumontanum cephalad, thus leaving the ejaculatory ducts exposed and extension into the bulbar urethra at least 5 mm, beyond the membranous urethra caudally. If necessary, an additional overlapping stent may also be placed to ensure complete bridging of the external sphincter. After confirming correct positioning, the prosthesis is released from the delivery device and self-expansion occurs. Inaccurate placement can be immediately corrected by slightly repositioning the device or withdrawing it completely through a resectoscope sheath with grasping forceps under endoscopic guidance. An effective point of technique is suprapubic catheter placement

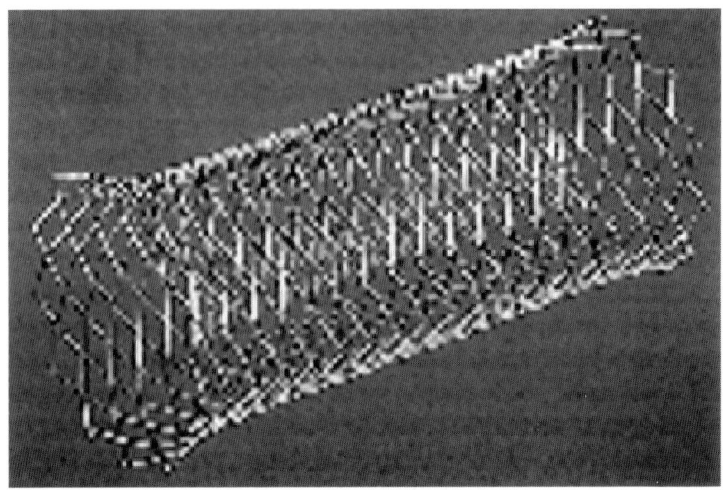

Fig. 1. The Urolume prosthesis.

to optimize visibility and postoperative urinary drainage. A condom catheter is secured at the end of the procedure. Urethral catheterization in the immediate and early postoperative period is contraindicated due to the risk of stent displacement. Postoperative plain X-ray further confirms correct stent positioning (*see* Fig. 2). Because an in-dwelling foreign material has been introduced into an already compromised urinary tract, intravenous antibiotic prophylaxis perioperatively and oral antibiotic coverage postoperatively is mandatory.

The first report on the effectiveness of urethral stents to treat DSD was by Shaw et al. in 1990, using the Urolume prosthesis *(20)*. Since then, several studies have confirmed the utility of stent placement in this clinical scenario.

Noll et al. reported that in 22 of 24 male patients with severe DSD, infravesical obstruction was effectively relieved by Medivent Wallstent placement *(21)*. The majority (71%) of these patients had previously undergone unsuccessful surgical external sphincterotomy.

McInerney et al. reported their series of 22 spinal cord-injured males with DSD in whom a Medinvent Wallstent was placed across the external sphincter *(22)*. Half of these patients had previously undergone repeated unsuccessful external sphincterotomy and three patients had artificial urinary sphincters *in situ*. Stents were placed at or immediately subjacent to the level of the verumontanum, dependent upon whether subsequent fertility was of importance. Fifteen (68%) patients were noted to have effective urinary drainage postoperatively, whereas 3 (14%)

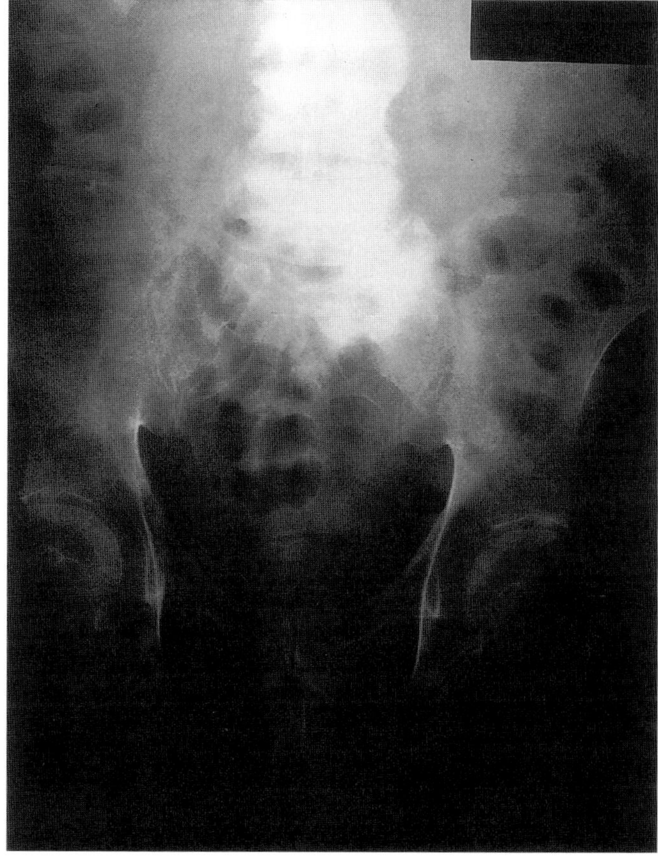

Fig. 2. Plain radiograph demonstrating a Urolume stent correctly positioned in a patient with extensive spinal injury.

developed bladder neck obstruction. None of the patients with artificial urinary sphincters drained adequately following stent placement.

In 1993, Chancellor et al. reported their experience with the Urolume device in 25 spinal cord-injured men with DSD *(23)*. One year following insertion, voiding pressures and residual urine volumes remained low and bladder capacity was unchanged. Early (within 6 wk) stent migration occurred in three (12%) patients and one patient developed pyelonephritis postoperatively. The authors concluded that this simple technique is an attractive alternative to formal surgical sphincterotomy.

In 1994, Rivas et al. compared Urolume™ implantation with surgical external sphincterotomy in 46 spinal cord-injured males with DSD over a follow-up period of 6–20-mo *(24)*. Both modalities were equally effective in reducing voiding pressures and residual urine volumes without adversely affecting bladder capacity. Surgical complication rates (approx 25% of patients) were also similar in the two groups. Stent placement was, however, less expensive, associated with less bleeding and had a significantly shorter operating time and hospital stay. Similar conclusions were reached by Chancellor et al. when they prospectively compared stent placement, external sphincter balloon dilatation and traditional surgical external sphincterotomy in 61 patients *(25)*. Juma et al. highlighted the simplicity of stent insertion, short hospital stay and low short-term morbidity in their cohort study of 10 patients *(26)*. In 1996, McFarlane et al. reported the results of Urolume implantation in 12 patients with 5-yr clinical follow-up, which included urodynamic and ultrasonographic studies *(27)*. Although stent migration, erosion or infection did not occur in this study, stent removal was necessary in two patients and 50% developed bladder neck obstruction, which required surgical intervention.

The first large clinical study on Urolume placement was the North American multicenter trial, which prospectively investigated the device's efficacy in 153 spinal cord-injured men with DSD over a follow-up period ranging from 2 to 33 mo *(12)*. Approx one-third of the patients had previously undergone surgical external sphincterotomy, but such a history did not affect the clinical results. A large portion (68.6%) of patients were managed with a single stent, and most of the remainder required two prostheses. The authors reported a statistically significant reduction in voiding pressures postoperatively, which remained low (< 40 cm H_2O) at 2 yr. Although residual urine measurements were similarly reduced, bladder capacity was not adversely affected. Stent epithelialization was observed to begin within 3 mo of insertion and was virtually complete by 2 yr. Hyperplasia was noted in one third of patients at 3 mo and one-half at 2 yr, although this was only regarded as being marked in a maximum of 10% of patients and, in no cases, did this cause urethral stenosis or urinary obstruction. Clinically significant urinary tract infection occurred in only four patients postoperatively and improvement or stabilization of preoperative hydronephrosis was virtually universal. Autonomic dysrreflexia was reported by approx 70% of patients preoperatively and 30–40% of patients postoperatively. Ten cases of stent explantation were performed, most commonly because of stent migration, of which half occurred in the immediate postoperative period and subsequent reimplantation was successfully performed in most cases. Only 8.5% of patients subsequently developed secondary bladder neck obstruction, which was effectively managed nonsurgically in half the patients. Complication rates were low, with no significant bleeding, tissue erosion or calculus formation. The authors conclude from these impressive results that Urolume stent placement is a simple and effective alternative to traditional sphincterotomy when managing these complex cases.

Further urodynamic data was published by Chancellor et al. in 1995 on a subset of 41 patients who had participated in the Multicenter North American Urolume Trial *(28)*. One-quarter of these patients had a previous history of failed external sphincterotomy. At 12 and 24 mo, voiding pressures remained significantly low (< 40 cm H_2O) as did residual urine volumes (< 100 mL), whereas bladder capacity was unaffected. Again, no differences were noted between patients with and without a history of previous external sphincterotomy. Sauerwein et al. also reported improved urodynamic, radiological, and clinical findings in 51 male spinal cord-injured patients with DSD at up to 3 yr follow-up *(29)*.

The long-term follow-up of the North American Multicenter Urolume Trial have been published recently *(30)*. Five-year follow-up results were available from 15 centers on a total of 160 spinal cord-injured men with DSD who had undergone Urolume stent placement in the original study. The overall results were again unaffected by a previous history of external sphincterotomy. Almost one-third of patients required at least two insertion procedures to achieve adequate external sphincter coverage, with a single stent being used in 52% of patients, two stents in 30%, and three stents in 6.9%. The previously noted significant reductions in mean voiding pressure and residual urine volumes were maintained at 5 yr postoperatively and bladder capacities remained unchanged. It is, however, worth noting that despite the significant reductions in residual urine following stent placement, the absolute postoperative volumes were still high throughout follow-up, averaging 132 cm^3 at 5 yr. Of the 115 (72%) patients who suffered from autonomic dysrreflexia prior to entering the study, this remained resolved in 70% at 1 yr and improvement was maintained at 5 yr. Sixty-three of eighty-six (85%) patients who required an in-dwelling urinary catheter preoperatively remained converted to condom catheter drainage following stent implantation. Preoperatively, hydronephrosis was present in 16% of a total of 320 renal units in 160 patients and this reduced to 4% of units at 1 through to 5 yr. Data on colonization and infection rates were unavailable for the preoperative and early postoperative periods, but for the remainder of the study, asymptomatic bacteriuria was present in over 90% of patients, although symptomatic urinary tract infection presented in only 3–12%. Erectile function and antegrade ejaculation remained unaffected by stent placement for the duration of the study. Regarding to the cystoscopic appearance of the implant site, complete urothelial stent coverage progressively increased from 49% of patients at 1 yr up to 96% at 5 yr. A moderate to severe intraluminal hyperplastic response was observed in 20% of patients at 1 yr and 7% at 5 yr. Intrastent stenosis developed in only 3% of patients, encrustation was evident in 6%, and calculus formation was not observed. Twenty-four (15%) patients underwent prosthesis explantation primarily for stent migration and four of these patients subsequently had a further stent placed successfully. Although significant bleeding or soft tissue erosion did not occur, 47 (26%) patients developed bladder neck obstruction, of whom less than half required surgical incision. Subjective improvement in bladder emptying was reported by 91% of patients at 1 yr and 74% at 5 yr, whereas physician's subjective perception of operative success was 94% at 1 yr and 98% at 5 yr. The authors concluded that Urolume stenting is an effective, potentially reversible alternative to surgical external sphincter destruction.

Chancellor et al. prospectively compared the results of Urolume placement with traditional external sphincterotomy in their recently published multicenter randomized trial *(31)*. Urodynamic data, voiding questionnaires, and quality-of-life measurements were analyzed over 2 yr. A significant reduction in maximum detrusor pressures was noted following both procedures, both performing equally well in this manner. Reductions in residual urine volumes following stent placement were, however, only significant at 3 mo postoperatively, although sphincterotomy continued to minimize postvoid residual at 2 yr. Bladder capacity was unaffected by either procedure. Postoperative bleeding was insignificant in both groups and hospital stay was generally shorter for stented patients. Although a significant improvement in bladder emptying was more commonly reported by patients with stents, there was a tendency for patients who had undergone sphincterotomy to report less worry, bother, hampering of daily activities and interference with social activities. The authors concluded that, overall, stent placement was as effective as traditional sphincterotomy, but preferable because of the shorter hospital stay and potential reversibility.

Urolume explantation has now been described in detail and the results studied by working members of the North American Study Group (Gajewski et al., personal communication). Removal is acheived by endoscopically grasping several rows of the prosthesis wire at least 2 mm from the distal end of the device. Gentle withdrawal permits stent elongation and narrowing, facilitating intact removal of the prosthesis. Failure to remove the device intact may occur if an insufficient number of wires are grasped initially, in which case piecemeal retrieval of the individual wires is required. If stent epithelialization is evident, preliminary endoscopic tissue resection is necessary to free the prosthesis prior to its withdrawal. Resection should be performed using low, brief, pure current settings to avoid thermal disruption of the wire components. Twenty-one (13%) patients in the original multicenter study required immediate prosthesis removal at the time of initial insertion, mainly because of misplacement or migration. Retrieval was reported to be easy to perform and a device was then correctly placed in the majority (90%) of the patients. In the longer term, formal explantation was necessary in 31 (20%) of the overall study group at a mean of 22 mo following stent placement, most prostheses being removed between 2–4 yr because of stent migration. Less common indications for removal included inadequate epithelialization, urinary tract infection, pain, and squamous metaplasia. Thirty (97%) of these patients had their devices removed successfully and 6 (4%) underwent successful stent replacement. Roughly half of the stents were removed intact, half were delivered piecemeal and open removal was necessary in one patient. The degree of urothelial trauma caused by stent removal was reportedly minimal, although more marked for piecemeal, removal. There were no lasting consequences of prosthesis explantation, demonstrating the potentially reversible role Urolume placement has in treating these patients.

Temporary Stents

Because permanent sphincter stenting is, by definition, irreversible, this may render implantation a somewhat less-attractive option for some patients. Permanent stents may also prove troublesome if epithelialization is poor and hyperplastic growth leads to urethral occlusion *(32)*. Concerns about fertility and the potential long-term risk of malignant transformation also need to be considered by both patient and physician. In an effort to circumvent these difficulties, some authors have investigated the Memokath temporary urethral stent (Engineers & Doctors A/S, Hornbaek, Denmark). This second-generation thermosensitive stent is composed of titanium nickel alloy with shape memory effect. Stent placement using a delivery catheter is controlled by fluoroscopy, ultrasonography, or flexible cystoscopy. After deploying and positioning the proximal end of the stent at the bladder neck, warm saline (45°C) is flushed through the stent to expand it's distal coils in the bulbar urethra, thus providing bridging of both internal and external sphincters. Stent replacement is required at 12–18 mo and is easily performed by cooling the stent with 4°C saline, which renders the stent supersoft, facilitating endoscopic removal.

Soni et al. deployed the device in 10 male spinal cord-injured patients with urinary retention *(33)*. Insertion was controlled by fluoroscopy in seven patients and by flexible cystoscopy in three. Immediate and early complications included autonomic dysreflexia, bleeding, and urinary tract infection in a total of four patients. Over a follow-up period of 3–7 mo, all patients were noted to have insignificant residual urine volumes and stent migration or occlusion did not occur.

Shah et al. studied the efficacy of the Memokath device in managing DSD *(34)*. Fourteen patients had stents inserted under cystoscopic guidance as an outpatient procedure. Both bladder neck and external sphincter were stented in 11 patients using 5–7-cm stents and the sphinter alone was stented with a 4-cm stent in three patients. Over the follow-up period, which extended to 2 yr, residual volume measurements remained significantly reduced whereas preoperative hydronephrosis and autonomic dysreflexia were effectively resolved. Regarding to optimizing bladder emptying, bridging both the external sphincter and bladder neck was considerably more effective than sphincteric stenting alone. The authors suggested that the Memokath stent should be the prosthesis of choice if fertility concerns or patient indecision may influence clinical decision-making.

As an alternative to formal external sphincterotomy, Low et al. implanted 26 Memokath stents in 24 high tetraplegic males with DSD who were unable to catheterise *(35)*. Disappointingly, implantation failed to improve emptying and 19 (79%) patients required prosthesis removal because of infection or stent migration.

The Memotherm prosthesis (Angiomed), originally developed as a permanent stent for the relief of benign prostatic obstruction, has since undergone modifications to become an essentially temporary device. This flexible wire mesh is composed of the thermoreactive material Nitinol, which gains its maximum expansion force at 37°C (*see* Fig. 3). This heat-sensitivity facilitates repositioning as for the Memokath prosthesis *(36)*.

Garcia et al. recently implanted the Memotherm prosthesis in 24 spinal cord-injured patients with DSD *(37)*. Over a mean follow-up of 15 mo, urodynamically demonstrated leak point pressures and residual urine volumes remained significantly low. Stent migration occurred in four patients and two patients developed infection and calculus formation, necessitating explantation.

CONCLUSION

DSD poses significant risks to the upper tracts of spinal cord-injured patients. Clinical management can be particularly difficult if the combination of intermittent catheterization and antimuscarinic therapy is not possible because of an individual patient's lack of manual dexterity,

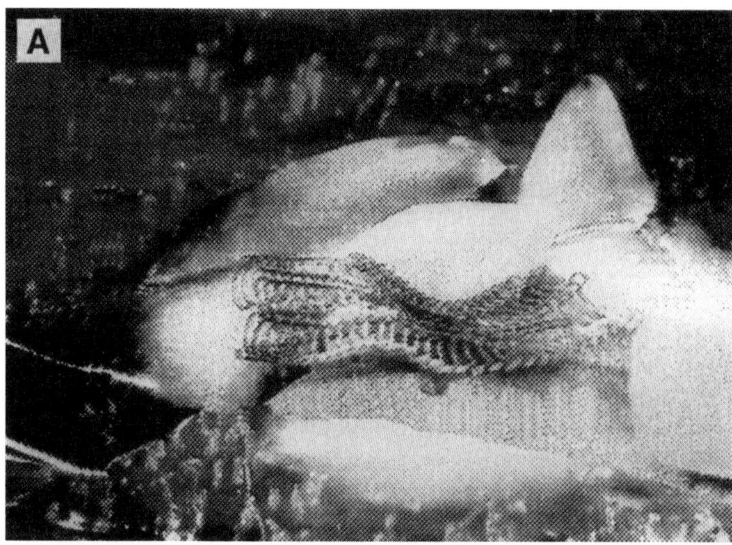

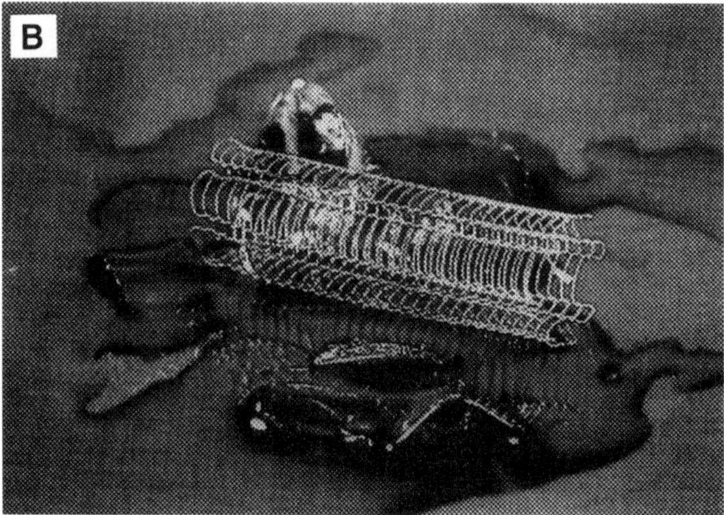

Fig. 3. Memotherm endoprosthesis at (**A**) 0°C and (**B**) after flushing with saline at 37°C.

poor social support or lack of compliance with treatment. Surgical external sphincterotomy was introduced as a means of circumventing this difficult situation. The initial enthusiasm for sphincterotomy has become tempered somewhat by the realization that, in the long term, this procedure is not as effective in eliminating residual urine as was originally thought. This realization, coupled with the observation that sphincterotomy is not free from surgical complications, has further encouraged neuro-urologists to look towards other means of ensuring effective low-pressure bladder emptying.

The introduction of external sphincter stenting as a treatment for potentially hazardous DSD in males with spinal cord injury represents a significant advance in urological practice, with clinical experience accumulating as time progresses, particularly with the Urolume prosthesis. Although initial reports were tempered with concerns about long-term safety, this would appear not to be a major concern at least at 5-yr follow-up. The results reported in several publications emerging from the North American Multicenter Trial appear conclusive that stenting is as effective as sphincterotomy. The advantages of sphincter stenting include ease of prosthesis placement which, if performed correctly, is associated with minimal complications and a short hospital stay.

It must be stated that residual urine is not eliminated by sphincter stenting and, whereas the figures reported in the literature are an improvement on preoperative values, it should be noted that the volumes themselves remain considerable. One-quarter to one-half of patients develop significant bladder neck obstruction following stent implantation and this may explain the persistence of inefficient emptying. The development of bladder neck obstruction would also suggest that the presence of a stent itself contributes to outlet obstruction, perhaps by intraluminal occlusion secondary to the hyperplastic tissue response described in 50% of patients. To date, the published reports remain unclear on this matter.

It has been suggested that Urolume prosthesis insertion is a potentially reversible procedure. Most Urolume stents are, however, virtually completely epithelialized as early as 6 mo after placement, which would be expected to render removal difficult. Formal explantation was necessary in 20% of the large group of patients in the North American Multicenter study, mainly because of prosthesis migration, although pain, inflammatory changes, and urinary tract infection also necessitated stent removal in some cases. Only 50% of stents were removed intact and, in the author's experience, stent removal can certainly be a difficult and time-consuming procedure. Only 4% of explanted patients have subsequently undergone successful reimplantation, further indicating that stent placement should not be considered a procedure which is easily revised.

Overall, placement of a permanent sphincter stent such as the Urolume is not superior to traditional sphincterotomy, merely equally effective. Although considerable experience has been gained with the use of the Urolume stent, placement of this prosthesis must still be regarded as being only potentially reversible, because the ease and safety of device removal remain undetermined. Knowing external sphincterotomy has been seen to perform poorly in the long term, the question arises as to the utility of a procedure that is similarly efficacious, but entails the essentially permanent placement of a foreign body in an already compromised lower urinary tract. The presence of a permanent prosthesis may additionally lead to the development of squamous metaplasia and the possibility of subsequent malignant transformation remains a concern. The thermosensitive temporary Memokath and Memotherm stents thus appear attractive by virtue of their removability, which is also a particularly important feature if patient indecision or concerns about fertility are major issues in management. To date, however, clinical experience with temporary stents is limited to only a few European studies, although these initial reports are certainly encouraging.

The gold standard of managing post-spinal cord-injury DSD remains the combination of an effective intermittent catheterization regimen (by patient or carer) together with antimuscarinic pharmacotherapy. In the authors' experience, most patients are able to cooperate with such an approach and alternative methods are only required in a small subpopulation. In the latter group, apart from stent implantation, current options include in-dwelling catheter, preferably via the suprapubic route (reversible), external sphincterotomy (irreversible), augmentation cystoplasty (irreversible and still reliant upon the need for catheterization), urinary diversion (irreversible), and incontinent ileo-vesicostomy (irreversible). The role of stent placement would appear to be as a suitable, but only potentially reversible alternative to the equally efficacious but irreversible external sphincterotomy, and should only be considered if the patient does not agree to the aforementioned alternatives. Growing experience with the development and employment of temporary prostheses may produce further clinical advances and allow for more routine use of such devices.

REFERENCES

1. Stover SL, Fine PR (1987) The epidemiology and economics of spinal cord injury. *Paraplegia* 25:225.
2. De Vivo MJ, Rutt RD, Black KJ, Go BK, Stover SL (1992) Trends in spinal cord injury demographics and treatment outcome between 1973 and 1986. *Arch Phys Med Rehab* 73:424.
3. Blaivas JG (1982) The neurophysiology of micturition: a clinical study of 550 patients. *J Urol* 127:958.
4. Bianchine J (1980) Drugs for Parkinson's disease: centrally acting muscle relaxants. In: Gilman AG, Goodman LS, Gilman, A, eds., *The Pharmocological Basis of Therapeutics.* New York: MacMillan, pp. 475–495.
5. Hackler RH, Broeker BH, Klein FA, Brady SM (1980) A clinical experience with dantrolene sodium for external urinary sphincter hypertonicity in spinal cord injured patients. *J Urol* 124:78.

6. Steers WD, Meythaler JM, Haworth C, Herrell D, Park TS (1992) Effects of acute bolus and chronic continuous intrathecal baclofen on genitourinary dysfunction due to spinal cord pathology. *J Urol* 148:1849.

7. Watkins RH (1936) The bladder function in spinal injury. *Br J Surg* 23:734.

8. Schellhammer PF, Hackler RH, Bunts RC (1973) External sphincterotomy: an evaluation of 150 patients with neurogenic bladder. *J Urol* 110:199.

9. Perkash I (1976) Modified approach to sphincterotomy in spinal cord injury patients: indications, technique, and results in 32 patients. *Paraplegia* 13:247.

10. Vapnek J, Couillard D, Stone A (1994) Is sphincterotomy the best management of the spinal-cord-injured bladder? *J Urol* 151:951.

11. Dykstra DD, Sidi AA (1990) Treatment of detrusor-sphincter dyssynergia with botulinum A toxin: adouble-blind study. *Arch Phys Med Rehab* 71:24.

12. Chancellor MB, Rivas DA, Linsenmeyer T, Abdill CA, Douglas Ackman CF, Appell RA, et al. (1994) Multicenter trial in North America of Urolume sphincter prosthesis. *J Urol* 152:924–930.

13. Fabian KM (1980) Der interprostatische "partielle Katheter" (Urologische Spirale). *Urologe* 19:236–238.

14. Walsh IK, Keane PF (1993) Malignant sphincter stricture treated by a permanent indwelling stent. *Br J Urol* 72(4):522.

15. Badlani GH (1997) Role of permanent stents. *J Endourol* 11(6):473–475.

16. Corujo M, Badlani GH (1997) Epithelialization of permanent stents. *J Endourol* 11(6):477–480.

17. Raillat C, Rousseau H, Joffre F, Roux D (1990) Treatment of iliac artery stenoses with the Wallstent endoprosthesis. *Am J Roentgenol* 154(3):613–616.

18. Roddie ME, Adam A (1992) Metallic stents in biliary disease. *Baillieres Clin Gastroenterol* 6(2):341–354.

19. Milroy EJG, Cooper JE, Wallsten H et al (1988) A new treatment for urethral strictures. *Lancet* 1:1424–1427.

20. Shaw PJR, Milroy EJG, Timoney AG, Mitchel N (1990) Permanent external sphincter stents in spinal injured patients. *Br J Urol* 66:297–302.

21. Noll F, Hoch V, Schreiter F (1992) Wall-stent for treatment of bulbar urethral stricture and DSD in spastic bladder. *Urologe A* 31(5):290–295.

22. McInernay PD, Vanner TF, Harris SA, Stephenson TP (1991) Permanent urethral stents for detrusor sphincter dyssynergia. *Br J Urol* 67(3):291–294.

23. Chancellor MB, Karusick S, Erhard MJ, Abdill CK, Liu JB, Goldberg BB, Staas WE (1993) Placement of a wire mesh prosthesis in the external urinary sphincter of men with spinal cord injuries. *Radiology* 187(2):551–555.

24. Rivas DA, Chancellor MB, Bagley D (1994) Prospective comparison of external sphincter prosthesis placement and external sphincterotomy in men with spinal cord injury. *J Endourol* 8(2):89–93.

25. Chancellor MB, Rivas DA, Abdill C, Ehrlich SM, Staas WE (1994) Prospective comparison of external sphincter balloon dilatation and prosthesis placement with external sphincterotomy in spinal cord injured men. *Arch Phys Med Rehabil* 75(3):297–305.

26. Juma S, Niku SD, Brodak PP, Joseph AC (1994) Urolume urethral wallstent in the treatment of detrusor sphincter dyssynergia. *Paraplegia* 32(9):616–621.

27. McFarlane IP, Foley SJ, Shah PJ (1996) Long-term outcome of permanent urethral stents in the treatment of detrusor-sphincter dyssynergia. *Br J Urol* 78(5):729–732.

28. Chancellor MB, Rivas DA, Abdill CK, Staas WE Jr, Bennett CJ, Finocchiaro MV, et al. (1995) Management of sphincter dyssynergia using the sphincter

stent prosthesis in chronically catheterized SCI men. *J Spinal Cord Med* 18(2):88–94.

29. Sauerwein D, Gross AJ, Kutzenberger J, Ringert RH (1995) Wallstents in patients with detrusor-sphincter dyssynergia. *J Urol* 154(2 Pt 1):495–497.

30. Chancellor MB, Gajewski J, Ackman CF, Appell RA, Bennett J, Binard J, et al. (1999) Long-term followup of the North American Mulricenter Urolume* trail for the treatment of external detrusor-sphincter dyssynergia. *J Urol* 161(5):1545–1550.

31. Chancellor MB, Bennett C, Simoneau AR, Finocchario MV, Kline C, Bennett JK, et al. (1999) Sphincteric stent versus external sphincterotomy in spinal cord injured men: prospective randomized multicenter trial. *J Urol* 161(6):1893–1898.

32. Corujo M, Badlani GH (1997) Epithelialization of permanent stents. *J Endourol* 11(6):477–480.

33. Soni BM, Vaidyanatham S, Krishnan KR (1994) Use of Memokath, a second generation urethral stent for relief of urinary retention in male spinal cord injured patients. *Paraplegia* 32(7):480–488.

34. Shah NC, Foley SJ, Shah PJ (1997) Use of Memokath temporary urethral stent in treatment of detrusor-sphincter dyssynergia. *J Endourol* 11(6):485–488.

35. Low AI, McRae PJ (1998) Use of the Memokath for detrusor-sphincter dyssynergia after spinal cord injury-a cautionary tale. *Spinal Cord* 36(1):39–44.

36. Osvaldo N, Iglegias Prieto JI, Mancebo Gomez JM, Massarra Halabi J, Cisneros Ledo J, Perez-Castro Ellendt E (1995) Memotherm as a therapeutic device in intravesical obstruction. *Arch Esp Urol* 48(9):933–936.

37. Juan Garcia FJ, Salvador S, Montoto A, Balvis B, Rodriguez A, Fernandez M, Sanchez J (1999) Intraurethral stent prosthesis in spinal cord injured patients with sphincter dyssynergia. *Spinal Cord* 37(1):54–57.

7

Urolume Stents in the Management of Benign Prostatic Hyperplasia

Christopher R. Chapple, MD,
J. C. Damian Png, MD, Jorgen Nordling, MD
and Euan J. G. Milroy, MD

CONTENTS

INTRODUCTION
HISTORY OF THE UROLUME STENT
STENT INSERTION
A RANDOMIZED CONTROLLED TRIAL
DISCUSSION
CONCLUSION
REFERENCES

INTRODUCTION

Benign prostatic hyperplasia (BPH) occurs histologically in approx 50% of men near the age of 60 and in nearly 100% of men by the age of 80 *(1)*. It has been estimated that the prevalence of "clinical" BPH, defined as an enlargement of the prostate gland >20 gm in the presence of symptoms and/or a urinary flow rate <15 mL/s and without evidence of malignancy was 253/1000 in a sample of 705 men aged 40–79 registered with a group general practice in Scotland *(2)*. In the United States, Glynn et al. calculated the chance of a 40-yr-old man subsequently requiring a prostatectomy as 29% *(3)*.

Transurethral resection of the prostate (TURP) is still the traditional therapy of choice for symptomatic BPH and represents the gold standard *(4,5)*, against which other therapies need to be judged. Although

From: *Urologic Prostheses:*
The Complete, Practical Guide to Devices, Their Implantation and Patient Follow Up
Edited by: C. C. Carson © Humana Press Inc., Totowa, NJ

mortality has been decreasing over the last decade from 1.2% in 1984 to 0.77% in 1990, it is still significant *(6–8)* and increases with age from 0.39% in the 65–69 age group to 1.1% in the 75–79 age group and 3.54% in those older than 85 yr of age *(9)*. This is associated with a significant morbidity of about 18% *(10)*, which includes a 1% risk of total incontinence; 2.1% risk of stress incontinence; 1.9% risk of urge incontinence; a 1.7% risk of vesical neck contractures, and a 3.1% risk of urethral strictures *(11)*. This, coupled with increased public awareness of alternative nonsurgical or minimally invasive treatment options, has raised a number of questions as to the appropriate therapy in contemporary practice.

One of these alternative surgical options is a minimally invasive approach using a permanent endoprosthetic stent to tackle the problem of bladder outlet obstruction, secondary to BPH. The use of such prostatic stents appear to have a number of advantages, namely: a short operating time, minimal blood loss, ease of insertion, a short hospital stay, no in-dwelling catheter post op, and the absence of any expensive equipment, which is often required in other alternative minimally invasive therapies.

An example of such a stent is the Urolume stent, which is a mesh of corrosion-resistant nickel superalloy wire woven into a flexible, expandable tube. It was originally developed for endovascular use by Hans Wallsten, a Swedish national, for the prevention of stenoses after transluminal angioplasty *(12,13)*, but has been used successfully in the urinary tract for the treatment of urethral strictures *(14,15)* and, more recently, for the treatment of BPH in patients not fit to undergo a TURP.

HISTORY OF THE UROLUME STENT

The Urolume stent was first used in urology for the treatment of bulbar urethral strictures that were unresponsive to urethrotomy by Milroy and Chapple with fairly good results *(14)*. Given its success with bulbar strictures, it was used for the treatment of 12 patients with prostatic outflow obstruction who were in a high risk group for surgery by the same authors *(16)*. This was successful in resolving the outlet obstruction in 11 patients with good re-epithelialization of the stent in 6–8 months. In five patients, some amount of stent protruded into the bladder giving rise to encrustations in two. This study was extended to include 54 unfit patients with prostatic outflow obstruction 3 yr later *(17)*. Four patients were unable to void postprocedure as a result of chronic retention, leaving 50 patients who could void immediately postop. A number of patients developed irritative urinary symptoms at

1–3 mo after the procedure but this resolved after 9 mo in the majority of the patients. Symptom scores and peak flows were also significantly improved after stent insertion by more than two times. Encrustation was a problem in 14 patients (25.9%) and occurred in those patients with either a protrusion of the stent into the bladder or when the re-epithelialization was incomplete. Only one patient developed incontinence as a result of stent encroachment over the distal sphincter mechanism. This was easily removed. In all, 6 (11.1%) stents had to be removed: 3 because of problems with positioning, 1 because of distal obstruction secondary to prostatic adenocarcinoma, and 2 because of severe urge incontinence in the presence of persistent detrusor instability.

Because of the relatively good results of the Urolume stent in unfit patients, a number of studies involving fit, healthy men with BPH were carried out both in Europe and in the United States.

A European series by Milroy et al. *(18)* in 140 patients with an 18-mo follow-up showed similar findings to the earlier studies by Milroy and Chapple. There were 94 patients with symptomatic BPH and 46 with acute urinary retention. Both groups showed significant improvements to their peak urine flows and their symptom scores from a preoperative mean peak flow of 9.3 mL/s to a postoperative mean peak flow of 17.3 mL/s in the symptomatic BPH group and 13.5 mL/s in the retention group. Symptom scores were similarly reduced to a mean of 7.6 and 3 (Madsen-Iversen), respectively. Fourteen patients *(10%)* had their stent removed: 11 for malposition and 3 for persistent symptoms related to the stent.

The North American Urolume Prosthesis Study Group's experience with the Urolume prostatic stent was reported by Oesterling et al. *(19)* and involved 126 men, of which 95 had symptomatic BPH and 31 had acute retention of urine. At 2-yr follow-up, symptom scores (Madsen-Iversen) decreased from a mean of 14.3 preinsertion to 5.4 postinsertion in the no-retention group and to 4.1 postinsertion in the retention group. Mean peak flows increased from 9.1 mL/s preinsertion to 13.1 mL/s postinsertion in the nonretention group and to 11.4 mL/s in the retention group. Residual urine volumes were similarly improved from 85 mL preinsertion to 47 mL postinsertion in the nonretention group to 46 mL in the retention group. Significant long-term complications that required stent removal was seen in 17 patients (13%). These were removed transurethrally without any subsequent effects. The most common causes of stent removal were stent migration (29.4%) and recurrent obstruction at the bladder neck or apex (29.4%). Two (11.8%) were removed for persistent irritative symptoms, two for perineal discomfort, and two for encrustations secondary to the exposed stents at the bladder neck.

Because of such complications regarding protrusion of the stent into the bladder neck, modification of the stent was carried out and studied in 135 fit men with prostate outflow obstruction by Guazzoni et al. *(20)* in a multicenter trial in Europe. The modifications carried out allowed a reduction of the amount of shortening that occurs when the stent expands. This was thought to facilitate proper stent placement and was achieved by altering the crossing angles of the wires from 142° to 110° and using a thicker wire diameter (0.17 mm–0.20 mm). However, it also resulted in a decrease in the applied pressure/mm of urothelium from 6972 Pa to 2941 Pa. Long-term results regarding improvements in symptom scores, uroflowmetry, and residual urine volumes at 18 mo were no different from the earlier studies, but the modified less-shortening (LS) Urolume stent had a much higher long-term complication rate (31.1%, *n*=42) when compared to the commercially available (CA) Urolume stent. These included 11 (26.2%) stent migrations, 17 (40.5%) under-stentings or malpositions, 4 severe epithelial hyperplasia, 2 persistent irritative symptoms, 2 subsequent regrowth of the median lobe, and 2 urethral strictures. These required the removal of the prostatic stents in 21 (15.5%) patients with the authors commenting that some of the complications, particularly stent migrations and epithelial hyperplasia, are related directly to the changes made in the modified LS Urolume stents. This stent was subsequently dropped from use.

STENT INSERTION

The Urolume stent is designed for use with an introducer that is designed to be used like a cystoscope. General, regional, or local anesthesia with urethral lignocaine and intravenous sedation are given and the patient is placed in the lithotomy position.

Based on our previous experience with prostatic stent insertion, we have introduced a number of modifications to the original technique used for device implantation *(16)* to ensure correct placement with maximum stenting of the prostatic urethra and, in particular ,to avoid protrusion of the stent into the bladder when the bladder neck is funneled open at the time of a full bladder.

A cystoscopy is carried out on the patient and, using a purpose-designed measurement catheter with a foley balloon at its proximal end, the length of the prostatic urethra is measured under direct vision from the bladder neck to the distal sphincter mechanism. A stent with a length 0.5 cm less than the measured length of the urethra is inserted. The stent-insertion device is inserted under direct vision and positioned at the bladder neck. The outer sheath is then withdrawn a bit, allowing partial opening of the stent, which is then withdrawn distally to ensure that the stent lies distal to the bladder neck itself; checking, in particular, that this is the case at the 12 o'clock position. The outer sheath is then removed completely to the safety-lock position, the position of the stent, in particular, relative to the bladder neck is then checked. At this stage, the stent can be retracted back into the device and repositioned as required. When the operator is happy with this, the safety lock is removed and the stent fully deployed.

The stent can be removed by retrograde displacement back into the bladder followed by extraction via a purpose-designed extraction device. In the initial series, we removed six stents, four at up to 1 mo, because of initial problems related to placement. In two patients at longer intervals—11 mo and 18 mo after insertion, in one case because of persisting incontinence in a patient with severe recalcitrant detrusor instability, the latter being a patient with Parkinson's disease. In these two patients, it was necessary to resect the covering urothelium prior to removal.

A RANDOMIZED CONTROLLED TRIAL

Because of the relatively good results with the Urolume stents in patients with symptomatic BPH who were unfit for a TURP and its perioperative advantages, namely: a short operating time, minimal blood loss, ease of insertion, a reduced hospital stay, and no in-dwelling catheter postoperatively, it would, by comparison, appear to provide a suitable treatment alternative to TURP for the management of symptomatic BPH, especially in older patients *(9)*. In order to evaluate the efficacy of a permanently implanted stent in the fit patient over age 65 with BPH, we conducted a randomized controlled trial to compare the Urolume Plus prostatic stent against standard TURP in 86 patients with symptomatic BPH.

Methods and Patient Data

This prospective randomized trial was carried out in three centers in the United Kingdom and Denmark, with full ethical committee approval.

Eighty-six surgically fit patients above age 65 on the waiting list for prostatic surgery with symptomatic and urodynamically proven bladder outlet obstruction caused by BPH were selected for treatment and randomized to either Urolume insertion or TURP.

Safety and efficacy data before, during, and up to 1 yr after treatment were collected and analyzed. Reviews were carried out at 1, 3, 6, and 12 mo regarding to urinary symptoms, pain and sexual function scores, urine flow rates (adjusted for voided volume), residual urine volumes, and pressure flow studies. An IPSS quality-of-life questionaire was administered at the 1- and 12-mo visits with a BPH impact index at the same time. Patients with known bladder cancer or intravesical stones, neurological disease affecting bladder function, urethral stricture disease, known or suspected prostatic cancer, prostate volume < 30 g, prostatic urethra < 2.0 cm in length, median lobe obstruction, and those on current pharmacotherapy for BPH were excluded.

Data was also collected on perioperative and post-operative complications, length of operating time, and length of postprocedure hospitalization. Potential risks identified with the endoscopic treatment of prostatic obstruction included risks associated with anesthesia, bleeding, infection, incontinence, sexual dysfunction, and urethral stricture formation. Specific risks identified with stent placement included misplacement or placement of an incorrect size stent requiring removal and replacement, urethral injury, encrustation, erosion, wire fracture, stent migration, stent shortening, and obstructive reactive hyperplasia. Specific risks identified with TURP included hemorrhage and clot retention, retrograde ejaculation, and the TUR syndrome.

Results

Ten patients dropped out of the study before treatment began and a further four in the TURP arm were found to have bladder neck obstruction and underwent a bladder neck incision instead of TURP and were excluded from the study. Of the remaining 72 patients, 14 had urinary retention and were excluded from the efficacy analysis, but were included in the safety analysis. Three patients from the Urolume arm failed stent insertion leaving a final 30 patients on the Urolume arm and 25 patients on the TURP arm with complete follow-up for a full analysis at 1 yr.

There were no significant differences between the two arms regarding age, IPSS scores, residual urine volumes, prostate-specific antigen (PSA) levels, prostate volumes, and length. There was, however, a difference between the peak urine flow rates between the two groups, which, on adjusting for voided volumes, showed a p value of 0.05 (student t-test), which just misses significance (*see* Table 1)

Data addressing the potential risks of the two treatments were analyzed in 72 patients from both nonretention and retention groups.

Procedure and Safety Results

The median operating time was 11.5 min (range: 10–40 min) for the Urolume arm compared to 37.5 min (range: 15–100) for the TURP arm. This was statistically significant ($p< 0.001$). Three patients out of 39 in the Urolume arm failed stent insertion because of difficulty in releasing the stent in two and a "tight" gland that squeezed onto the stent in one.

Table 1
BPH Impact Index (BII)

	None	*A little*	*Some*	*A lot*
1. Over the past month, how much physical discomfort did any urinary problems cause you?		0	1	2
2. Over the past month, how much did you worry about your health because of any urinary problems?	0	1	2	3
3. Overall, how bothersome has any trouble with urination been during the past month?	*None at all* 0	*Bothers me a little* 1	*Bothers me some* 2	*Bothers me a lot* 3
4. Over the past month, how much of the time has any urinary problem kept you from doing the kinds of things you would usually do?	*None of the time* 0	*A little of the time* 1	*Some of the time* 2	*Most of the time* 3	*All of the time* 4

Total
BII
score =

Four patients out of the 33 undergoing TU resection experienced severe bleeding requiring transfusion intraoperatively during the TURP. There were three documented capsular perforations.

The median days of hospitalization were 1 (0–10 d) and 4 (2–9 d) days for stent insertion and TURP, respectively, and the difference was statistically significant (p=0.001). All patients with a TURP were catheterized compared to two Urolume patients who had a suprapubic catheter inserted after failing to void. However, the duration of an in-dwelling catheter was a median of two days for the TURP arm compared with the 5.5 d for the Urolume arm.

Three patients developed nausea and vomiting in the immediate postoperative period after TURP compared to none in the Urolume arm. Early postop hematuria was present in four patients after stent insertion and four after TURP. All four patients on the TURP arm required blood transfusions, whereas the hematuria poststent insertion was milder and required no action.

Five patients on the Urolume arm and 8 patients on the TURP arm had repeated positive urine cultures during the 1-yr follow-up. One patient on the Urolume arm developed epididymoorchitis. All patients were treated with antibiotics and the infections duly resolved with no further complications.

Two patients on the TURP arm developed persistent hematuria and one had gross hematuria requiring emergency admission and transfusion 6 wk after the procedure. Two patients on the Urolume arm developed persistent hematuria. One had a urethral stone on the bare stent at the 6-mo visit and the other patient had marked intrastent reactive hyperplasia.

Three patients in each arm required a second intervention during the 1-yr follow-up. Two patients with stents inserted required a second stent as a result of shortening discovered during follow-up at 3 and 6 mo. One recovered uneventfully, whereas the other who initially presented with acute retention required intermittent self-catheterization for large residual urine volumes. The third had marked intrastent reactive hyperplasia, which required a TU resection. The three patients on the TURP arm with reintervention included a repeat TURP for residual gland at 3 mo follow-up, a urethrotomy for a urethral stricture at 6-mo follow-up and a bladder neck incision for a bladder neck stenosis at 12 mo.

Three patients died during the course of the study. One patient committed suicide a month after his TURP. Another patient with a Urolume stent died of acute renal failure secondary to ischemic bowel at 3-mo follow-up and the third patient died of severe pneumonia and GI hemorrhage 8-mo post-Urolume stent insertion. One patient in the retention group who had a Urolume stent inserted was discovered at 3-mo follow-up to have prostate cancer on a third set of prostatic biopsies with the previous two having been reported as normal.

Pain

Data was collected on urethral pain and pain associated with both erection and ejaculation.

Urethral Pain

Six patients in the Urolume arm and one in the TURP arm had urethral pain pretreatment (*see* Fig. 1). At the one month follow-up, patients with urethral pain increased significantly to 13 in the Urolume arm and 11 in the TURP arm, respectively. Although there was statistical significance

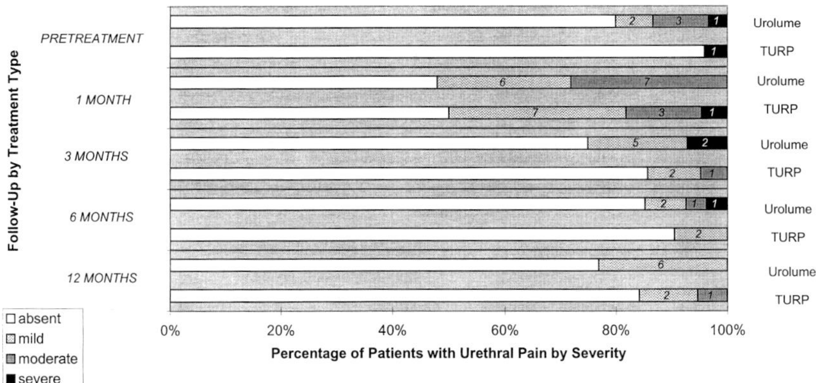

Fig. 1. Urethral pain by treatment type and length of follow-up.

in both groups ($p=0.013$ and $p=0.001$, respectively) at 1 mo and pretreatment, no statistical difference between the two groups was seen. The number of patients with urethral pain then reverted back to baseline values at 6 and 12 mo in both arms of the study.

ERECTION PAIN

One patient in the Urolume arm and two patients in the TURP arm had mild pain on erection before treatment (*see* Fig. 2). This did not change significantly with time. At the end of 12 mo, one further patient in each treatment group experienced moderate pain on erection.

PAIN WITH INTERCOURSE

One patient in the Urolume arm and three patients in the TURP arm had mild to severe pain on intercourse before treatment (*see* Fig. 3). Patients who have not had intercourse were excluded from the statistical analysis. At 3 mo, one patient had severe pain and two had mild pain during intercourse in the Urolume arm compared to none in the TURP arm. This was statistically significant. ($p<0.05$) This improved to three experiencing mild pain at 6 mo in the Urolume group and both groups having three patients at 12 mo follow-up with mild pain during intercourse.

Sexual Function

ERECTION

There was no significant change in the number of patients and strength of erection in both groups before and after treatment (*see* Fig. 4). They were approx divided into three equal groups with a third having no erections, a third having partial erections, and a third having full erec-

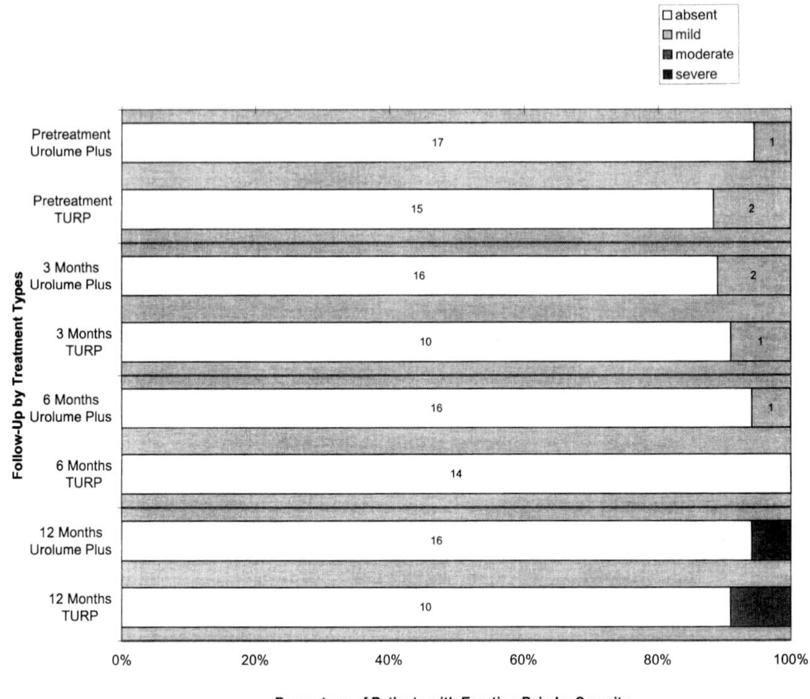

Fig. 2. Erection pain by treatment type and time after procedure.

tions. No difference was noted between the two arms before treatment and at 12 mo.

No difference was also noted in erection frequency between the two groups.

EJACULATION

In the Urolume and TURP arms, 77.8% and 83.3% of patients, respectively, had the ability to ejaculate before treatment (*see* Fig. 5). This decreased slightly to 64.7% and 72.7%, respectively, at 3 mo and 75% and 60%, respectively, at 12 mo. Although there appeared to be a trend toward decreased ejaculatory ability with time in the TURP group, it did not approach statistical significance. There was no significant change in the Urolume group.

Regarding the nature of ejaculation, 92.9% and 100% of patients in the Urolume and TURP groups, respectively, had antegrade ejaculation prior to treatment (*see* Fig. 6). Although there was a statistically significant increase in the numbers with retrograde ejaculation before treatment: -7.1% and 0%, respectively, to 50% and 50%, respectively, at 12 mo

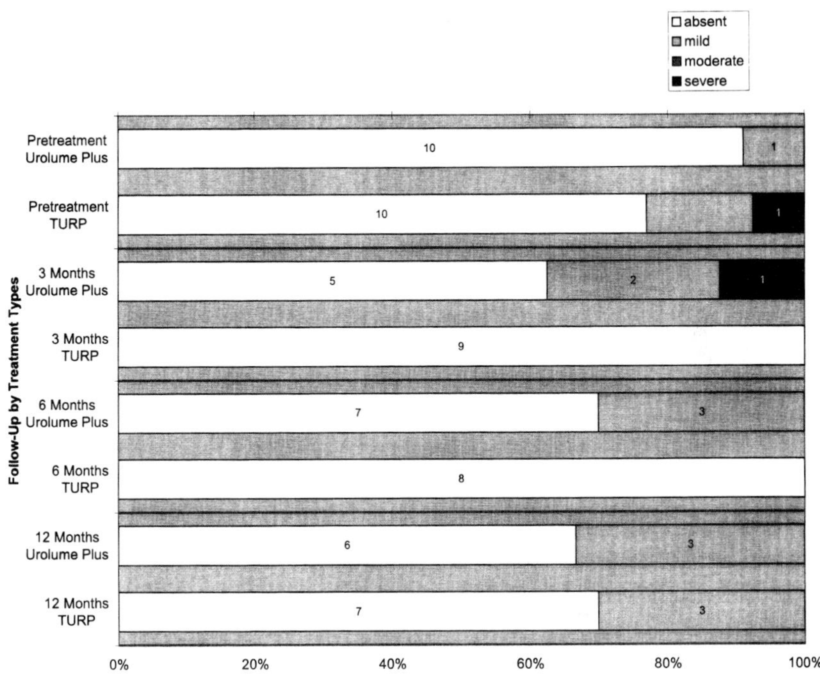

Fig. 3. Pain during intercourse by treatment type and time after procedure.

after treatment in both groups, there was no statistical difference between the changes between the two arms of the study.

Endoscopic Follow-Up of Patients

EPITHELIALIZATION

Of the 20 Urolume patients assessed by cystourethroscopy at 12 months postprocedure, 75% of the patients had 90–100% epithelialization of the stent. Ninety percent had at least 70% epithelialization and one patient had less than 50% epithelialization (*see* Fig. 7).

ENCRUSTATIONS

Four (20%) patients with the Urolume stents developed encrustations on their stents. The majority were small calcifications, but one had a stone sized 1 cm in diameter in midurethra arising from an exposed area of the stent. The stone was easily removed endoscopically during the cystoscopic evaluation. There were no intravesical protrusions of the stents identified at 12 mo.

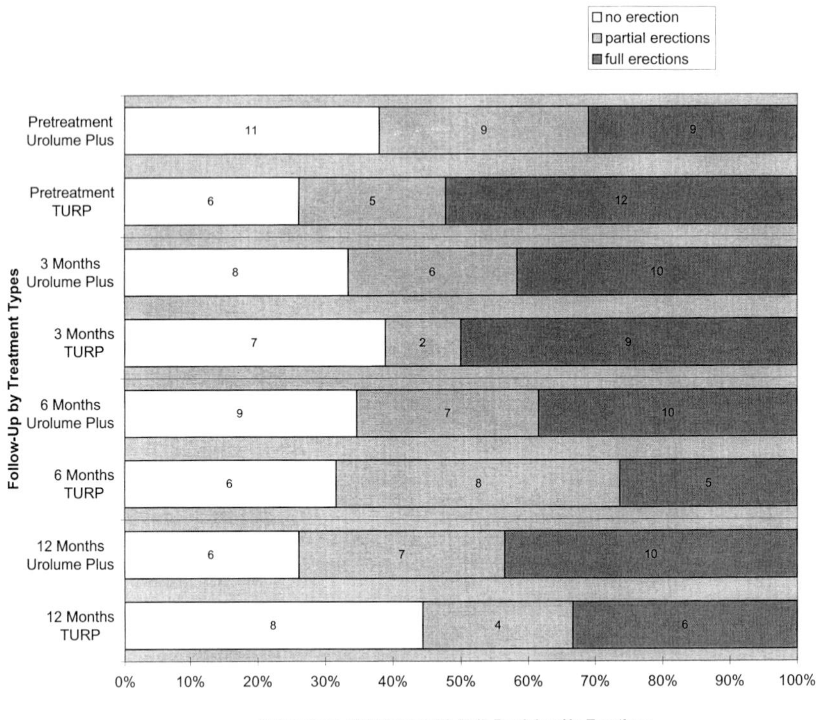

Fig. 4. Potency by treatment type and time after procedure.

HYPERPLASIA

Thirteen patients (65%) developed intrastent reactive hyperplasia at 12 mo. Of these, three (15%) had marked hyperplasia with one requiring TU resection of the hyperplastic tissue. This recurred at 12 mo. The other two did not require further intervention. It was interesting to note that neither of these two had any bare wires visible, although one had encrustations seen within the hyperplastic tissue.

STENT MIGRATION

There was one stent migration identified at the 12-mo follow-up. This was found in the bladder and was completely encrusted. It was removed transurethrally and a TURP was subsequently carried out.

RESIDUAL HYPERTROPHIC TISSUE

There were 6 patients with residual hypertrophic tissue after TURP out of the 12 assessed cystoscopically. Of these, one required a repeat TURP on the basis of urodynamically proven bladder outflow obstruction.

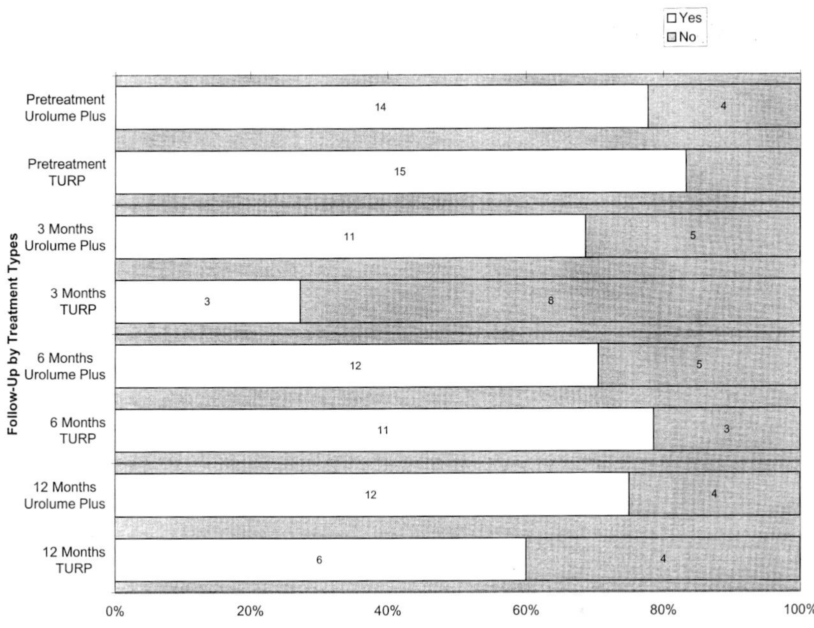

Fig. 5. Ejaculatory ability by treatment type and time after procedure.

Efficacy Data

PEAK FLOW RATES

Baseline peak flow rates was 9.2 mL/s (SD:2.61) and 7.6 mL/s (SD:2.19) for the Urolume and TURP arms, respectively. Both improved significantly ($p<0.001$) to 12.7 mL/s (SD:7.60) and 16.1 mL/s (SD: 8.2), respectively, at 3 mo and 12.8 mL/s (SD: 6.04) and 19.3 mL/s (SD: 8.7), respectively, at 12 mo after treatment (*see* Fig. 8). The TURP group also had significantly better peak flow rates ($p=0.028$) as compared to the Urolume group over time. Similar results were obtained with the adjusted peak flow rates.

If one looks at success rates by percentage improvement (*see* Fig. 9), 75% of patients after TURP had a 77.8% improvement to their peak flow rates at 1-yr follow-up, compared to only 30.8% of patients in the Urolume arm. In the Urolume arm, 57.7% had at least a 25% improvement to the peak flow rates, compared to 94.4% in the TURP arm.

RESIDUAL URINE VOLUME

Residual urine volumes were both significantly reduced from a median baseline of 77.5 mL (range: 0–400 mL) to 35.5 mL (range: 0–177 mL) at

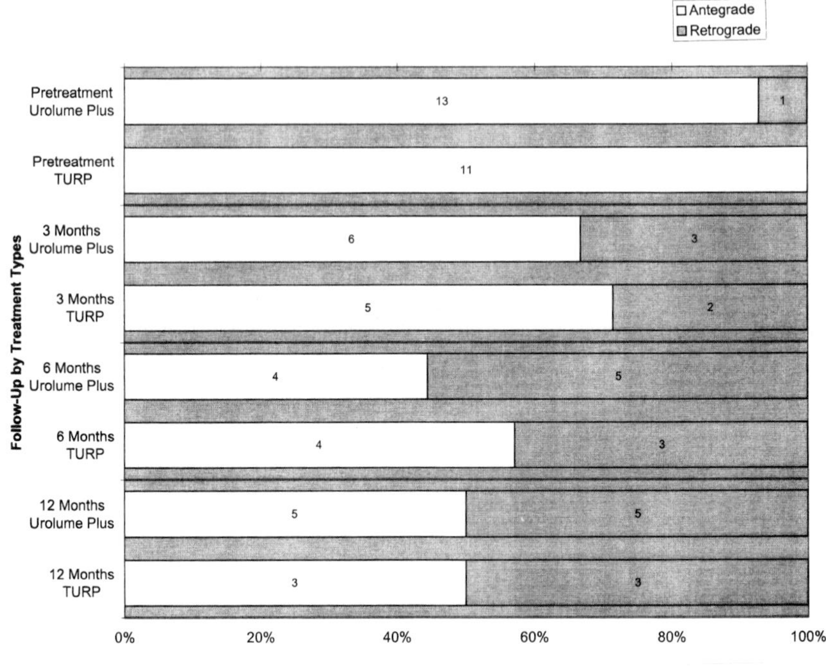

Fig. 6. Type of ejaculation by treatment type and time after procedure.

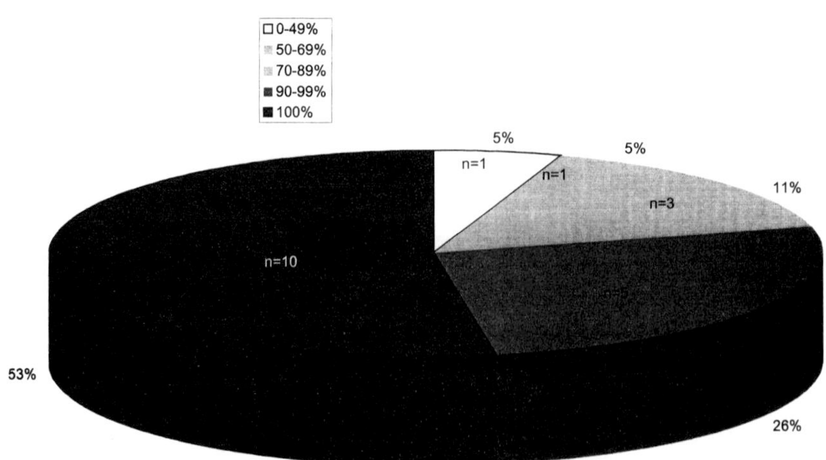

Fig. 7. Epithelialization of the Urolume Plus at 12-mo follow-up.

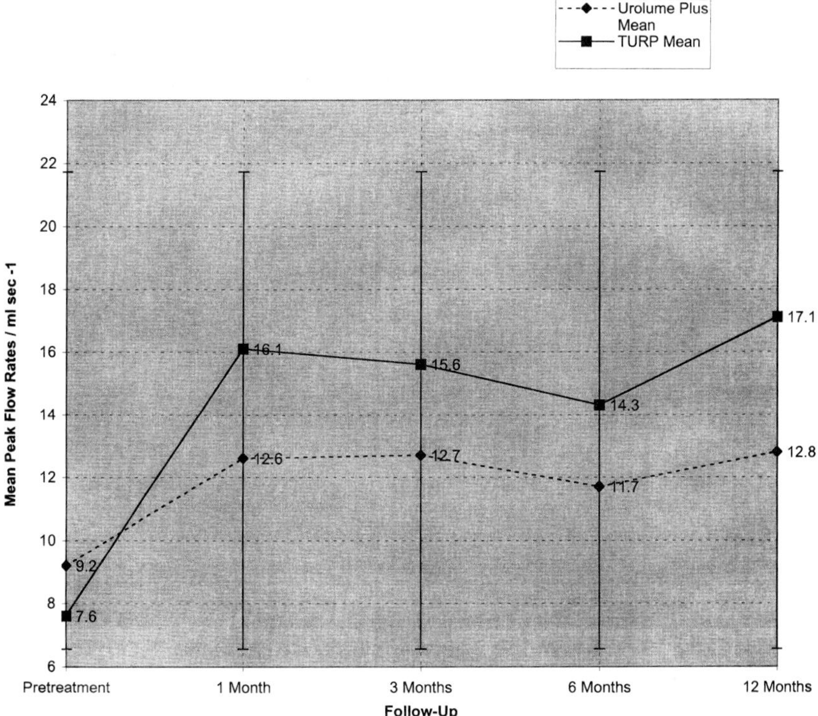

Fig. 8. Mean peak flow rates by treatment type and time after procedure.

12 mo for the Urolume arm and 50 mL (range: 0–600 mL) to 10 mL (range: 0–99 mL) at 12 mo for the TURP arm. Although there appears to be a significant difference between residual urine volumes for the TURP and Urolume arms at 12 mo ($p=0.002$), there was no significant difference between the two groups if the degree of improvement between the baseline and 1-yr residual volumes was used ($p=0.94$). The difference being a result of the initial difference of the baseline residual volumes between the two groups, rather than a true difference as a result of treatment.

If one looks at percentage improvement of residual volumes, 72.7% in the Urolume arm and 82.4% in the TURP arm had at least a 25% improvement to their residual urine volumes. There was no statistical difference between the two groups. More than half (58.8%) of patients after TURP had a 75% improvement to their residual urine volumes at 1 yr. This is fairly similar to the 50% of patients in the Urolume arm who also had a 75% improvement to their residual urine volumes.

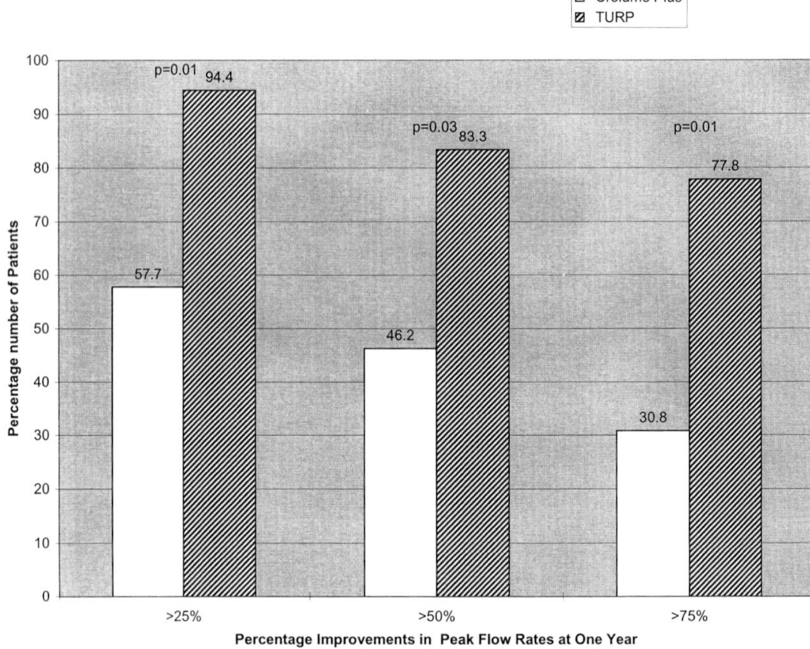

Fig. 9. Success rates by percent improvement of peak flow rates at 1 yr.

PRESSURE FLOW STUDIES

Mean detrusor pressures at peak flow decreased significantly from 98.1 (SD:6.5) cm H_2O to 42.9 (SD:5.3) cm H_2O for the TURP arm, and from 89.6 (SD:5.4) cm H_2O to 56.1 (SD:6.9) cm H_2O for the Urolume arm at the 6-mo follow-up (*see* Fig. 10). Although there was a significant difference in the pre- and posttreatment detrusor pressures in both groups, there was no significant difference between the detrusor pressures of the two groups following treatment.

IPSS SYMPTOM SCORES

AUA symptom scores showed a significant drop from a mean baseline value of 20.4 (SD:7.36, *p*=0.001) in the Urolume arm and 19.8 (SD:5.39, *p*=0.001) in the TURP arm to a mean value of 13.6 (SD:7.12) and 12.3 (SD:6.39), respectively, during the first month after treatment. This value then decreased gradually to a score of 10 (SD:5.19) and 7.8 (SD:6.41), respectively, at 12 mo (*see* Fig. 11). There was no significant difference between the two treatment arms in the ANOVA analysis (*p*=0.459).

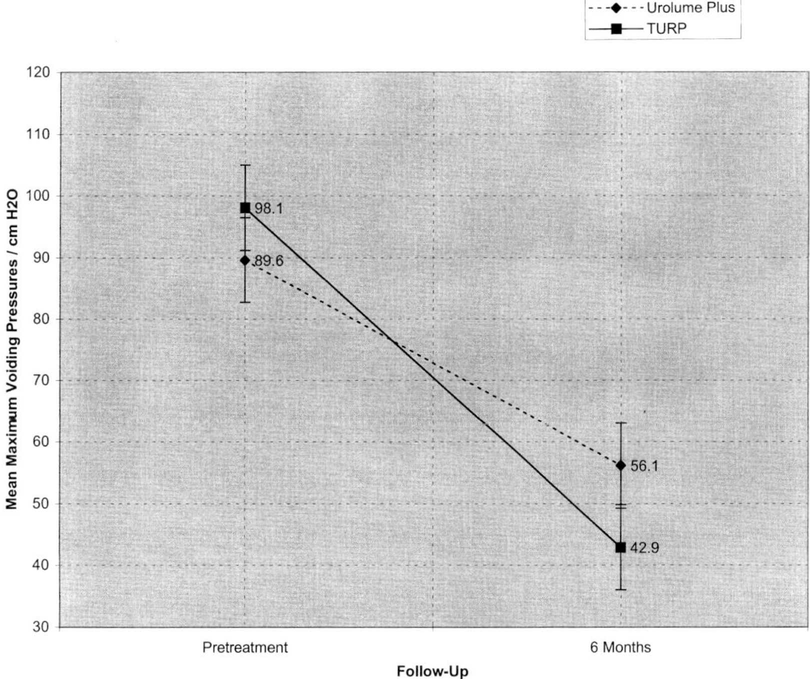

Fig. 10. Comparison of mean maximum voiding pressures by treatment type at 6 mo.

Quality-of-Life (QOL) Scores

The QOL score owing to urinary symptoms revealed 73.3% of the Urolume arm and 79.2% of the TURP patients who were "mostly dissatisfied," "unhappy," or "feel terrible" before treatment, compared to 42.3% and 33.3% at 1 mo after treatment and 8% and 10% at 12-mo follow-up, respectively (*see* Fig. 12). There was no significant difference in QOL scores between both arms.

Only two patients (6.7% and 8.3%) in each arm were either "pleased" or "mostly satisfied" before treatment, compared to 38.5% of the Urolume arm and 52.4% of the TURP arm at 1 mo after treatment. This improved to 68% for the Urolume arm at 12 mo and 80% for the TURP arm. Although the mean values and the median scores (*see* Table 2) for the TURP arm was better at 1 and 12 mo compared to the Urolume arm, there was no statistical difference between the two groups.

BPH Impact Index

This is a QOL index that measures how much the urinary symptoms affect the various domains of health.

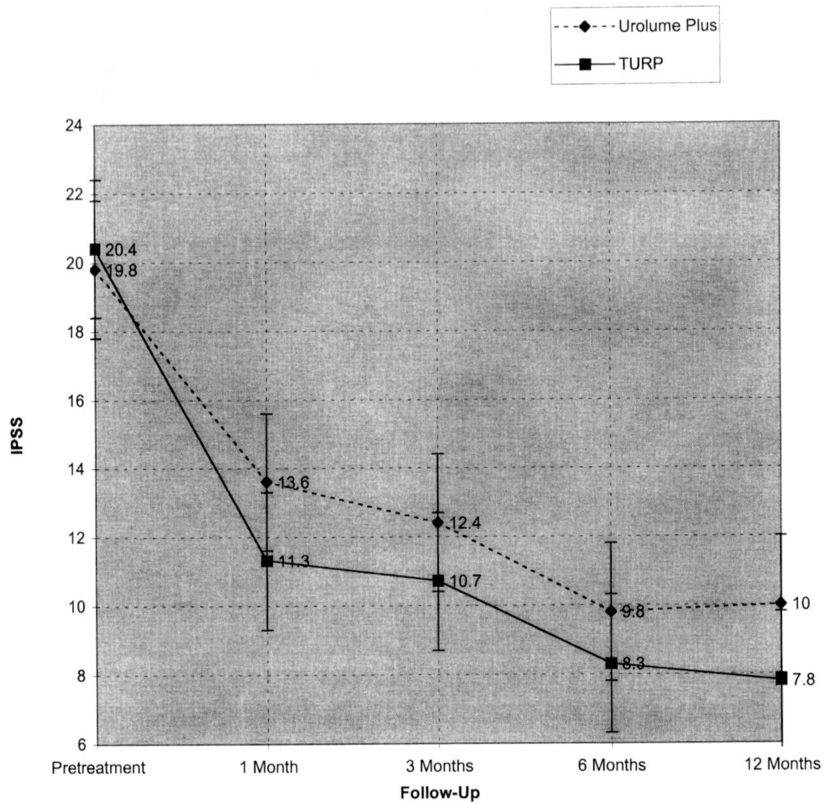

Fig. 11. Follow-up comparison of mean AUA symptom scores by treatment type.

The mean BPH Impact Index decreased from 6.5 before treatment to 1.8 at 12 mo in the Urolume arm. This was not significantly different from the decrease seen in the TURP group with a pretreatment value of 5.8 changing to 1.8 in 12 mo. No difference between treatment types (p=0.314) was found in the ANOVA analysis, but there was a significant difference in both the groups before and after treatment (p=0.001).

DISCUSSION

Since the use of Urolume urethral stents in the treatment of benign prostatic hyperplasia was first reported in 1989 *(21)*, its use has been advocated by a number of authors in unfit patients undergoing prostatic surgery *(16,22,23)*. The Urolume stent has been evaluated in a number of studies of unfit patients. In a collaborative study involving 96 unfit

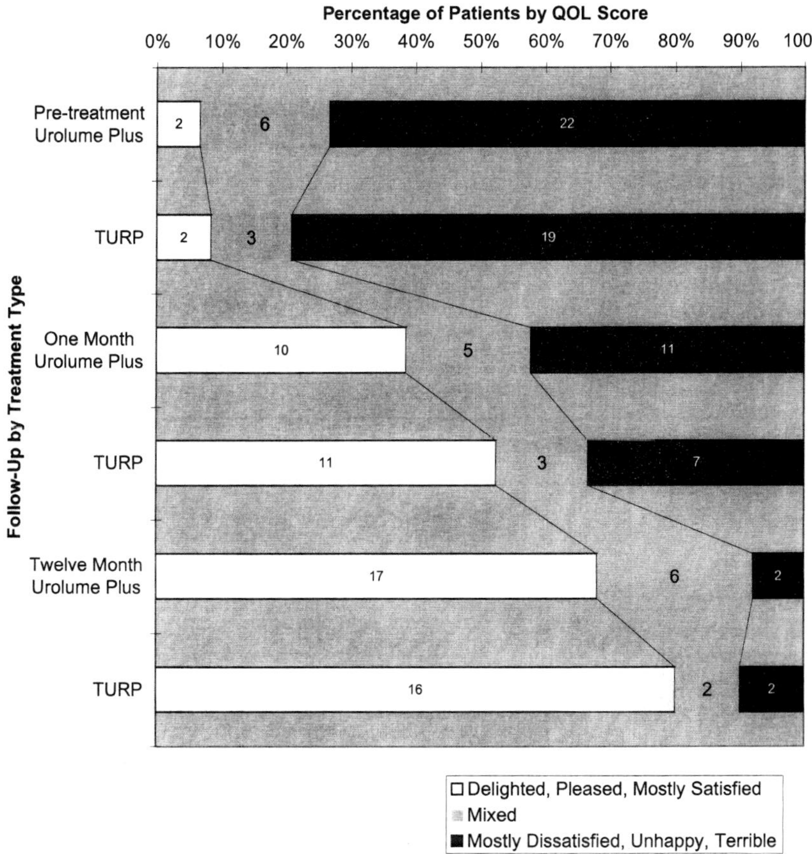

Fig. 12. QOL scores by treatment type and follow-up.

men from five European centers, Williams et al. *(24)* showed that objective and symptomatic evidence of relief of the bladder obstruction was evident throughout the 12 mo of the study. Complications included irritative symptoms in the first 3 mo postinsertion requiring removal in three patients and encrustations that developed in 14 patients, with 9 of these resulting in urinary infection. To deal with this, modifications of the insertion technique have been developed as aforementioned.

In this study, which represents the first randomized study against TURP involving 86 patients included in the two treatment groups, we found that the Urolume stent had a distinct advantage over a standard TURP when the operative procedure and the perioperative course was reviewed. It only took about 11.5 min to employ a urethral stent, compared to 37.5 min for a TURP. Blood loss was minimal compared to the four patients who required blood transfusion during the resection.

Table 2
Baseline Characteristics of Patients Randomized Trial Receiving Either
UroLume Insertion or TURP, in Three Centers in the UK and Denmark

Characteristic	Urolume Plus	Group	TURP	tValue	pValue
Age at insertion	n	30	25		
(yr)	Mean	72.5	72.3		
	SD	+/–6.73	+/–4.90		
	Range	62.0–90.0	63.0–84.0	0.14	0.89
AUA Symptom	n	28	24		
Score	Mean	19.8	20.4		
	SD	+/–7.36	+/–6.08		
	Range	5.0–30.0	11.0–33.0	–0.31	0.76
Peak flow (ml/s)	n	30	25		
	Mean	9.2	7.6		
	SD	+/–2.61	+/–2.19		
	Range	3.9–15.0	4.2–11.7	2.31	0.03
Adjusted peak	n	30	25		
flow (ml/s)	Mean	0.71	0.58		
	SD	+/–0.27	+/–0.23		
	Range	0.32–1.39	0.27–1.28	1.97	0.05
Volume voided	n	30	25		
(ml)	Mean	191.6	209.5		
	SD	+/–91.1	+/–107.8		
	Range	69.0–413.0	48.0–456.0	–0.67	0.51
Residual urine	n	28	23		
volume (ml)	Mean	77.5	50.0		
	Range	0.0–400.0	0.0–600.0	NA*	0.63*
Length of prostate	n	30	22		
(cm)	Mean	2.5	30		
	Range	2.0–4.0	2.0–6.0	NA*	0.05*
Prostate-specific	n	25	22		
antigen (ng/mL)	Mean	4.65	4.65		
	Range	0.6–17.8	0.7–38.5	NA*	0.91*
Obstruction	minor	1(3.3)[†]	1(4.2)		
	partial	16(53.3)	9(37.5)		
	major	13(43.3)	14(58.3)		
	Total	30(100.0)	24(100.0)	—	0.32*
Prostate weight (g)	20–30	1(3.4)	1(4.0)		
	31–40	13(44.8)	14(56.0)		
	41–50	5(17.2)	3(12.0)		
	50–60	4(13.8)	3(12.0)		
	61–70	6(20.7)	3(12.0)		
	71–80	0(0.0)	1(4.0)	—	0.48*
	Total	29(100.0)	25(100.0)	—	0.48*

*Mann-Whitney U-test used for non-normal data
[†]Percentages in parentheses

Hospital stay was 1 d, compared to 4 d for a TURP, and only two patients required a urinary catheter.

However, postoperatively both procedures were equally affected by complications abeit differing in terms of their nature and severity. Three patients developed nausea and vomiting after the TURP, compared to none in the Urolume arm. This may be more related to the length of anesthesia, rather than the effects of the surgery. It was, however, interesting to note that four patients on each arm developed bleeding with the four from the TURP arm requiring intraoperative blood transfusion. This is probably the greatest problem with the TURP. One patient who developed clot retention after the stent insertion, required a bladder washout via the suprapubic catheter. This was removed after 4 d and the patient was discharged after voiding normally. Although the Urolume stent is a foreign body in the urethra and needs time for epithelialization, there was no difference in urinary infection rates between the two groups. All infections resolved with antibiotics. Urinary infections have previously been reported in association with stent encrustation *(25)*, but this association was not found in our study.

Persistent hematuria without pyuria was another problem that occurred in both groups. For those in the TURP arm this was probably related to a raw resected surface that had not yet fully epithelialized. The two patients in the Urolume arm with persistent hematuria were found to have a urethral stone and marked intrastent reactive hyperplasia, respectively.

There was also no difference regarding the reintervention rates in both arms although the types of reintervention were quite different. TURP had problems with residual gland, urethral strictures, and bladder neck stenosis, whereas the Urolume arm had problems with intrastent reactive hyperplasia and shortening of the stent. Whether this is a result of incorrect selection of the stent length during the procedure or due to a true shortening of the stent is unclear.

Urethral pain was a significant problem in both groups with the 1-mo follow-up with the Urolume arm having nearly twice the number of patients with moderate or severe urethral pain compared to the TURP arm. There was no significant difference regarding the frequency of urethral pain in both groups, although most studies involving stents do report this to be a problem. Urethral pain decreased markedly at 3 mo and resolved spontaneously by the 12-mo follow-up in both arms of the study. No patient required removal of the stent as a result of urethral pain in this study. There was no significant pain on erection between the two groups, but at the 3-mo follow up, there were significantly more patients with pain during intercourse in the Urolume group compared to the TURP group (p=0.05). The pain on intercourse in the Urolume arm improved to a mild pain at 6 mo to baseline at 12 mo.

Where the strength and frequency of erection was concerned, there was no significant difference between the two groups. There was also no statistical difference in the ability to ejaculate in both groups. However, both TURP and stents resulted in retrograde ejaculation in about 50% of patients treated in each arm at the end of 12 mo. There was no statistical difference between the two groups.

Cystoscopic follow-up showed that 25% of patients with the Urolume stent had <90% epithelization after 1 yr of follow-up. This led to asymptomatic encrustations in four patients (20%). None were related to urinary infections. Some degree of intrastent hyperplasia was present in 65% of patients with the Urolume stent inserted with 15% showing marked hyperplasia. One patient required a transurethral resection of the hyperplastic tissue. The cause of the hyperplasia is still not fully understood. Whether it is because of the intrinsic reaction of the urothelium to the stent material or secondary to chronic irritation as a result of encrustations or infection or a combination of the two is still open to debate. Stent migration occurred in one patient (3.3%) and was thought to be caused by an incorrect implantation technique. Residual hypertrophic tissue after TURP was seen in six patients.

Regarding the efficacy of both treatments, peak and adjusted peak flow rates were improved significantly after both types of treatment. Where the peak flow rates after Urolume tended to plateau off 1 mo poststent insertion, peak flow rates after a TURP continued to improve with time to give a significantly much better flow rate at 12 mo, compared to the Urolume stent. Using percentage improvements to the flow rates as an index, 80% of patients had a 50% improvement to their flow rates compared to only 46.2% in the Urolume arm.

Although the improvement in flow rates in the TURP group were greater, there was no greater reduction in the mean voiding detrusor pressures at peak flow in the TURP group compared to the stent group. Improvements in the residual urine volumes in both groups were also noted after treatment but there was no difference in the reduction of the residual urine volumes between the two groups.

When one looks at symptom scores, both treatments had significant improvement to their scores as a result of treatment. This improved over the 12 mo, with no statistical difference between the two groups.

QOL scores in both groups were similarly improved after treatment significantly. Both groups also saw their scores improve over the 12 months with the TURP arm suggesting a marginal advantage. However there was no statistical difference between the two groups. The same results were found with the BPH impact indices.

CONCLUSION

These results and the results of earlier studies suggest that a permanently implanted Urolume prostatic urethral stent, with its low morbidity via a reduced operating time and hospital stay, is a safe alternative to TURP. It appears to produce only slightly more postprocedure discomfort and pain during intercourse than a TURP and the majority of such symptoms resolve eventually. Erection and ejaculatory dysfunction are also not dissimilar.

The improvement in symptoms and QOL are identical with both treatments at 1-yr follow-up, but TURP produces a significantly better flow rate compared to the Urolume stent. However, residual urine volumes and mean detrusor pressures were not significantly different. It may well be in this assessment that the Urolume stent, because it is associated with less morbidity, has a distinct perioperative advantage over a TURP for the elderly fit patient. However, unlike a TURP, its use is limited by the anatomy of the prostatic enlargement which can be associated with technical failure, for instance in the wide or short prostatic urethra and the presence of an obstructing median lobe hyperplasia. In the longer term, intrastent hyperplasia and calcifications do occur in an unpredictable fashion and together with the failure of epithelialization, represent a problem for use of stents for BPH. For unlike many post-TURP complications, such complications after stent insertion may necessitate stent removal.

TURP should still remain as the standard treatment for BPH in the fit nongeriatric patient until such time when the problems of intrastent hyperplasia and epithelialization failure are resolved and probably when longer term results, with up to 5-yr follow-up, of the Urolume stents are available.

REFERENCES

1. Isaacs JT (1990) Importance of the natural history of benign prostatic hyperplasia in the evaluation of pharmacologic intervention. *Prostate* Suppl 3:1–7.
2. Garraway WM, Collins GN, Lee RJ (1991) High prevalence of benign prostatic hypertrophy in the community. *Lancet* 338:469–471.
3. Glynn RJ, Campion EW, Bouchard GR, Silbert JE (1985) The development of benign prostatic hyperplasia among volunteers in the normative aging study. *J Epidemiol* 121:78–82.
4. Chilton CP, Morgan RJ, England HR (1978) A critical evaluation of the results of transurethral resection of the prostate. *Brit J Urol* 50:542–546.
5. Abrams PH, Farrar DJ, Turner-Warwick RT (1979) The results of prostatectomy: a symptomatic and urodynamic analysis of 152 patients. *J Urol* 121:640–642.
6. Roos N, Wenneburg JE, Fisher ES (1989) Mortality and reoperation after open and transurethral resection of the prostate for benign prostatic hyperplasia. *N Engl J Med* 320:1120–1124.

7. Evans JWH, Singer M, Chapple CR, Macartney N, Coppinger SWV, Milroy EJG (1991) Haemodynamic evidence of per-operative cardiac stress during transurethral prostatectomy: preliminary communication. *Br J Urol* 67:376–380.

8. Evans JWH, Singer M, Chapple CR, Macartney N, Coppinger SWV, Milroy EJG (1992) Haemodynamic responses and core temperature changes during transurethral prostatectomy and non-endoscopic general surgical procedures in age matched men. *Br Med J* 304:666–671.

9. Lu-Yao G, Barry MJ, Chang CH, Wasson JH, Wennberg JE (1994) Transurethral resection of the prostate among Medicare beneficiaries in the United States: Time trends and outcomes. *Urology* 44(5):693–699.

10. Mebust WK, Holtgrewe HL, Cockett ATK, Peters PC (1989) Transurethral prostatectomy: Immediate and postoperative complications. A cooperative study of 13 participating institutions evaluating 3885 patients. *J Urol* 141:243–247.

11. McConnell J, Barry M, Bruskewitz R (1994) *Benign Prostatic Hyperplasia: Diagnosis and Treatment. Clinical Practice Guidelines, No 8.* AHCPR Publication 940582. Rockville, MD, Agency for Health Care Policy and Res, Public Health Serv, US Dept of Health Human Serv.

12. Sigwart U, Puel J, Mirkovitch V, et al. (1987) Intravascular stents to prevent occlusion and rectenosis after transluminal angioplasty. *N Engl J Med* 316:701–706.

13. Rousseau H, Puel J, Joffre F, et al. (1987) Self-expanding endovascular prosthesis: an experimental study. *Radiology* 164:709–714.

14. Milroy EJG, Chapple CR, Cooper JE, et al. (1988) A new Treatment for urethral strictures. *Lancet* 1:1424–1427.

15. Sarramon JP, Joffre F, Rischmann P, et al. (1989) Prosthese endourethrale Wallstent dans les stenoses recidivantes de l'urethre. *Ann Urol* 23:383–387.

16. Chapple CR, Milroy JG, Rickards D (1990) Permanently implanted urethral stent for prostatic obstruction in the unfit patient. *Br J Urol* 66:58–65.

17. Milroy E, Chapple CR (1993) The Urolume stent in the management of benign prostatic hyperplasia. *J Urol* 150:1630–1635.

18. Milroy E, Coulage C, Pansadoro V, et al. (1994) The Urolume permanent prostatic stent as an alternative to TURP: long-term European results. *J Urol* 151:396A.

19. Oersterling JE, Fefalco AJ, and the North American Study Group: (1994) The North American experience with the Urolume endoprosthesis as a treatment for benign prostatic hyperplasia: Long term results. *Urology* 44:353–362.

20. Guazzoni G, Pansadoro V Montorsi F, et al. (1994) A modified prostatic Urolume wallsten for healthy patients with symptomatic benign prostatic hyperplasia: A European multicentre study. *Urology* 44:364–374.

21. Williams G, Jager R, McLoughlin J, El Din A, Machan L, Gill K, Asopa R, Adam A (1989)Use of stents for treating obstruction of urinary outflow in patients unfit for surgery. *Br Med J* 298:1429.

22. Gabellon S, Wisard M, Leisinger HJ (1994) A prospective clinical study of the Urolume endoprosthesis for the treatment of benign prostatic hyperplasia in inoperable patients. *J Urol* 151:396A.

23. Guazzoni G, Bergamaschi F, Montorsi F. et al. (1993) Prostatic Urolume wallsten for benign prostatic hyperplasia patients at poor operative risk: Clinical uroflowmetric and ultrasonographic patterns. *J Urol* 150:1641.

24. Williams G, Coulange C, Milroy EJG, Sarramon JP, Rubben H (1993) The Urolume, a permanently implanted prostatic stent for patients at high risk of surgery: Results from 5 collaborative centres. *Br J Urol* 72:335–340.

25. Holmes SA, Miller PD, Crocker P, et al. (1992) Encrustation of intraprostatic stents—a comparative study. *Br J Urol* 69:383–387.

8 Testicular Prostheses

Timothy P. Bukowski, MD

CONTENTS

INTRODUCTION
HISTORY OF PROSTHESIS
CURRENT TESTICULAR IMPLANTS
INDICATIONS FOR PLACEMENT
SURGERY
MORBIDITY
PATIENT FOLLOW-UP
CONCLUSION
REFERENCES

INTRODUCTION

Testicular prostheses are used in scrotal reconstruction for multiple diagnoses, including replacement following orchiectomy for prostate cancer, traumatic loss, congenital absence, testicular torsion, infection, or testicular tumor. The ideal testicular prosthesis should conform to the size, shape, and consistency of the normal testis. It should be made of a biochemically inert substance, producing little tissue reaction, and noncarcinogenic. For practical purposes it should be easily sterilizable, and not change size or shape with time *(1)*.

HISTORY OF PROSTHESIS

The first report of the use of a testicular prosthesis was in 1941 by Girsdansky and Newman who used a vitallium implant *(2)*. Since then, others materials have been used including Lucite, glass, Gelfoam,

From: *Urologic Prostheses:*
The Complete, Practical Guide to Devices, Their Implantation and Patient Follow Up
Edited by: C. C. Carson © Humana Press Inc., Totowa, NJ

Dacron, polyethylene, and silicone rubber *(3)*. A prosthesis made of a silicone rubber bag filled with silicone gel became available in 1973, and was used until 1992.

In 1976, Congress passed an amendment providing the FDA with the authority to regulate medical devices. Preamendment devices were those that had been used prior to the creation of the FDA, such as the testicular prosthesis, and had escaped regulatory scrutiny. In 1990, Congress passed the Safe Medical Devices Act, which gave the FDA (until 1995) to review the safety and efficacy of preamendment devices. The act also mandated that manufacturers of high-risk devices keep easily obtainable records of the identity and location of patients using these devices. Silicon gel-filled prosthetics were included on the high-risk list *(4)*.

In 1992, because of this regulatory action, and probably because of the question of silicon gel leakage from breast implants and its question of association with systemic disease, manufacturers halted production of gel-filled testicular implants. (In spite of the fact that no patient with a gel-filled testicular prostheses had been reported to develop systemic disease.) In its 1992 policy statement, the AUA recommended that physicians weigh individual risks, benefits, and informed desires in consideration of implantation or removal of testicular prostheses *(5)*.

Silicon Controversy Regarding Testicular Prostheses

There is a paucity of data implicating silicone implants in the development of alleged human adjuvant disease. Human adjuvant disease is manifested by symptoms and serological disorders of autoimmune disease. Rheumatoid arthritis, scleroderma, systemic lupus erythematosus, and other connective tissue diseases have been linked to human adjuvant disease. The development of human adjuvant disease has been linked to silicone gel breast implants, but not yet to gel-filled testicular implants. Locoregional diseases, such as Kikuchi's disease, lymphadenopathy and lymphoma, which have been associated with breast implants, have not been linked to testicular implants *(6)*. Moreover, silicone materials are worldwide, and its exposure is almost universal, yet the development of these diseases has not been widespread.

What causes the purported immune reaction? There are a few theories. It may be that the silicone gel, which leaks from the envelope, acts as an antigen. Alternatively, macrophages may convert silicone to silica, which is also an antigen. Silica has been found in the area around various silicone implants. The silicone itself may block the clearance of normally produced cellular debris to allow an autoimmune reaction. Unfortunately, the exact mechanism is unknown.

Pidutti and Morales reported on 51 patients receiving 63 gel-filled prostheses between 1978–1991, of which 34 were available for follow-up. They reviewed hospital admission charts for any problem the patients encountered since placement of the prosthesis. After a mean follow-up of 5 yr, they found no evidence of disease linked to human adjuvant disease *(7)*. Henderson et al. went one step further by giving follow-up patients a detailed health profile questionnaire, physical exam, and serologic testing (sedimentation rate, rheumatoid factor, C3, C4, IgA, IgE, IgG, IgM). Of 48 patients, 35 had an undescended testicle, and 13 testicular torsion, with implant surgery during the years 1979–1992. Seven patients agreed to follow-up studies, with a mean surgical age of 14 yr, and follow-up range of 1–7 yr. None of these patients had human adjuvant disease, but five of seven had one or more abnormal serologic tests. Their patient population seems younger than women who had breast implants, so longer follow-up will be necessary before any real conclusion can be obtained.

CURRENT TESTICULAR IMPLANTS

Currently, there are a couple of types of implants that are worth reviewing. Silimed, Inc. markets an oval carving block of solid silicon elastomer, historically used for facial reconstruction. It has a mesh button that can be used for an anchoring stitch. It is available in five sizes [*see* Figs. 1(A), (B)]. Although it is solid, it is relatively soft. As it is a carving block, it can be made smaller, if needed.

Mentor has a saline-filled model, which is marketed internationally, but at the current time is under experimental review in the United States. The Mentor Saline-Filled Testicular Prosthesis (SFTP) is a Class III product, requiring a human clinical trial for market clearance. This trial, called an Investigational Device Exemption, follows patients who have been implanted with the prosthesis. Once clinical data are collected on these core trial patients, a premarket approval is submitted to the Food and Drug Administration, reporting on the safety and effectiveness of the device. Mentor has completed the enrollment into the core study. There is currently an adjunct study to allow patients access to the device while the core study data are being reviewed

The Mentor SFTP approximates the weight, shape, and feel of a normal testicle. The prosthesis is available in four sizes; extra small, small, medium, and large. The implant consists of a molded silicone shell, approx 0.035-in thick, with a self-sealing injection site located on one of the prosthesis. The injection site allows the surgeon to fill the implant with sterile, pyrogen-free sodium chloride solution. On the end

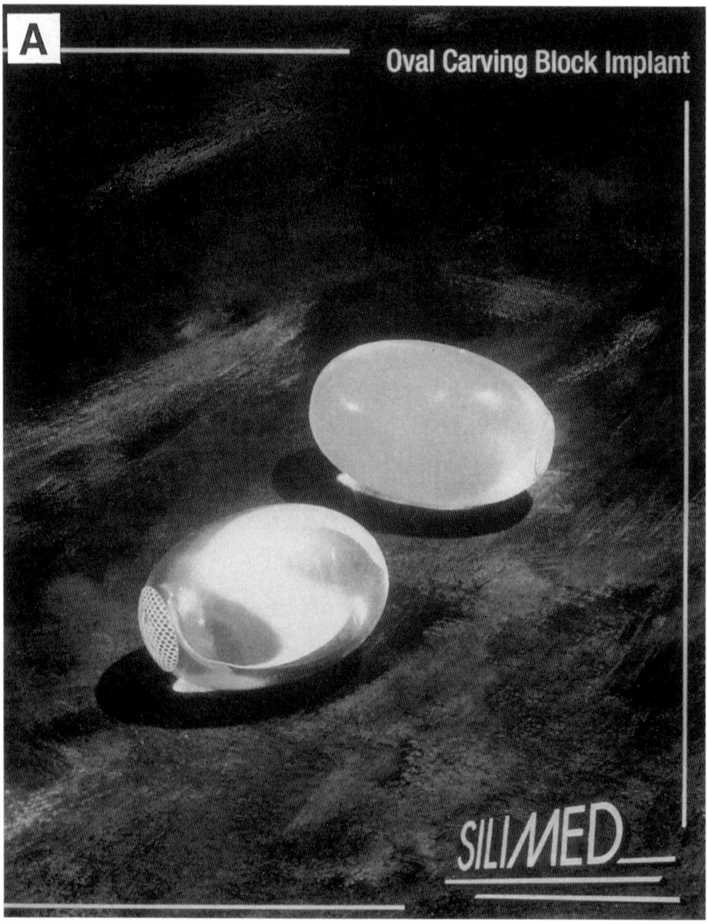

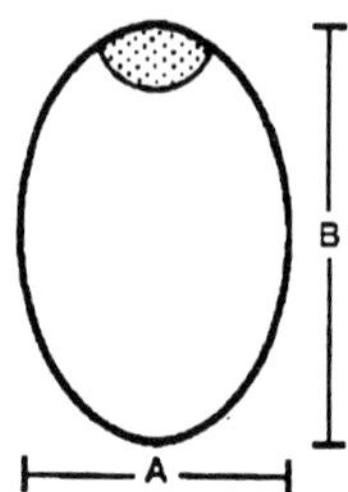
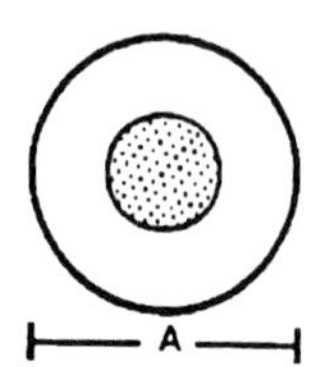

B

SILICONE ELASTOMER

Catalog Ordering Information

REFERENCE	VOLUME cm³	DIMENSIONS cm	
		A	B
3210-023	5,3	2,0	2,3
3210-034	12,7	2,5	3,4
3210-042	22,6	3,0	4,2
3210-047	28,6	3,2	4,7
3210-050	45,8	4,0	5,0

Fig. 1. (**A**) Silimed oval carving block is a solid silicone elastomer. (**B**) Silimed—catalog ordering information.

opposite of the fill site is a silicone elastomer tab for suturing the prosthesis in place if desired. For study sites, call Mentor at *(800) 525–8773 (8)*.

INDICATIONS FOR PLACEMENT

The major benefit of testicular implants used in scrotal reconstruction is to restore the appearance of a man's testicles, and provide psychosocial sexual well-being. Certainly in an adult, who previously had testicles, such as in patients with prostate cancer, insertion of prostheses may be an easy decision, as they can know if they experience a change in body image with orchiectomy. It may be that coping mechanisms are established in mature males. Some may feel that it is somehow unnatural to place prostheses, and they have to learn to live without anything in their scrotum. Others may feel that it is important to make use of what is available to make them feel whole again.

Unfortunately, not much is known on the role of the testes in male psychosocial development. It is possible that school-age children do feel anxiety, and may experience the absence of testicles as a phallic defect. Placement of prostheses was helpful in various psychiatric reports *(9)*. Money reports on a patient with Kallman's syndrome who waited until age 30 to have implants because he felt he was not ready. In retrospect, the patient writes that he "spent a lot of (his) youth on needless depression . . . now he felt part of the human race" and . . . the prostheses "became a natural part of him," allowing him to be more secure in his role as a male, both sexually and socially *(10)*. In dealing with children and adolescents, it is important to support their decision, and if needed, seek counseling to help them sort through the options.

Bracka evaluated long-term psychosexual findings in boys who had hypospadias repair, and found that genital appearance was much more important in their teenage years than in boyhood *(11)*. He also found, however, that those with less initial deformity and those with a better-looking penis had better self-esteem with more sexual partners. Those with a more severe initial deformity or ultimately worse-looking penis had poor self-esteem, and fewer sexual partners. In a similar report on hypospadias follow-up, Berg et al. reported on 39 men who underwent hypospadias repair between age 3 and 9 yr. Overall, the group tended to have fewer coital partners, and a later age at initiation of sexual activity, compared to an age-matched control group *(12)*.

An important part in dealing with a child with a genital anomaly psychosexual identity depends not only on appearance, but also on how the parents deal with the problem. In general, not focusing on the genitals is important, but parents can be sensitive to when it seems problems arise. Offering children and adolescents educational support with professional counseling by surgeons and psychiatrists is important.

Exclusion from Implant

In general, any patient with an intrascrotal neoplasm or infection, infection or abscess anywhere in the body, or uncontrolled diabetes or other wound-healing impairment should not have an implant. Patients with tissue damage from radiation, or compromised vascularity are at higher risk of surgical failure. Until more is known about the relationship of autoimmune diseases to silicone, prosthetics should not be placed in patients with systemic lupus, discoid lupus, scleroderma, rheumatoid arthritis, or other connective tissue disorders. Finally, any patient with severe psychological instability may be better served not having an implant placed, particularly if he is at risk of poor follow-up.

SURGERY

When the scrotum is small from disuse or previous infection, it can be difficult to place a prosthesis. One method is to place a small prosthesis at first, and steadily increase the size with subsequent operations over a number of years. This method can be cumbersome for the patient, as well as costly. In addition, Marshall found the inadequate scrotal distention and wound dehiscence were common problems, especially if orchiectomy had occurred because of inflammatory conditions. In children, even if the small prosthesis is placed during infancy, scrotal stretching is needed after puberty to accommodate an adult size. In addition, if a solitary testis undergoes compensatory hypertrophy, increasing the size of the prosthesis will need to be if symmetry is desired *(13)*.

Lattimer and Stalnecker suggested tissue expansion may be a satisfactory alternative to multiple prostheses. Tissue expansion minimizes additional scar from multiple operations. It slowly distends the scrotum, minimizing pain, and fluid can be withdrawn if the patient is too uncomfortable. Expanding the skin beyond the size needed for the implant allows a more relaxed fit, preventing the implant from overriding the normal testis. For a successful tissue expansion of the scrotum, they suggested:

1. Use a 75–100-cm^3 expander, rather than overfilling a smaller bag.
2. Place the filling port suprapubically in the midline, so that it is easily accessible, and tolerated.
3. Use adjustable-length tube to attach the filling port.
4. Use an even larger implant when compensatory hypertrophy has occurred *(14)*.

A common problem of placement is extrusion of the prosthesis through the suture line. A high scrotal or low inguinal incision is best used to keep the suture line from the prosthesis. If the patient lost the testicle as a result of inflammatory reasons or cancer, it may be best to wait 6 mo for the scrotum to soften up after initial orchiectomy *(15)*.

I prefer to use a low inguinal incision at the level of the pectineal line for placement of the prosthesis. Just lateral to the pubic tubercle is a shallow groove in which the spermatic cord lies. The transverse incision is made here, which will allow the surgeon to remain outside the external inguinal ring, but along the natural path of the spermatic cord. Dissection through the superficial fat and Scarpa's layer allows exposure to the floor, so that a direct path to the scrotum is facilitated. Invaginating the scrotum may help with determination of the inguinal path. Dissection of the scrotum with a finger, then a Kelley instrument, allows the surgeon to thin the dartos. One must be careful not to break through the skin. A sizer is introduced to evaluate symmetry. Rinse with antibiotic solution, both soaking the implant and washing the wound regularly. I prefer to suture the mesh button to the superior portion of the dartos for two reasons. First, it allows the testicle to "hang," and will prevent it from flopping sideways. Second, one is less likely to stitch through the skin, and one can incorporate this as a first closure of the dartos. Closure of the fatty pad prevents migration into the inguinal canal. Pursestring may be the best option (*see* Fig. 2). Patients are kept on broad-spectrum perioperative parenteral antibiotics with bedrest and scrotal elevation for 1 d to minimize edema, and then sent home on broad-spectrum antibiotics for 3 wk. Activity is restricted for 1 mo to allow resolution of swelling, and capsule formation (*see* Fig. 3).

Infant Placement

Placement at the time of inguinal exploration in an infant for whom one finds an atrophied or vanished testicle may be useful. Because the testicle does not grow much throughout childhood, it may be reasonable to insert a prosthesis to allow the child to develop a normal body image. The testicle grows from 1.6 to 2.9 × 1.0 to 1.8 cm from age 2 to 10 yr. The adult testicle is around 5 cm, larger if solitary. Until the late 1980s the smallest prosthesis available was 2.7 × 4.1 cm, creating an asymmetric appearance in infants and school-age boys *(16)*. Now Silimed's smallest is 2.0 × 2.3 cm, and Mentor's smallest is 1.7 × 2.5 cm for infants.

Placement of a small testicle may not help much to preserve space for placement of a larger one after puberty, because the size needed in adulthood is so great. Placement of adult size prosthesis in an infant is grotesque. The small prosthesis may be useful for normal psychosocial

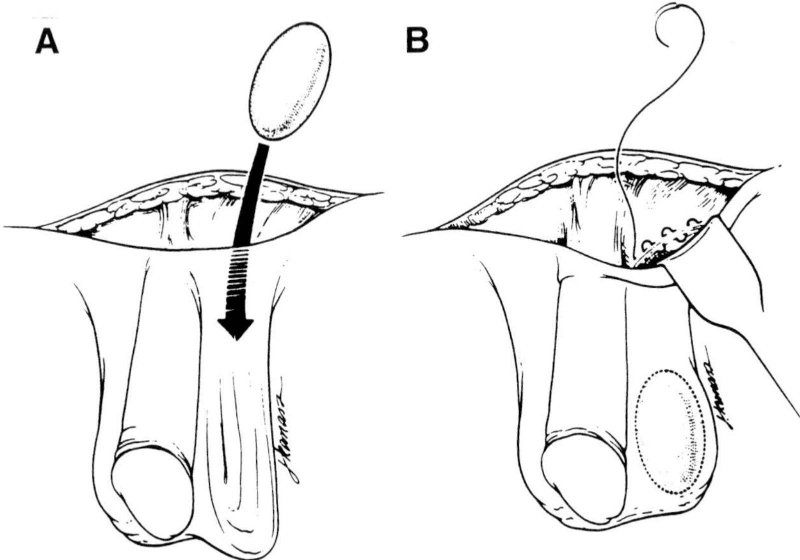

Fig. 2. Insertion technique (as described by Klein) provides for a cosmetic incision with access to bilateral inguinal cords if bilateral orchiectomy is performed for prostate cancer (Klein). I prefer an incision this low, but bilaterally in adolescents for insertion of prosthesis.

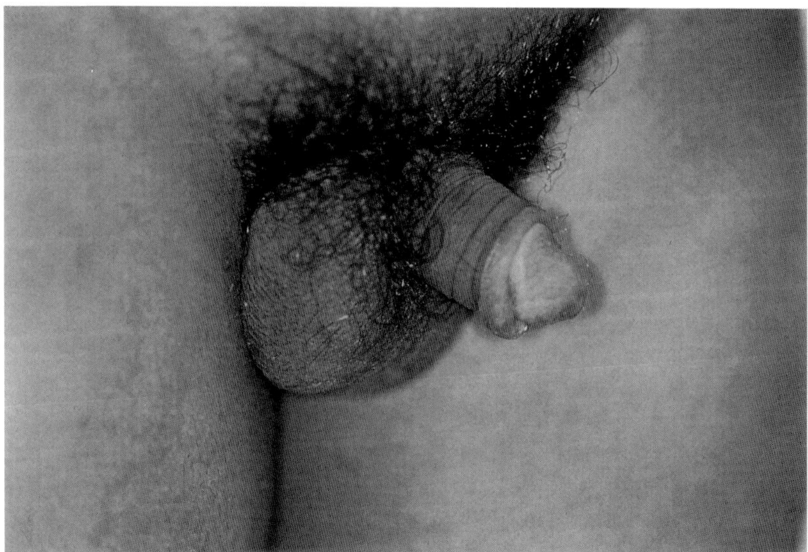

Fig. 3. 6-mo postoperative appearance of 12-yr-old patient with bilateral prostheses placed for scrotal reconstruction. This patient had bilateral incarcerated hernias as newborn, with subsequent anorchia. Notice low inguinal incision.

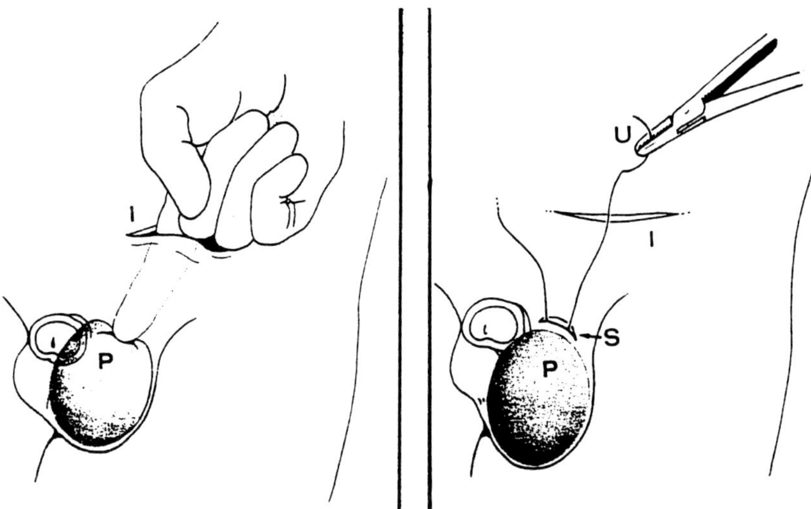

Fig. 4. Insertion technique in infant (Ferro). This is particularly useful if surgery includes inguinal exploration for nonpalpable testicle. A second small incision allows placement of a pursestring suture in the Dartos muscle which prevents migration or extrusion of the implant.

development, though. Elder et al. reported insertion of a gel-filled prosthesis in 40 children aged 9 mo to 4 yr. After insertion into the scrotum, the scrotal outlet was closed with a pursestring of nonabsorbable suture and the prosthesis sutured to the scrotal wall. They had one complication of a wound infection that did not involve the prosthesis. In a follow-up phone survey, 94% of the families were happy the prosthesis had been inserted. Nearly half believed that the child would require a larger prosthesis at puberty, whereas one-third had no opinion and felt that the decision would be left up to the child at adolescence.

Ferro et al. suggested that rather tan struggling to use a pursestring deep through an inguinal incision in a child, making a second small incision in the high scrotum for the pursestring is simpler *(17)* *(see* Fig. 4).

Adult Placement

In adults with metastatic prostate cancer, a number of options exist. One option is placement of an intracapsular testicle prosthesis following subcapsular orchiectomy *(18)*. After curettage of the testicular tissue, and cauterization of the arteries and remnant seminiferous tubules, a prosthesis is placed inside, and a running suture closes the capsule. Mentor used to manufacture a smaller device with a Dacron mesh running along the side. Inclusion of the suture line with the imbedded

Dacron mesh could stabilize the implant. Although a simple subcapsular orchiectomy has an advantage of leaving palpable tissue in the scrotum, it is a much less significant mass than with the addition of a prosthetic device.

Another option at elective orchiectomy is to free the native testicle from the epididymis, and suture a solid silicone testicle in its place *(19)*. This requires a trans-scrotal incision, as its main benefit is to leave the epididymis and gubernaculum *in situ*, ultimately limiting mobility of the prosthetic device. It runs the risk of hematoma from the cord, and scrotal wound opening.

A suprapubic approach for simultaneous orchiectomy and placement of testicular prosthesis is useful in patients with advanced prostate cancer. A subcutaneous approach to the scrotum keeps the incision away from the prosthesis. This option is quick and cosmetic, as the incision is hidden in a lower abdominal crease and covered by pubic hair *(20)*.

Placement at the time of the initial surgery is a good option for patients undergoing orchiectomy for prostate cancer, because one can clearly explain the risks and benefits of the prosthesis, and expect the patient to understand with reasonable consent. It is not as clear for patients with more urgent disorders, however.

Patients with a testicle tumor may need chemotherapy and radiation, which may predispose to wound breakdown. As well, it is an emotionally difficult time for the patient, and obtaining consent may be difficult. Commonly, patients found to have torsion of the testis are typically emergent, and consent may also be an issue. With epididymitis, one is concerned with infection. Marshall showed that complications were more likely to occur in patients with an underlying inflammatory condition of the scrotum *(13)*.

MORBIDITY

Marshall surveyed 488 surgeons for their experience with complications following placement of a testicle prosthesis. Three-hundred eighty-seven surgeons reported placing 3031 over a 10-yr period. Reasons for placement are in Chart 1 (*see* Fig. 5). (UDT 35%, tumor 23%, torsion 17%, CaP 16%, orchitis/epididymitis 8%, trauma 1%.) In general, most complications occurred in patients with a history of epididymitis, or if there was a history of inflammation due to prolonged torsion. In short, those patients with a reason for scrotal scar were most likely to have problems with placement of a prosthesis. Overall complications (transient scrotal contraction 4.2%, persistent scrotal contraction 3.2%,

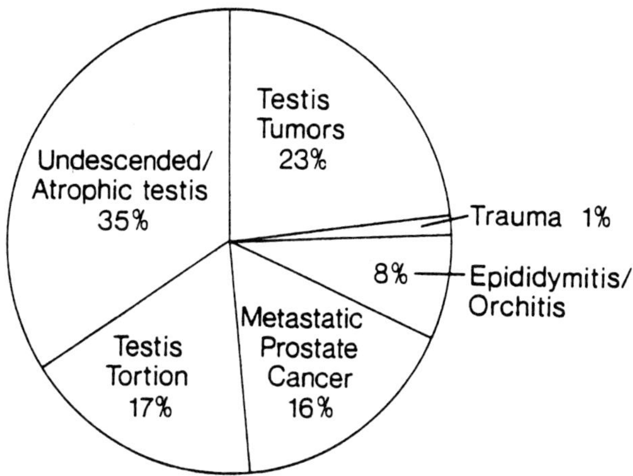

Underlying diagnosis for testicular re-
moval before prosthesis insertion.

Fig. 5. Diagnoses as percentage of 2533 patients with 3,031 testicular prostheses over a 10-yr period (*see* ref. *13*).

wound dehiscence/extrusion 4.1%, infection 1.0%, hematoma 0.8%, pain 1.3%) are listed in (*see* Fig. 6).

Infection

Infection can occur with any foreign body. Elsahy reported one patient who developed severe scrotal and penile lymphedema after chronic, recurrent infection of a testicular prosthesis *(21)*.

Deflation/Rupture of the Implant

Five cases have been reported of silicon gel leakage following rupture of the implant, up to 10 yr after implantation. One may have been associated with a needle stick during a penile operation. Three patients had a history of excessive pressure on the prosthesis (one racing cyclist, one jumping on horseback, and one with an elastic device use during sex). Patient may have pain and deformity of the hemiscrotum. Most were intracapsular ruptures, facilitating excision and replacement. Silicone may be found outside the capsule, but was not associated with adenopathy, nor was it associated with systemic disease in any of these patients (22,6).

The patient may present with pain, without trauma. In an intact device, ultrasound should show a smooth, homogenous, echo-free space. Rupture causes septation within the device owing to infolding of the outer shell, with internal echoes. Ultrasonically, this may be referred to as the

Complications of testicular prosthesis insertion in 2,533 patients[*]

Diagnosis (No. of Patients)	Transient Scrotal Contraction	Persistent Scrotal Contraction	Complication[†] Wound Dehiscence/Prosthesis Extrusion	Infection	Hematoma	Pain	Total Complication Rate (%)
Epididymitis/ orchitis (231)	22 (9.5)	11 (5)	18 (8)	5 (2)	6 (3)	7 (3)	31
Torsion (527)	22 (4)	16 (3)	27 (5)	7 (1)	9 (2)	6 (1)	16
Undescended/ atrophic/absent testis (1,079)	44 (4)	29 (3)	42 (4)	7 (0.6)	3 (0.3)	11 (1)	13
Testicular tumor (696)	18 (3)	24 (3)	18 (3)	4 (0.6)	2 (0.3)	10 (1)	11

[*]Complications of prosthesis insertion in patients with trauma and cancer of the prostate are not included in this table. The overall complication rate was highest in situations of previous scrotal inflammation (epididymitis/orchitis and delayed testicular torsion). It should be noted that many patients had more than one complication.
[†]Figures in parentheses indicate per cent.

Fig. 6. Complications following placement of prosthesis in relation to diagnoses (*see* ref. *13*).

stepladder sign, most likely because of the crumpled edges of the implant *(6)*. As well, hypoechoic areas can also be seen surrounding the device *(22)*. Magnetic resonance imaging (MRI) may show the linguini sign, again representing the edge of the crumpled implant. Although a MRI is very useful in breast implant evaluation, the size and subcutaneous position of the testicular implant allow easy evaluation by ultrasound.

The scrotum may be at lower risk for leakage than the chest wall for breast implants. In women presenting for complaints of psychological or physical breast implant discomfort, about half were found to have a ruptured envelope at 15 yr. This number is certainly much lower in patents with testicular prostheses, as prior to 1992 there were probably 3000 implants placed per year, and so few have been reported *(4)*. The scrotum is a low-tension area, has less vascularity, and a lower temperature. Testicle prostheses may also be more mobile, less vulnerable to pressure injury *(23)*.

Extrusion/Migration of Implant

Gordan described a patient whose testicular implant extruded 2 yr after surgery, presumably because of skin erosion of a Dacron tab used for an anchor stitch on earlier models. Since then, the Dacron mesh has been imbedded in the wall of the prosthesis *(3)*.

Other Problems

Other problems such as hematoma formation and fluid accumulation around the prosthesis can also occur. Calcium deposits have been noted, and in general do not cause a problem unless the prosthesis is mistaken for a real testicle, and biopsy is performed. Capsule contracture can occur around any prosthetic device, which may alter its position and softness. Unresolved issues remain for the very long term, including the impact of silicone particle shedding, carcinogenesis, and the development of autoimmune diseases, none of which have been problematic as of this writing.

PATIENT FOLLOW-UP

It is important to follow-up for wound check within a month postoperatively, and then at 6 mo to look for capsule contraction or implant migration. Patients should be instructed that any sudden pain or discomfort should bring them in for an exam.

Prior to the availability of a gel-filled implant, solid elastomer implants were occasionally mistaken for testicular tumors. Making sure an adolescent knows he had a prosthesis placed as a child is important to avoid this embarrassment. As well, as adolescent visit allows the patient to educate himself about his condition, as he may otherwise be too insecure to ask his parents *(11)*. He has the right of assent to having the prosthesis upsized, removed, or left alone if it had been placed as an infant.

If a question exists regarding rupture of a gel-filled prosthesis, ultrasound may be useful, as aforementioned. MRI of testicular prosthesis has been documented *(24)*. On T1 weighted images, both solid and liquid filled prostheses demonstrated homogeneous low signal intensity; on T2 weighted images, the fluid implants had a uniformly low signal intensity, and the solid implants had a uniformly high signal intensity.

CONCLUSION

Testicular prosthesis can be placed successfully in infancy, childhood, or adulthood with good success, and minimal morbidity. Market scare of the gel-filled breast implant has resulted in minimal current available options for testicle prosthetics.

REFERENCES

1. Puranik SR, Mencia LF, Gilbert MG (1973) Artificial testicles in children: a new silastic gel testicular prosthesis. *J Urol* 109(4):735, 736.
2. Girsdansky J, Newman HF (1941) Use of a vitallium testicular implant. *Am J Surg* 53:514.
3. Gordon JA, Schwartz BB (1979). Delayed extrusion of testicular prosthesis. *Urology* 14(1):59, 60.
4. Randall T (1992) Penile, testicular, other silicone implants soon will undergo FDA review. *JAMA* 267(19):2578, 2579.

5. Silicon Testicular Implants. Policy statement of American Urological Association, Inc., 4:33. October 1992.

6. Hage JJ, Taets van Amerongen AH, Van Diest PJ (1999) Rupture of silicone gel filled testicular prosthesis: causes, diagnostic modalities and treatment of a rare event. *J Urol* 161(2):467–471.

7. Pidutti R, Morales A (1993) Silicone gel-filled testicular prosthesis and systemic disease. *Urology* 42(2):155–157.

8. C Kline, private communication, mentor communication Feb 24: 2000.

9. Schiffman A, Straker N (1979) The psychological role of the testicles. A case report of a 9-year-old boy with agenesis of the testicles. *J Am Acad Child Psych* 18(3):521–526.

10. Money J, Sollod R (1978) Body image, plastic surgery (prosthetic testes) and Kallmann's syndrome. *Br J Med Psychol* 51(1):91–94.

11. Bracka A (1989) A long-term view of hypospadias. *Br J Plastic Surg* 42:251–255.

12. Berg G, Berg R (1983) Castration complex. Evidence from men operated for hypospadias. *Acta Psychiatrica Scandinavica* 68:143–153.

13. Marshall S (1986) Potential problems with testicular prostheses. *Urology* 28(5):388–390.

14. Lattimer JK, Stalnecker MC (1989) Tissue expansion of underdeveloped scrotum to accommodate large testicular prosthesis. A technique. *Urology* 33(1):6–9.

15. Lattimer JK, Vakili BF, Smith AM, Morishima A (1973) A natural-feeling testicular prosthesis. *J Urol* 110(1):81–83.

16. Elder JS, Keating MA, Duckett JW (1989) Infant testicular prostheses. *J Urol* 141(6):1413–1415.

17. Ferro F, Caterino S, Lais A (1991) Testicular prosthesis in children: a simplified insertion technique. *Euro Urol* 19(3):230–232.

18. Merrill DC (1991) Intracapsular testicular prosthesis. *Urology* 37(1):78, 79.

19. Solomon AA (1972) Testicular prosthesis: a new insertion operation. *J Urol* 108(3):436–438.

20. Klein EA, Herr HW (1990) Suprapubic approach for bilateral orchiectomy and placement of testicular prostheses. *J Urol* 143(4):765, 766.

21. Eisahy NI (1972) Scrotal and penile lymph edema as a complication of testicular prosthesis. *J Urol* 108(4):595–598.

22. Twidwell J (1994) Ruptured testicular prosthesis. *J Urol* 152(1):167, 168.

23. Henderson J, Culkin D, Mata J, Wilson M, Venable D (1995) Analysis of immunological alterations associated with testicular prostheses. *J Urol* 154(5):1748–1751.

24. Semelka R, Anderson M, Hricak H (1989) Prosthetic testicle: appearance at MR imaging. *Radiology* 173(2):561, 562.

9

Current Status and Future of Penile Prosthesis Surgery

Culley C. Carson, III, MD

CONTENTS

INTRODUCTION
RECONSTRUCTION USING PENILE PROSTHESIS
PEYRONIE'S DISEASE
CORPUS CAVERNOSUM FIBROSIS AND PRIAPISM
PENILE PROSTHESIS IMPLANTATION AFTER RADICAL
    PROSTATECTOMY
PENILE PROSTHESIS AND SPINAL CORD INJURY
PENILE RECONSTRUCTION
ARTIFICIAL URINARY SPHINCTER
CONCLUSION
REFERENCES

INTRODUCTION

Since the implantation of rib cartilage for reproducing penile rigidity in a fashion similar to the os penis or baculum of lower animals in the 1930s and 40s, surgeons and urologists have pursued the implantation of penile prostheses for the production of erections satisfactory for normal coitus. The development of newer synthetic materials associated with the space program in the 1950s and 1960s allowed advances in human prosthetic devices to include the treatment of chronic erectile impotence. The silicone-based prosthetic materials introduced during that time revolutionized the science of human prosthetics and, subsequently, urologic penile prosthetic devices. The era of modern penile

From: *Urologic Prostheses:*
The Complete, Practical Guide to Devices, Their Implantation and Patient Follow Up
Edited by: C. C. Carson © Humana Press Inc., Totowa, NJ

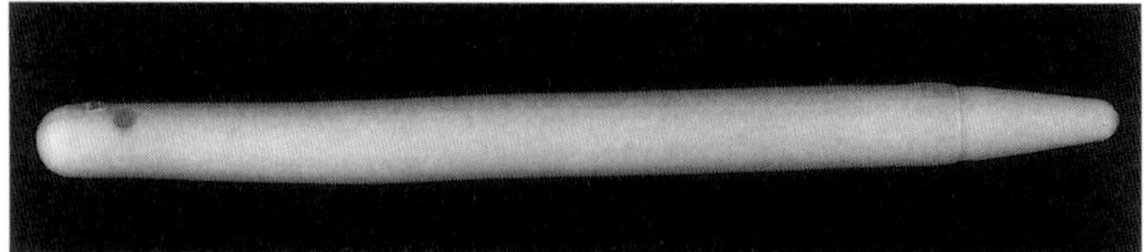

Fig. 1. AMS 600 malleable penile prosthesis.

prosthetic surgery began with the reports of Small et al. and Scott et al. in 1973 *(1,2)*. These surgeons introduced new prostheses which were the results of the development of penile prostheses, by earlier pioneers.

Small et al. and Scott et al., however, defined the two current classes of penile prosthetic devices with their reports more than 25 yr ago. Small et al. described a pair of silicone cylinders comprised of a silicone elastomer outer sheath covering a silicone-filled sponge sized to fill the corpora cavernosa from the glans penis to the crura *(1)*. These implants, which decreased the previously noted prosthetic migration and recreated a physiologic erection, could be sized to the individual patient with two different girths and four different lengths. Semirigid rod penile implants, whose successors continue to be implanted today, are sufficient in size and rigidity and simulate the normal erection and provide stability adequate for coitus *(see* Fig. 1). Since its introduction, the Small Carrion penile prosthesis has been the most widely implanted semirigid rod prosthesis. Initial results from the Small Carrion penile prosthesis, the archetype of semirigid rod prostheses, were successful in 72–91% of patients in whom they were implanted *(1)*.

The second group of penile prostheses introduced in 1973 were designed as inflatable penile prostheses and were developed by Scott et al. *(2)*. Because the inflatable design promised a more physiologic erection and a more natural-appearing flaccid penis, the Scott inflatable penile prosthesis has been widely used. Since implementation of improved designs with decreased mechanical malfunction rates, its use has surpassed the semirigid rod penile prosthesis in popularity. A recent statewide study in North Carolina has documented a more than threefold prevalence of inflatable penile prosthesis implantation to semirigid rod devices *(3)*. Whereas the original inflatable penile prosthesis had an inflate and a deflate pump, the combined inflate/deflate pump in the current inflatable penile prosthesis has been the design of both Mentor and American Medical Systems devices for more than two decades. These inflatable prostheses consist of three components, including paired silastic or bioflex corporal cylinders that are hollow and can be sized to the individual patient. These corporal cylinders are connected

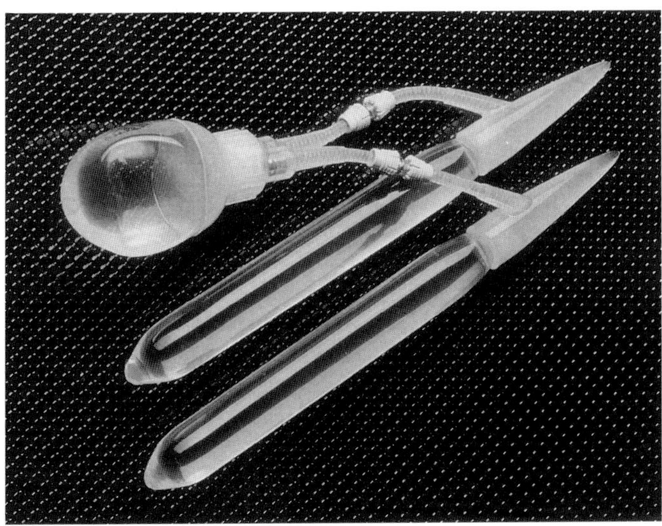

Fig. 2. Mentor 2-piece inflatable penile prosthesis.

to a fluid-filled reservoir placed beneath the anterior abdominal rectus muscle. The third component consists of a pump mechanism that was initially designed as two pumps and subsequently united into a single scrotal pump. The patient can activate this device by palpation of the pump mechanism in the scrotum and by depressing the inflation portion to transfer fluid from the reservoir to the cylinders creating a normal appearing, feeling, and functioning erection. On deflation of the device, the cylinders empty and a flaccid penis results. The components of this prosthesis are connected by kink-free silicone tubing tailored and connected by connectors that were first made of stainless steel and currently of a softer, plastic material. Subsequent designs have introduced connector-free inflatable penile prostheses. Although initial results demonstrated excellent erections, mechanical malfunction rates varied and were frequently reported in excess of 60% *(4)*. Multiple design and material changes over the past two decades have resulted in mechanical malfunction rates of less than 10% over 5 yr *(5–7)*. Complications, such as infection, can now be managed with prosthesis-preserving techniques, which include salvage protocols designed for acute replacement and irrigation *(8)*.

Current prosthetic devices include the inflatable variety, which can be divided into multiple component inflatable prostheses of which there are two- and three-piece models available *(see* Fig. 2–4). There are also single-rod inflatable prostheses which have also been termed the hydraulic hinge penile prostheses *(see* Fig. 5). These prostheses are

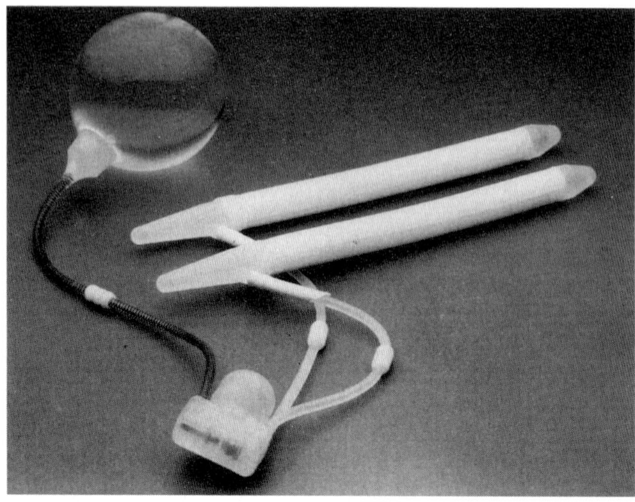

Fig. 3. AMS 700CX inflatable penile prosthesis (American Medical Systems Inc., Minnetonka MN).

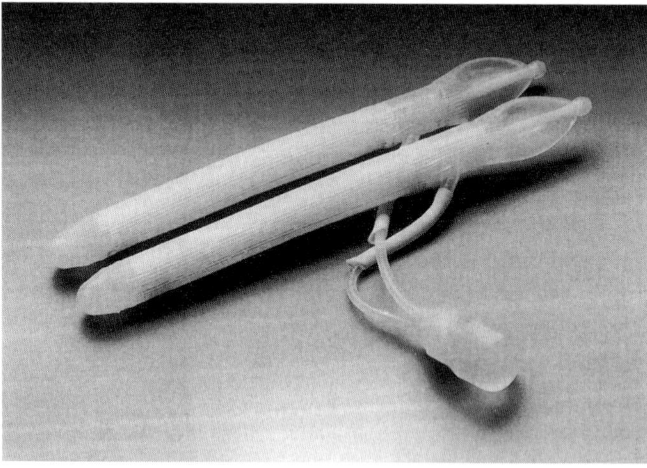

Fig. 4. Ambicor 2-piece inflatable penile prosthesis (American Medical Systems Inc., Minnetonka MN).

rarely used and are of limited availability in the twenty-first century *(9,10)*. Semirigid prostheses are also available and can be grouped as malleable, mechanical, and semirigid. The former contain a central metal wire for improved positioning and the latter, such as the Dura II prosthesis (Timm medical, Augusta, GA), and finally, the original semirigid rod penile prostheses is still implanted.

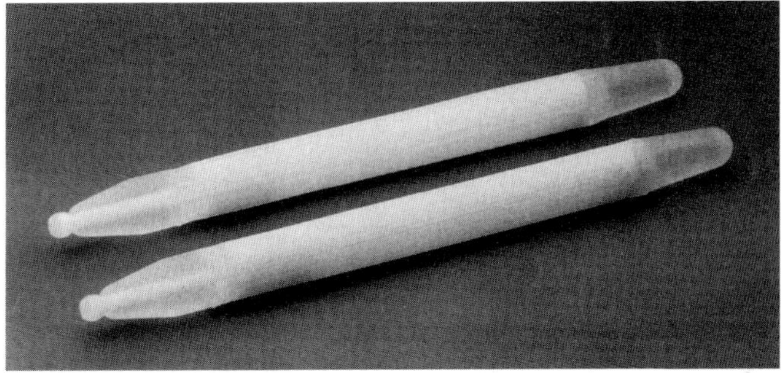

Fig. 5. Dynaflex inflatable penile prosthesis (American Medical Systems Inc., Minnetonka MN).

RECONSTRUCTION USING PENILE PROSTHESIS

In the era of oral agents and minimally invasive treatment options for erectile dysfunction, most patients with organic and psychogenic erectile dysfunction undergo penile prosthesis implantation when less-invasive options have been unsuccessful. Penile prostheses, however, are widely used in patients who require complex reconstruction of the genitalia.

PEYRONIE'S DISEASE

Penile prostheses have been used for patients with Peyronie's disease since their introduction in the 1970s. Peyronie's disease with penile curvature or penile deformity associated with erectile dysfunction are successfully treated with penile implants. Many patients with inadequate erections will not respond adequately to penile straightening alone because inadequate erectile function will compromise their ability to perform coitus satisfactorily. Straightening alone may be difficult in patients with severe penile curvature. Severe penile shortening and penile prostheses have been successfully used to rehabilitate these complex patients, especially when associated with erectile dysfunction. In counseling patients about surgical treatment of severe Peyronie's disease, however, it is critically important to include the option of penile prosthesis because this single surgical procedure has excellent success rates, low morbidity, and correct both penile deformity and potential erectile dysfunction. Expected infection rates are no different from those of patients with penile prosthesis implantation and no Peyronie's disease *(12)*. Excellent results have been reported by many investigators using penile prosthesis implantation, both with and without corpus cavernosum reconstruction. Although corpus cavernosum reconstruction is occasionally required to produce penile straightening, the recent introduction of penile modeling has reduced the number of incisions for reconstruction of these complex patients. The inflatable penile prosthesis has been demonstrated to have the best long-term patient satisfaction in the treatment of patients with penile curvature and Peyronie's disease. Although functional results are satisfactory with both inflatable and semirigid rod prostheses, Montorsi et al. reported poor patient satisfaction with semirigid rod penile prosthesis implanted for Peyronie's disease compared with excellent patient and partner satisfaction in a similar group of patients undergoing inflatable prostheses from the same urologic practice *(13,14)*.

Prior to the introduction of penile modeling as a penile-straightening technique, the most common method for surgical correction of penile curvature after penile prosthesis implantation was incision or excision of the plaque or curvature area with or without grafting. In 1994, Wilson and Delk first proposed the technique of penile modeling to eliminate or modify penile curvature after prosthesis implantation *(15)*. This technique requires a high pressure inflatable penile prosthesis cylinder such as the AMS 700CX or Mentor α-1 prosthesis cylinders. Once penile prosthesis cylinders are implanted, many patients will have penile straightening with corpus cavernosum dilation alone. Those with continued penile curvature after prosthesis insertion, however, can undergo penile modeling. Modeling procedures can be performed for other causes of penile deformity from corpus cavernosum fibrosis or other abnormalities. The AMS 700 Ultrex cylinders are less satisfactory and modeling pressure and implantation of these cylinders may result in aneurysmal dilation or S-shaped deformity. Similarly, high-pressure stress on the Mentor Bioflex cylinders has been reported to result in aneurysmal dilation.

Modeling begins with full inflation of the prosthetic cylinders and clamping the inflate tubing to protect the inflatable pump. The curved penis is then grasped with both hands bending the penis over the fully inflated cylinders of the prosthesis at the area of maximum curvature. Deflection is maintained for 90 s and reevaluation of the shape is carried out after straightening and further cylinder inflation. Repeated modeling can be carried out until full straightening is obtained. Results of the modeling procedure have been reported in several series with success rates in excess of 85% *(15–17)*. Complications are no greater in penile prosthesis implantation without modeling and plaque incision is reduced to less than 10% of patients.

In those patients in whom modeling is inadequate for penile shortening, plaque excision or incision may be necessary. Igner et al. reported an 88% satisfaction rate with plaque incision after prosthesis implantation *(18)*. Patients were able to engage actively in sexual intercourse during a mean follow-up of 6.9 yr. If a significant defect results from this straightening procedure, patching with material such as Gortex (WL Gore & Associates) may be necessary for improved cosmetic results and penile shaft support. The use of an additional foreign body for these support grafts, however, may lead to increase in infection risks in some patients. Severe penile shortening may be improved using a circumferential corpus cavernosum incision with grafting with or without a penile implant *(19)*.

CORPUS CAVERNOSUM FIBROSIS AND PRIAPISM

Dense fibrosis of the corpus cavernosum may be a result of conditions such as penile prosthesis infection, repeated intracavernosal injections, especially with Papaverine, diabetes mellitus, Peyronie's disease, and priapism. This intense corpus cavernosum fibrosis may be severe and result in severe changes in corpus cavernosum tissue compliance with an increased incidence of venous leak, decreased penile turgidity, and penile shortening. Implantation of a penile prosthesis is the most often used and most successful method for rehabilitating patients with these disabling fibrotic conditions *(20)*. Although an infrapubic incision is most amenable to penile reconstruction using penile prosthesis, Carbone et al. reported a series of 26 men implanted with AMS 700CXM prostheses with severe corpora fibrosis through a transverse scrotal approach *(21)*. Although this approach is reasonable, flexibility, the use of multiple corporotomies and creative surgical incisions may be necessary in these complex cases. In corpus cavernosum fibrosis, which is mild or moderate, dilation may be carried out in a standard fashion but may require advanced surgical techniques to create a channel satisfactory for penile prosthesis implantation. These techniques may include the use of an Otis urethrotome, Rosillo cavernotome, and sharp scissor dissection of the corpora cavernosa. If duration or calcification makes dilator introduction difficult, sharp dissection using scissors may provide initial tunneling followed by excision of the scarred corpus tissue, direct dilation, and multiple corporotomy incisions to dilate under direct vision. When attempting penile prosthesis cylinder placement in these difficult conditions, it is critical to have available the downsized inflatable penile prosthesis cylinders. These devices are available from both Mentor and American Medical Systems and include the AMS 700CXM.

The use of a vacuum erection device prior to surgical implantation has been reported to improve penile length and assist in softening corporal fibrosis *(22)*. Patients are asked to apply the device 2–3 times weekly without a constriction ring for 8–12 wk. Use of a vacuum erection device after prosthesis implantation has been reported, but may result in damage to an implanted device. If all dilation attempts are unsuccessful, a longitudinal incision of the corpus cavernosum can be carried out with dissection of the fibrotic tissue from the corpus cavernosum. This is a difficult procedure and requires significant care to avoid the urethra and other penile structures. Once performed, however, a prosthetic cylinder may be placed in an open dissected area and covered with tunica albuginea, Gortex graft, or other packaged materials *(23)*. If inflation of the prosthesis is unsuccessful, however, the use of a semirigid rod device may be necessary to permit satisfactory prosthesis function.

Penile prostheses and implants have been successfully implanted in patients with sickle cell priapism with excellent results. Monga et al. reported the use of penile prosthesis implantation after sickle cell associated priapism *(24)*. They suggested an advantage maintaining penile size and corpus cavernosum compliance by early prosthesis implantation in patients with severe and repeated sickle cell priapism.

PENILE PROSTHESIS IMPLANTATION AFTER RADICAL PROSTATECTOMY

Although nerve-sparing radical prostatectomy has improved the erections postoperatively in many patients surgically treated for prostate cancer, as many as 40% of patients who undergo radical prostatectomy will suffer from post operative erectile dysfunction. Although many of these men can be managed with oral, intraurethral, or injectable agents, some patients will require penile prosthesis implantation. Specifically, those patients who undergo radical prostatectomy without nerve-sparing procedures may not respond to less-invasive techniques for restoration of erectile function. In a subgroup of patients with preoperatively placed penile prosthesis, the prosthesis can be maintained during radical prostatectomy with excellent function and healing following surgery. There is no increase in infection rates and prosthetic function is maintained *(5)*. There is no clear indication for removal of a preexisting penile prosthesis during or before radical prostatectomy. Some investigators have suggested the immediate and simultaneous placement of a penile prosthesis along with radical prostatectomy. Khoudary et al. report 50 men undergoing a combination nerve-sparing radical retropubic prostatectomy and penile prosthesis implantation *(25)*. In comparing these men with 72 men undergoing radical prostatectomy without penile prosthesis implantation, the authors report a mean return to successful satisfactory coitus of 12.7 wk with no patients suffering penile prosthesis infection and an 8% revision rate, similar to that of patients without simultaneous radical prostatectomy.

Similarly, patients have excellent function and penile prosthesis satisfaction after definitive radiation therapy for prostatic carcinoma. Dubocq et al. reported 35 patients undergoing radiation therapy alone and eight patients undergoing radiation therapy after radical prostatectomy who also received penile prosthesis for rehabilitation *(26)*. None of the patients in this series had infection or erosion and 71% of the patients used their prosthesis at least once weekly, 17% twice a month, whereas only 12% remain sexually active without penile prosthesis implantation.

PENILE PROSTHESIS AND SPINAL CORD INJURY

Although many patients have successful restoration of erectile function with Sildenafil and other minimally invasive treatment alternatives following spinal cord injury, there is a substantial number of these usually young men who have erectile dysfunction refractory to simpler restorative techniques. Results of penile prosthesis implantation in patients with spinal cord injury assists in both physical and psychological rehabilitation. Gross et al. reported 209 paraplegic men who underwent penile prosthesis implantation for erectile dysfunction *(27)*. Infection rates in their patients were equivalent to those of nonparaplegic men and men who underwent penile prostheses exhibited improved self-confidence and facilitated condom urinary collection. Watanabe et al. also reported patients undergoing penile prosthesis implantation after spinal cord injury *(28)*. Of those undergoing penile prosthesis implantation, no patients had a prosthesis infection or malfunction and all used their prosthesis at least five times monthly. Frequency of use was greater than that for patients with injection therapy or vacuum erection device therapy.

PENILE RECONSTRUCTION

One of the most difficult groups of patients to treat are those patients with penile loss secondary to congenital absence, trauma avulsion, or penectomy for cancer of the penis. A variety of phallic reconstruction techniques are available, the most common currently used is the innervated vascularized pedicle flap from the forearm. After phallic reconstruction, penile prosthesis implantation permits a functional penis.

Reconstruction with a neourethra allows for more normal voiding and a penile prosthesis permits sexual activity. Because these phallic reconstructive techniques involve nerve reconstruction, sensation can be expected in the majority of patients. Alter et al. describe the use of inflatable and semirigid rod penile prostheses after phallic reconstruction. Semirigid penile prostheses have also been successfully used to create rigidity in these neophalluses.

Difficult penile-prosthesis implantation using reinforcement material whether natural or artificial, especially in patients with significant immunocompromise may result in increased infection rates. Jarow et al. report the risk of penile prosthesis infection at 21.7% in patients requiring penile reconstruction compared with an overall infection rate of 1.8% *(29)*. Similarly, Carson reports an increased infection rate in patients requiring Gortex grafts for reconstruction of patients with severe corporal fibrosis *(30)*. Although this increased infection rate is evident for complex reconstructions that involve longer operative times, more incisions and additional foreign bodies, the further increased risk of diabetes with penile implants does not appear to be significant.

ARTIFICIAL URINARY SPHINCTER

The first hydraulic artificial urinary sphincter was developed in the mid-1970s as an outgrowth of the development of the inflatable penile prosthesis. Because of significant mechanical reliability concerns and urethral erosion, multiple redesigns and mechanical improvements have taken place over the past two decades. The current artificial urinary sphincter available as the American Medical Systems AS800 device consists of an inflatable cuff sized to the individual patient and placed around the urethra or bladder neck *(31)*. Associated pressure balloons provide periurethral pressure to the implantable cuff and the device is deflated actively by the patient through a scrotally placed deflation pump. Newer devices are being modified to be used with colonic implantation for fecal incontinence. The advantage of the current device include the ability to deactivate the cuff at the pump level without surgical intervention to allow for urethral healing and revascularization prior to the application of periurethral pressure. Additionally, the current device permits constant urethral pressure with patient activation to decrease urethral compromise and free voiding.

The artificial urinary sphincter is widely used in both adults and children, men and women to restore urinary continence. The reliability of these devices has been consistently reported. Elliott and Barrett report 323 patients in the largest current series, 72 of whom required only a single surgical intervention with a mean follow-up of 68.8 mo *(32)*.

Their study examined 272 sphincters placed around the urethra and 51 at the bladder neck. With the newer design artificial urinary sphincter, mechanical failure occurred in 7.6% of patients with nonmechanical complications identified in only 9% of patients.

These devices improve the quality of life of both men and women treated for urinary incontinence. They are most commonly used to treat incontinence after prostatectomy. Haab et al. reviewed the records of 68 men who underwent artificial urinary sphincter placement for postprostatectomy incontinence or neurogenic disease with a mean follow-up of 7.2 yr *(33)*. Quality of life was assessed in 52 of these patients by incontinence impact questionnaires and a urogenital distress inventory. The authors document a decrease in pads per day from 2.75 to 0.97 after surgery. Revisions for mechanical failure and urethral atrophy were required in 25% of patients and four patients required permanent removal of the prosthesis. By subjective improvement and overall satisfaction, ratings were 4.1 and 3.9, respectively, on a scale of 5. These authors concluded that patient quality of life is positively impacted by the implantation of an artificial urinary sphincter. Griebling et al. compared collagen injection with artificial urinary sphincter for the treatment of postprostatectomy incontinence *(34)*. Of 25 men undergoing collagen injection for postradical prostatectomy incontinence, only two men received significant improvement with 5 of 25 subsequently undergoing artificial urinary sphincter with subsequent satisfactory control.

Newer concepts in artificial urinary sphincter implantation includes the use of double-cuff artificial urinary sphincters. This double-cuff technique has been successfully used in patients with high-pressure bladders and failed artificial urinary sphincter. Kabalin reported five men with stress urinary incontinence after artificial urinary sphincter placement *(35)*. Using a stainless steel T-shaped connector, a second artificial urinary sphincter cuff was placed distal to the previously placed cuff. Four of five patients obtained satisfactory continence with the second cuff, although one man continued to be incontinent. Kowalczyk et al., however, report a higher erosion rate in those patients with double cuff artificial urinary sphincters *(36)*. Of 95 patients implanted with double cuffs, 10 patients sustained erosion of which four were considered to be caused by the second-cuff implantation. Second-cuff implantation may be appropriate, however, in those patients who are physically active and suffer stress incontinence with physical activity. Placement of a second cuff distal to an initial cuff appears to increase outlet resistance and increase continent rates in patients undergoing artificial urinary sphincter placement.

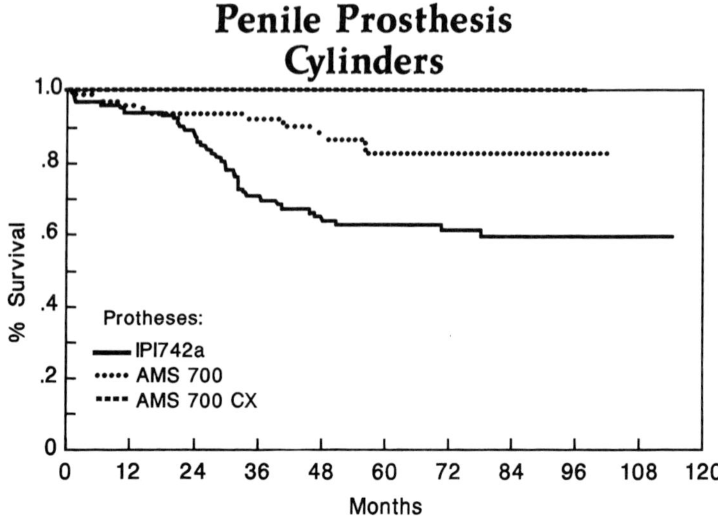

Fig. 6. Penile prostheses cylinders longevity (Kaplan Meier Curve). Comparing cylinder design and survival *(4)*.

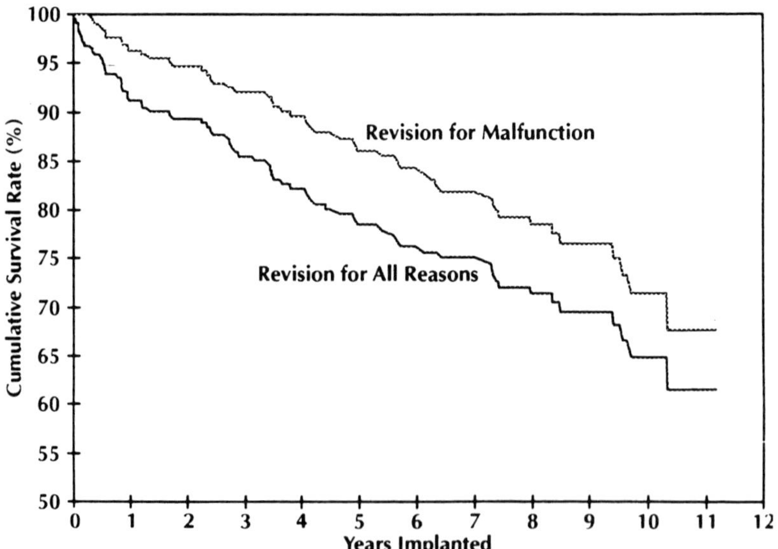

Fig. 7. Long-term actuarial survival of AMS 700CX penile prostheses implanted for treatment of erectile dysfunction *(5)*.

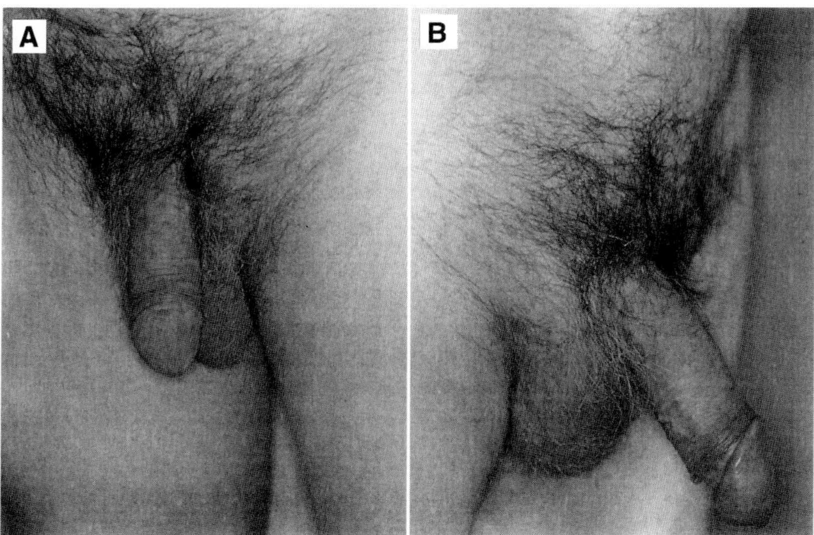

Fig. 8 (**A**) Malfunctioned penile prosthesis *in situ*. (**B**) Penis rigidity and elongation following insertion of MUSE, 250 mcg 30 min prior. (Note: penile elongation compared with inferior scrotal border, penile glans engorgement, and penile rigidity.)

CONCLUSION

In the beginning of the 21st century, urologists and surgeons have significant numbers of prosthetic devices available for reconstruction and improvement in patients lives. Prosthetics as simple as the testicular prosthesis restore the body image and psychological well being of many young men who have lost a testicle to trauma or malignancy. Patients with erectile dysfunction who fail less invasive alternatives can be reconstructed and return to normal sexual function with penile prosthesis implantation using either inflatable or noninflatable devices. Patient and partner acceptance, use, and satisfaction have been reported better than other alternatives including pharmacologic injection *(37,38)*. Inflatable devices are more frequently used than semirigid rods, their complication rates continue to decline and patient satisfaction rates continue to rise (*see* Fig. 6, 7). Now, as many as 90% of patients would recommend a penile prosthesis implantation to both friends and relatives as a result of excellent mechanical function and reliability (*see* Fig. 8). The artificial urinary sphincter which has been developed and redesigned over the past three decades now provides reliable restoration of continence in patients with difficult to manage stress and total urinary incontinence.

The introduction of standardized pressure and deactivation concept has improved the mechanical and physical reliability of these prosthetic devices. Currently, patients with significant incontinence, which impacts on their lifestyle and life satisfaction, can be improved with the implantation of an artificial urinary sphincter with expected function and satisfaction. The 21st century will continue to experience additional prosthetic devices to assist urologic surgeons and patients. These devices may include an artificial bladder, dissolvable ureteral, and urethral stents, and prosthetic replacements for both urethra and ureter in patients with traumatic iatrogenics or malignancy resulting in ureteral injury damage or loss.

REFERENCES

1. Small MP, Carrion HM, Gordon JA (1975) Small Carrion penile prosthesis: a new implant for the management of impotence. *Urology* 5:479–586.
2. Scott FB, Bradley WE, Timm DW (1973) Management of erectile impotence: use of implantable inflatable prosthesis. *Urology* 2:80–83.
3. Jhaveri FM, Rutledge R, Carson CC (1998) Penile prosthesis implantation surgery: a statewide population based analysis of 2354 patients. *Int J Impot Res* 10:251–254.
4. Carson CC (1999) Reconstructive surgery using urological prostheses. *Curr Opin Urol* 9:233–239.
5. Carson CC, Mulcahy JJ, Govier FE (2000) Efficacy, safety, and patient satisfaction outcomes of the AMS 700CX inflatable penile prosthesis: results of a long term multicenter study. *J Urol* 164:376–380.
6. Goldstein I, Newman L, Baum N, et al. (1997) Safety And efficacy outcome of Mentor Alpha-1 inflatable penile prosthesis implantation for impotence Treatment. *J Urol* 157:833–839.
7. Wilson SK, Cleves MA, Delk JR (1999) Comparison of mechanical reliability of original and enhanced Mentor alpha-1 penile prosthesis. *J Urol* 162:715–718.
8. Mulcahy JJ (2000) Long term experience with salvage of infected penile implants. *J Urol* 163:481–482.
9. Anafarta K, Yamaan O, Aydos K (1998) Clinical experience with dynaflex penile prosthesis in 120 patients. *Urology* 52:1098–1100.
10. Kabalin JN, Kuo JC (1997) Long term follow-up of and patient satisfaction with the Dynaflex self-contained inflatable penile prosthesis. *J Urol* 158:456–459.
11. Kearse WS, Sago AL, Peretsman SJ (1996) Report of a multicenter clinical evaluation of the Dura-II penile prosthesis. *J Urol* 155:1613–1616.
12. Carson CC, Mulcahy JJ, Govier FE (2000) Mechanical and satisfaction results of penile prosthesis implantation in patients with Peyronie's Disease: results of a multicenter study. *J Urol* 154A:464.
13. Montorsi F, Quazzoni G, Barbieri L, Maga T, Rigatti P, Graziottina, et al. (1996) AMS 700CX penile implants for Peyronie's Disease: functional results, morbidity and patient-partner satisfaction. *Int J Impot Res* 8:81–85.
14. Montorsi F, Quazzoni G, Bergamaschi F, Rigatti P (1993) Patient-partner satisfaction with semi-rigid penile prosthesis for Peyronie's Disease: a five year follow-up study. *J Urol* 150:1819–1821.
15. Wilson SK, Delk JR (1994) A new treatment for Peyronie's Disease: modeling penis over an inflatable penile prosthesis. *J Urol* 152:1121–1123.

16. Montague DK, Angermeier KW, Lakin MM, Ingoeright BJ (1996) AMS 3-piece inflatable penile prosthesis implantation in men with Peyronie's disease: comparison of CX and ultrex cylinders *J Urol* 156:1633–1635.

17. Carson CC (1998) Penile prosthesis implantation and the treatment of Peyronie's disease *Int J Impot Res* 10:125–128.

18. Eigner EB, Kabalin JN, Kessler R (1991) Penile implants and the treatment of Peyronie's disease. *J Urol* 145:69–71.

19. Lue TF, L-Sakka AI (1999) Lengthening shortened penis caused by Peyronie's disease using circular venous grafting and daily stretching with vacuum erection device. *J Urol* 161:1141–1144.

20. Ragpurkar A, Li H, Dhabuwala CB (1999) Penile implant success in patients with corporal fibrosis using multiple incisions and minimal scar tissue excision. *Urology* 54:145–147.

21. Carbone DJ, Daitch JA, Angermeier KW, Lakin MM, Montague DK (1998) Management of severe corporal fibrosis with implantation of prosthesis via transverse scrotal approach. *J Urol* 159:125–127.

22. Soderdahl DW, Betroski RA, Mode D, Schwartz BF, Thrasher JB (1997) The use of an external vacuum device to augment a penile prosthesis. *Tech Urol* 3:100–102.

23. Landman, Bar-Chama N (1999) The initial experience with processed human cadaveric allograft skin for reconstruction of the corpus cavernosum in repair of distal extrusion of a penile prosthesis. *Urology* 53:1222–1224.

24. Monga M, Broderick GA, Hellstrom WJ (1996) Priapism in sickle cell disease: the case for early implantation of penile prostheses. *Eur Urol* 30:54–59.

25. Khoudary KP, DeWolf WC, Bruning CO, Morgantaler A (1997) Immediate sexual rehabilitation by simultaneous placement of penile prosthesis in patients undergoing radical prostatectomy. *Urology* 50:395–399.

26. Dubocq FM, Bianco FJ, Maralani SS, Forman ID, Dhabwalla CD (1997) Outcome analysis of penile implant surgery after external beam radiation for prostate cancer. *J Urol* 158:1787–1790.

27. Gross AJ, Saverwein DH, Kutzenburg RJ, Ringent RH (1996) Penile prosthesis in paraplegic men *Br J Urol* 78:262–264.

28. Watanabe T, Chancellor MD, Riras DA, Hirsch IH, Bennett CJ, Finnochiaro MV, et al. (1996) Epidemiology of current treatment of sexual dysfunction in spinal cord injured men in the USA. Model Spinal Cord Injury Centers. *J Spinal Cord Med* 19:186–189.

29. Jarow JP (1996) Risk factors for penile prosthetic infection. *J Urol* 156:402–404.

30. Carson CC (1996) Increased infection risks with corpus cavernosum reconstruction and penile prosthesis implantation with corporeal fibrosis. *Int J Impot Res* 8:155.

31. Leibovich BC, Barrett WM (1997) Use of the artificial urinary sphincter in men and women *World J Urol* 15:316–319.

32. Elliott DS, Barrett DM (1998) Mayo Clinic long term analysis of the functional durability of the AMS 800 artificial urinary sphincter: a review of 323 cases. *J Urol* 159:1206–1208.

33. Haab F, Trockman BA, Zimmern TE, Leach GE (1997) Quality of life incontinence assessment of the artificial urinary sphincter in men with minimum of 3.5 years follow-up. *J Urol* 158:435–439.

34. Griebling TL, Kreder KJ, Williams RE (1997) Transurethral collagen injection for treatment of post prostatectomy urinary incontinence in men. *Urology* 49:907–912.

35. Kabalan JN (1996) Addition of a second urethral cuff to enhance the performance of the artificial urinary sphincter. *J Urol* 156:1302–1304.
36. Kowalczyk JJ, Spicer JDL, Mulcahy JJ (1996) Erosion rate of the double cuff AMS 800 artificial urinary sphincter: long term follow-up. *J Urol* 156:1300–1301.
37. Sexton WJ, Benedict JF, Jarow JP (1998) Comparison of long term outcomes of penile prosthesis and intracavernosal injection therapy. *J Urol* 159:811–815.
38. Tefilli MB, Dubocq F, Ragpurkar A, et al. (1998) Assessment of psychological adjustment after insertion of inflatable penile prosthesis. *Urology* 52:1106–1112.

10 Semirigid, Malleable, and Mechanical Penile Prostheses

Survey and State of the Art

Roy A. Brandell, MD,
and J. Brantley Thrasher, MD, FACS

CONTENTS

INTRODUCTION
DEVICES
GENERAL CONSIDERATIONS
PATIENT SELECTION
DISADVANTAGES
CONCLUSION
REFERENCES

INTRODUCTION

The first penile implants were performed following World War II for plastic surgical reconstruction of the penis in soldiers who had sustained destructive injuries to the genitalia, usually from land mines and burns. Autologous cartilage and bone grafts were fashioned for internal penile splinting, but long-term results were poor, partly because of reabsorption of the material over time *(1)*. These techniques were later expanded to the treatment of impotence, and the first use of synthetic materials (acrylic rods) was described by Goodwin and Scott in 1952 *(2)*.

From: *Urologic Prostheses:*
The Complete, Practical Guide to Devices, Their Implantation and Patient Follow Up
Edited by: C. C. Carson © Humana Press Inc., Totowa, NJ

Few advances in the field were forthcoming until the late 1960s when silicone-based materials were developed as part of the space program. Borrowing from this technology, the modern era of penile prosthetic surgery began in the early 1970s as Scott et al. reported on the successful placement of an inflatable device into the corpora cavernosa *(3)*. The Small-Carrion penile prosthesis, introduced soon thereafter, served as a prototype for the many malleable devices marketed over the next quarter century *(4)*. At one time, rod-like devices outsold multicomponent inflatables by a 3-to-1 margin as a result of their ease of placement and mechanical reliability. Today, the market has shifted, heavily favoring the three-piece inflatable devices viewed as "more physiologic" by urologists and patients alike. Manufacturers have improved the design and construction of inflatables, whereas urologists have gained confidence in their ability to safely place the pump and reservoir.

Nevertheless, certain clinical situations remain where implantation of a semirigid device is preferable to an inflatable prosthesis. This chapter provides a survey of the semirigid devices currently available, their indications, advantages, and disadvantages.

DEVICES

Although the terms "semirigid" and "malleable" are often used interchangeably in the medical literature, there are actually two types of semirigid rods: malleable and mechanical. American Medical Systems (AMS) and Mentor each produce malleable systems, whereas Dacomed is the only manufacturer of a mechanical device.

AMS Products

AMS offers two malleable prostheses, the 600M and the 650. Both have a stainless steel, woven-wire core redesigned several years ago to incorporate more numerous and thinner strands. This made bending easier and reduced the spring-back angle to 45 degrees. The core is surrounded by a three-layer polyester covering enclosed within a solid silicone body. Surrounding the body is a trimmable silicone elastomer jacket. The 650 cylinders measure 13 mm in diameter and are supplied in a variety lengths with rear-tip extenders for accurate sizing. If needed, the jacket can be removed, reducing the cylinder diameter to 11 mm *(see* Fig. 1). The 600M is a narrower version of the 650 supplied in a 11.5-mm width that reduces to 9.5 mm when the outer jacket is trimmed.

Mentor Products

Mentor also offers two bendable devices, the Malleable and the AccuForm. They both have a silver-wire core, but differ in its configu-

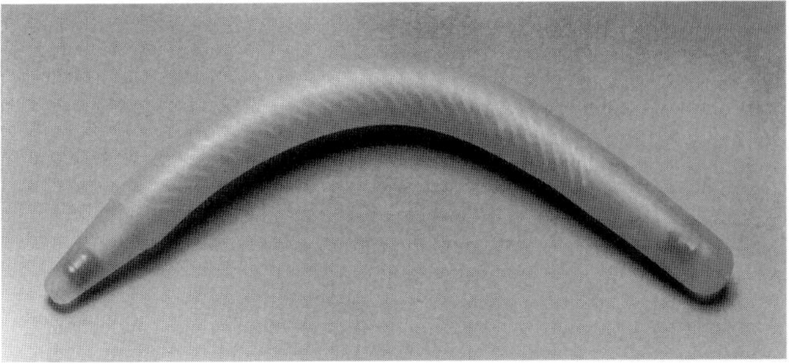

Fig. 1. The AMS 650 penile prosthesis.

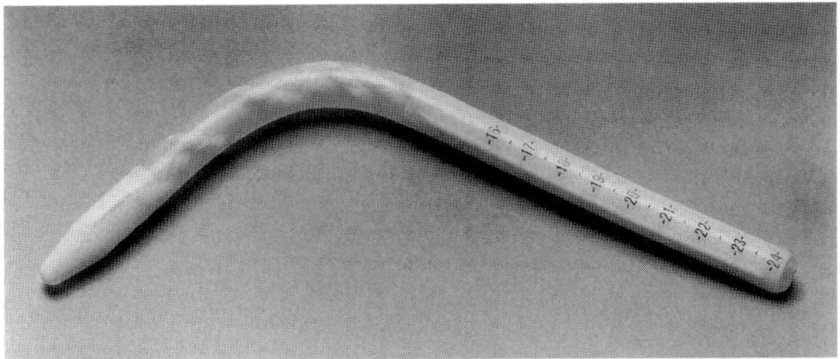

Fig. 2. The Mentor AccuForm penile prosthesis.

ration. The Malleable has a single spiral, whereas the AccuForm design employs a helical wire surrounding a central-wire core that provides greater flexibility with less springback after ventral positioning. Both versions are covered by a silicone elastomer with the silver segment positioned at the bend angle in the penis. A variety of lengths are available and precise sizing can be achieved by cutting the proximal end of the rod and attaching a tapered cap (*see* Fig. 2). Each Mentor device comes in three widths, 9.5 mm, 11 mm, and 13 mm.

Dacomed Product

Dacomed manufactures the only mechanical semirigid device currently available. It is marketed by Timm Medical Technologies. The Dura II is composed of articulating segments of high molecular-weight polyethylene. A stainless steel cable composed of seven wires containing 19 strands each runs through the segments and attaches to fixed posts on either end by a spring mechanism. The articulating segments are housed in a polytetrafluoroethylene (Teflon) sleeve coated with a thin membrane of silicone to prevent tissue ingrowth. The body of the cyl-

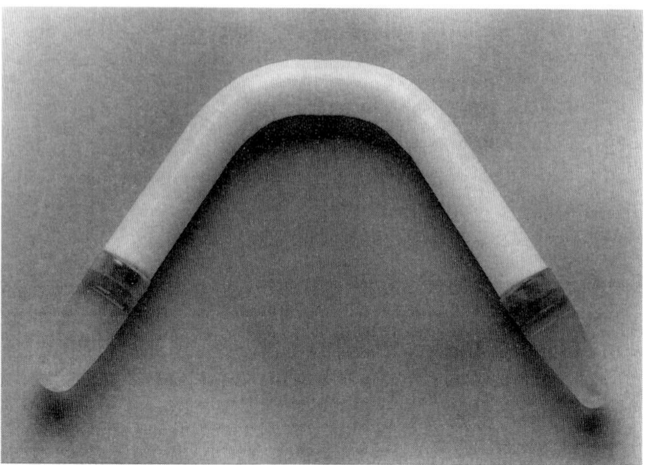

Fig. 3. The Dacomed DuraII penile prosthesis.

inder comes in one length, 13 cm, and sizing is achieved by adding proximal and distal tips to achieve the desired length. The shortest total length possible is 15 cm, making this device a poor choice for patients with a very short penis or those with extensive scarring. Two diameters are offered—10 mm and 13 mm. The device is capable of bending more than human penile anatomy will allow (*see* Fig. 3) and there is no springback.

GENERAL CONSIDERATIONS

The advantage of semirigid penile implants stem primarily from their ease of insertion by the urologist, ease of operation by the patient, and an excellent history of mechanical reliability, superior to that of the inflatables.

Semirigid penile prostheses can be inserted using either a subcoronal (circumcising) incision or a ventral penile approach. Some authors advocate a penoscrotal or infrapubic technique, but these incisions require a substantially larger corporotomy for safe insertion of the device. One should avoid "hyperflexing" the cylinder or handling it with surgical instruments in an attempt to force it through a small corporatomy. These maneuvers can damage the prosthesis and thus reduce its long-term reliability.

Inadvertent puncture of a semirigid rod while closing the corporotomy is not the disaster that is is with inflatables. In fact, sutures can be safely placed through most of these devices to anchor them to the corpus in cases where a proximal crural perforation has occurred. Salvage or "rescue" procedures are also easier with semirigid devices as there are fewer components, and the scrotal and retroperitoneal spaces have not been violated.

Malleable and mechanical prostheses can readily be placed in an ambulatory surgery center under local anesthesia. One simply infiltrates the base of the penis circumferentially with anesthetic as in performing a penile block for circumcision. A tourniquet is then placed around the base of the penis and 25 mL of 0.5% lidocaine without epinephrine is injected through a 21-gage butterfly needle into the corporal body, as if creating an artificial erection. After 2 or 3 min, the tourniquet is released and the anesthetic is allowed to migrate into the rest of the corpora proximally. Only plain lidocaine should be used as other local anesthetics can be cardiotoxic when given systemically in high doses.

All of the semirigid devices reported herein have an outstanding record of reliability. In fact, the authors are not aware of any reports describing spontaneous breakage of the semirigid prostheses currently available on the market. Manufactures have been quick to identify problems in earlier models and make the necessary changes in design and materials to ensure long-term reliability.

PATIENT SELECTION

There is no single penile implant that can be considered the best choice for all patients. Although the urologist is probably best able to determine which prosthesis is most suitable for a given patient, it is important to involve the patient in the decision-making process. Operation of an inflatable implant requires a certain degree of manual dexterity and mental capability. Semirigid devices may be a better choice for patients with neurologic disease (Parkinson's, multiple sclerosis), severe arthritis, missing limbs or fingers, and for some elderly patients. In addition, patients for whom cost is an overriding concern may be better served by a less-expensive semirigid device.

Although spinal cord-injured men typically respond very well to sildenafil, some will still require implantation of a penile prosthesis. Penile retraction, causing difficulty with condom catheter wear, is another potential indication for prosthetic insertion in this patient population. Men with spinal cord injuries have a much higher incidence of prosthetic infection compared to other patient groups, even diabetics *(5)*. It is tempting to use semirigid rods to potentially decrease the incidence of postoperative infection. Unfortunately, paraplegics also have a higher-than-average rate of device erosion, presumed secondary to diminished penile sensation. Instrumentation of the penis and urethra for bladder management may also be a factor. Thus, paraplegics with good upper extremity function are probably better suited to inflatable devices. Either way, consideration should be given to suprapubic catheter use for perioperative drainage of urine in these patients.

Semirigid devices have been advocated for patients with extensive corporal fibrosis, for whom insertion and adequate inflation of a hydraulic device is difficult. Monga et al. suggested that early placement of a semirigid device may be the optimum management for sickle cell patients with recurrent episodes of ischemic priapism *(6)*.

The use of semirigid devices in patients with Peyronie's disease is controversial. Ghanem et al. obtained good cosmetic results without the need for plaque surgery in 65% of cases with a patient satisfaction rate of 88% at 1 yr *(7)*. Adequate penile straightening was also reported by Montorsi et al., but they observed diminishing patient satisfaction with time *(8)*. At a minimum of 5 yr postoperatively, only 48% of their patients were totally satisfied and would repeat the same operation again. Sixteen percent of their patients chose to substitute the semirigid implant with a 3-component inflatable prosthesis.

Reports indicate that semirigid devices are a poor choice for patients with a long penis *(9,10)*. Adequate rigidity and concealment have been a problem. If capable, these men are probably better served by an inflatable device. In all patients, careful sizing of the cylinders is critical for optimizing concealment and decreasing the incidence of dreaded complications such as erosion and chronic penile pain.

DISADVANTAGES

Patients and their partners may become dissatisfied with a semirigid device for a variety of reasons, usually stemming from inability of the implants to adequately mimic a normal, physiologic erection. Reasons for dissatisfaction include chronic penile pain, numbness, diminished quality of orgasm, suboptimal penile length and/or girth, difficulty with concealment, and inadequate rigidity. Contrary to inflatable devices, difficulties with operating the semirigid prostheses are rarely reported even in patients with very poor manual dexterity. Autoinflation is also nonexistent with semirigid devices. Potential reasons for partner dissatisfaction include insufficient penile size, sensation of a cold penis, sensation of unnatural intercourse, and dyspareunia. Some reports have suggested that patient and partner satisfaction diminishes with time after implatation *(8)*, although others have shown just the opposite *(11)*.

Because the various semirigid devices are redesigned or modified every 5–8 yr, long-term data on a particular device usually becomes available just as it is replaced by a new, "improved" model. Kearse et al. recently reported a multicenter evaluation of the Dacomed Dura II prosthesis up to 2 yr after implantation *(11)*. Patient satisfaction was in the 85% range and adverse events (usually infection) occurred in only 8% of patients. Dorflinger and Bruskewitz published their results several years ago using the AMS 600 malleable device, predecessor of the AMS 650 *(12)*. They reported a 90% satisfaction rate, adverse events in 9%, and in 66% no difficulty with concealment was encountered. Virtually identical results were also obtained by Moul and McLeod *(10)*. Several authors have published their personal experience using a variety of semirigid devices (including the Mentor products) in a broad range of patients *(13–15)*. Results are remarkably consistent, with satisfaction rates in the 85 to 95% range and complication rates substantially lower than those reported for inflatable devices.

CONCLUSION

In order to optimize success, surgeons who perform prosthetic surgery need to be familiar with all the various devices currently available. Each model has its own unique set of advantages and disadvantages. Overwhelmingly, the key factors for achieving consistent positive outcomes are meticulous operative technique, careful patient selection, and thorough preoperative patient education. Other than infection or mechanical failure, the primary reason for patients' and partners' dissatisfaction is unrealistic expectations as to what the prosthesis will do. Semirigid devices provide adequate erections for most patients. They are easier to implant and manipulate, cost less, and have a lower mechanical failure rate than inflatable devices. With this in mind, semirigid penile prostheses are an excellent alternative for some men with end-stage organic erectile dysfunction.

REFERENCES

1. Bergman RT, Howard AH, Barnes RW (1948) Plastic reconstruction of the penis. *JAMA* 59:1174.
2. Goodwin WE, Scott WS (1960) Phalloplasty. *J Urol* 84:559.
3. Scott EB, Bradley WE, Timm GW (1973) Management of erectile impotence. *Urology* 2:80.
4. Small MP, Carrion HM, Gordon JA (1975) Small-Carrion penile prosthesis. *Urology* 2:479.
5. Collins KP, Hackler RH (1988) Complications of penile prostheses in spinal cord injured patients. *J Urol* 140:984.
6. Monga M, Broderick GA, Hellstrom WJG (1996) Priapism in sickle cell disease: the case for early implantation of the penile prosthesis. *Eur Urol* 30:54.
7. Ghanem HM, Fahmy I, El-Meliegy A (1998) Malleable penile implants without plaque surgery in the treatment of Peyronie's disease. *Int J Impot Res* 10:171.
8. Montorsi F, Guazzoni G, Bergamaschi F, Rigatti P (1993) Patient-Partner satisfaction with semirigid penile prostheses for Peyronie's disease: a 5-year followup study. *J Urol* 150:1819.

9. Chen GL, Kowitz AS, Berger RE (1997) Reinforcement of semirigid penile implant. *J Urol* 157:2258.
10. Moul JW, McLeod DG (1986) Experience with the AMS 600 malleable penile prosthesis. *J Urol* 135:929.
11. Kearse WS Jr, Sago AL, Peretsman SJ, et al. (1996) Report of a multicenter, clinical evaluation of the Dura II penile prosthesis. *J Urol* 155:1613.
12. Dorflinger T, Gruskewitz R (1986) AMS Malleable penile prosthesis. *Urology* 28:480.

11 Inflatable Penile Prostheses

*The American Medical
Systems' Experience*

Drogo K. Montague, MD
and Kenneth W. Angermeier, MD

CONTENTS

> HISTORY
> PENILE PROSTHESIS IMPLANTATION
> SUMMARY
> REFERENCES

HISTORY

Three Piece Inflatable Penile Prostheses

THE FIRST INFLATABLE PENILE PROSTHESIS

Until the early 1970s, most impotence, or what is now known as erectile dysfunction (ED), was assumed to be of psychogenic origin, and even urologists had little interest in its treatment. F. Brantley Scott, a urologist from the Baylor College of Medicine; William E. Bradley, a neurologist; and Gerald W. Timm, a biomedical engineer (both from the University of Minnesota) collaborated to develop an artificial urinary sphincter and an inflatable penile prosthesis. Together with a businessman, Robert Buuck, Drs. Scott, Bradley, and Timm formed American Medical Systems (AMS) to manufacture and market these devices.

From: *Urologic Prostheses:*
The Complete, Practical Guide to Devices, Their Implantation and Patient Follow Up
Edited by: C. C. Carson © Humana Press Inc., Totowa, NJ

The first inflatable penile prosthesis, made from Dacron-reinforced silicone elastomer, consisted of four parts: an inflation pump, a deflation pump, paired nondistensible cylinders, and a rectangular fluid reservoir. In their initial report, they described its use in five patients *(1)*. This first inflatable penile prosthesis, used from February 1973 to August 1974, was implanted in 12 patients with success in 9 *(2)*.

The first prosthesis to reach the market in 1974 was a modification of this original four-piece device. It had the following design changes: the Dacron reinforcement was eliminated and a single inflation-deflation pump was developed. The reservoir was round, flat, and had a peripheral seam. The cylinders were changed to expandable, single-ply silicone elastomer tubes. Two subsequent modifications to this device were later introduced: a seamless, spherical reservoir in 1978 and rear-tip extenders in 1980. This prosthesis remained in use from 1974 to 1983, and its availability rapidly sparked urologists' interest in ED.

Furlow reported on 63 men implanted with this prosthesis who had follow-up ranging from 6 to 24 mo. Seventeen (27%) experienced mechanical failures in this relatively short period of time *(3)*. Later, he updated his series with reports on 175 implant recipients followed for 6 to 42 mo. Mechanical failures occurred in 37 (21%) *(4)*. Scott et al. reported on 245 men implanted with this device between 1973 and 1977. The implant procedure was successful in 234 cases (96%) and 102 of these patients (44%) subsequently underwent repeat operation because of surgical complications, mechanical failures, or patient request for a new model *(5)*. Malloy et al. reported on implants in 93 men followed from 6 mo to 4 yr. Complications leading to 31 secondary procedures occurred in 27 (29%) of the patients *(6)*. Fallon et al. reported on 95 men implanted with these devices between 1977–1983. Of these, 48% had been revised, removed, or failed during follow-up *(7)*. We reported on 121 implant recipients. The first 70 patients implanted through a lower abdominal incision, had a total of 63 revisions in 34 patients. The next 51 implants, through a penoscrotal incision, using rear-tip extenders had revisions in only 4 patients *(8)*.

THE AMS 700 INFLATABLE PENILE PROSTHESIS

A new model of the inflatable penile prosthesis, the AMS 700 Inflatable Penile Prosthesis, was introduced in 1983. It included the following design changes: kink-resistant tubing, thicker cylinders with redesigned front and rear tips, polytetrafluoroethylene sleeves over the tubing to prevent cylinder wear, and a redesigned pump to permit easier deflation. A sutureless connector system was introduced in 1985. This model remained in use from 1983 to 1987.

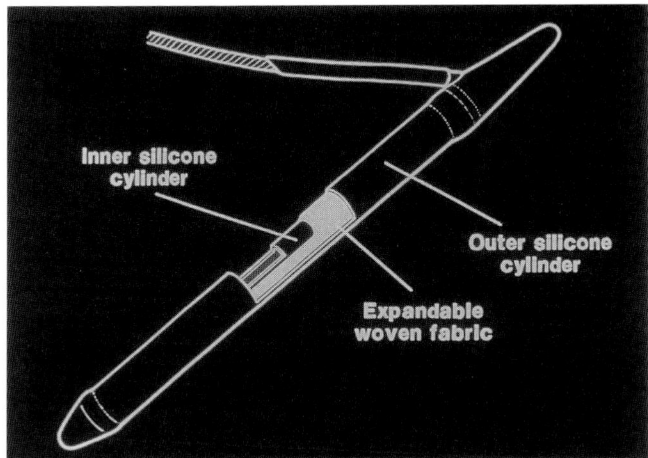

Fig. 1. The triple-ply cylinder design used in the AMS Three-Piece Inflatable Penile Prostheses. Courtesy of American Medical Systems, Inc., Minnetonka, MN.

Malloy et al. reported 290 men implanted with the AMS 700 prosthesis who were followed for at least 1 yr. There were three cylinder failures and eight leaks from kink-resistant tubing. No pump or reservoir failures occurred. Life table analysis showed a probability of device survival of 97.9% at 3 yr *(9)*. Gregory and Purcell reported on 131 implant recipients. Cylinder survival was 98% at 1 yr and 92% at 3 yr. Tubing leaks occurred in nine patients *(10)*. Scarzella reported on 325 implant recipients. Three-year cylinder survival was 72% for cylinders manufactured from 1974 to 1983 and was 86% for cylinders manufactured after 1983 (AMS 700 cylinders) *(11)*. Wilson et al. reported on 395 patients implanted since 1977. In patients implanted before 1983, there was a 61% complication/revision rate with follow-up of 3–11 yr. In patients implanted after 1983, only 13% required revision with follow-up to 4 yr *(12)*.

The expansion of these single-ply AMS 700 cylinders was determined primarily by the elastic characteristics of the recipients' corpora cavernosa. Because this varied from patient to patient, cylinder aneurysms with this device were common *(13)*.

The AMS 700CX™ Penile Prosthesis

The first triple-ply cylinders were introduced in 1987 *(see* Fig. 1). Fluid pumped into an inner silicone elastomer tube expanded against a middle woven fabric layer. An outer silicone covering prevented tissue growth into the fabric layer. The woven fabric controlled expansion of these cylinders; thus, cylinder expansion was no longer dependent on the elastic characteristics of recipients' tissues. The cylinders of this AMS 700CX prosthesis have diameters of 12 mm when deflated and diameters of 18 mm when inflated. This implant continues to be used today.

Furlow and Motley reported 63 men implanted with the AMS 700CX device with follow-up ranging from 8 to 38 mo (average 20 mo). There were no cylinder aneurysms and only 1 cylinder leak *(14)*. Quesada and Light reported 214 men who were implanted with the AMS 700CX prosthesis. Follow-up ranged from 18 to 84 mo with a mean follow-up of 55 mo. The probability of survival without revision to 6 yr was 97% for the cylinders and 90% for the device as a whole. Cylinder leaks occurred in 0.7% and there were no cylinder aneurysms *(15)*. Nickas et al. reported on 55 implant procedures using the AMS 700CX device and compared them to 252 implants with earlier AMS models of the inflatable penile prosthesis *(16)*. Actuarial 4-yr survival for the AMS 700CX prosthesis was 85% compared to 46% for the earlier devices. This difference was primarily a result of lower cylinder complications with the CX device. We reported 111 CX/CXM implants with follow-up ranging from 1 to 112 mo (mean 47 mo). There were 10 mechanical failures (9%) *(17)*. This prosthesis is now available in a model containing paired cylinders connected to a pump (the AMS 700CX Preconnected Penile Prosthesis).

The AMS 700CXM™ Penile Prosthesis

The AMS 700CXM prosthesis was originally developed for implantation in men with smaller penises; however, its main use now is in prosthesis implantation men with fibrotic penises *(18)*. This is a smaller version of the AMS 700CX prosthesis. Its pump and reservoir are smaller, and the cylinders have deflated diameters of 9.5 mm and inflated diameters of 14.2 mm. It was introduced in 1990 and remains in use today.

The 700 Ultrex™ Penile Prosthesis

This prosthesis (*see* Fig. 2) has triple-ply cylinders with the same deflated and inflated diameters as the AMS 700CX device (12 and 18 mm). The middle fabric layer of the Ultrex cylinders; however, expands in two directions; thus, these cylinders not only increase in diameter with inflation, they also increase in length. Outside the body, these cylinders are capable of increasing 20% in length. The amount of penile length achieved after implantation is determined primarily by the elasticity of the recipient's penis. This prosthesis was introduced in 1990 and remains in use. In 1992, the 700 Ultrex™ Plus Penile Prosthesis was developed. This device consists of prefilled Ultrex cylinders connected to a prefilled

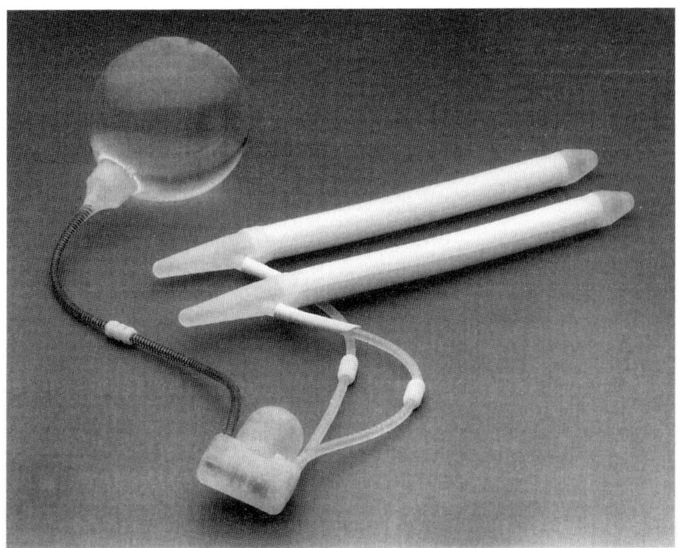

Fig. 2. The 700 Ultex™ Penile Prosthesis. Courtesy of American Medical Systems, Inc., Minnetonka, MN.

pump. The reservoir is implanted separately and a single connection is made between the reservoir and the pump.

We reported on the length expansion obtained following implantation of the Ultrex prosthesis. In 50 patients, the intraoperative penile-length measurement between deflation and inflation increased 1 to 4 cm (mean 1.9 cm). Postoperative measurements were obtained in 46 patients at a mean of 4 mo. In 28 patients, the intraoperative length expansion was maintained, whereas in six patients, it decreased by 1 cm, and in 12 patients, it increased by 1 cm *(19)*.

Holloway and Farah reported 145 patients implanted with the 700 Ultrex device. Follow-up ranged from 6 to 62 mo (mean 42 mo). There was a 13% reoperation rate and an 8% mechanical failure rate *(20)*. We reported on 152 Ultrex implant recipients with a follow-up of 0.7 to 71.5 mo (mean 34 mo). Mechanical failures occurred in 26 patients (17%) *(17)*. We found that this was primarily because of cylinder failure resulting from tearing of the middle fabric layer. In 1993, the middle fabric layer of the Ultrex cylinders was strengthened to increase device longevity, while still permitting the same degree of girth and length expansion. Published reports of cylinder survival with the modified Ultrex cylinder are not yet available. We have implanted 142 Ultrex devices containing modified cylinders with only three known cylinder failures; however, further follow-up is needed to

Table 1
Current AMS Three-Piece Inflatable Penile Prostheses

Model	Date introduced	Deflated diameter	Inflated diameter	Length expansion	Connections
700CX	1987	12 mm	18 mm	no	3
700CXM	1990	9.5 mm	14.2 mm	no	3
Ultrex	1990	12 mm	18 mm	yes	3
Ultrex Plus	1992	12 mm	18 mm	yes	1

determine the reliability of these cylinders. The three-piece AMS devices currently in use are shown in Table 1.

One-Piece Inflatable Penile Prostheses

THE AMS HYDROFLEX™ PENILE PROSTHESIS

The AMS Hydroflex prosthesis, used from 1985 to 1990, was developed to produce a device that would be rigid when inflated and, when deflated, would lose some of its rigidity. This device consisted of paired cylinders implanted in both corpora. A small pump in the distal cylinder was used to transfer a small volume of fluid from a rear-tip reservoir into a central nondistensible chamber. This device achieved rigidity without girth or length expansion. Deflation was obtained by pressing a release valve just proximal to the pump.

Mulcahy reported on 100 patients implanted with the AMS Hydroflex penile prosthesis *(21)*. Follow-up was from 1 to 3.5 yr. There were six mechanical failures and 15 patients had difficulty learning how to inflate and deflate the device. Kabalin and Kessler reported on 51 Hydroflex implant recipients followed from 6 to 33 mo (mean 20 mo) *(22)*. There were no mechanical failures and 81% of the patients were satisfied with the device.

THE AMS DYNAFLEX™ PENILE PROSTHESIS

The Dynaflex prosthesis was introduced in 1990 as a modification of the Hydroflex device. Deflation with the Dynaflex prosthesis was achieved by bending the device to increase pressure for 10 s. When the bend in the device was released, deflation occurred. This modification resulted in a prosthesis that was easier to deflate. The central nondistensible chamber was also longer, resulting in improved rigidity with inflation. Kabalin and Kuo reported on 62 Dynaflex implant recipients followed for a minimum of 24 and a mean of 50 mo *(23)*. There were six mechanical failures (9.7%), and 16.1% of the patients were dissatisfied

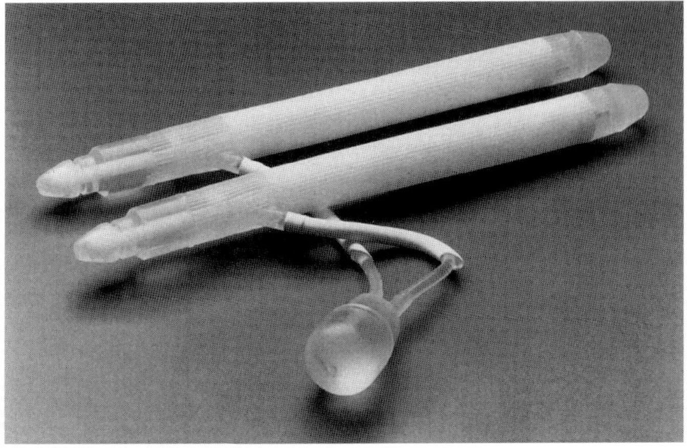

Fig. 3. The AMS Ambicor® Penile Prosthesis. Courtesy of American Medical Systems, Inc., Minnetonka, MN.

with the device. Anafarta et al. reported 120 men implanted with the Dynaflex device *(24)*. Follow-up ranged from 2 to 80 mo (mean 42 mo). The mechanical failure rate was 7.5%, and 16.7% were dissatisfied because of difficulty using the device. The AMS Hydroflex and the AMS Dynaflex prostheses, having been replaced by the Ambicor prosthesis (*see* next section), are no longer available in the United States.

Two Piece Inflatable Prostheses

THE AMS AMBICOR® PENILE PROSTHESIS

The Ambicor penile prosthesis consists of paired cylinders connected to a small scrotal pump (*see* Fig. 3). Like the Dynaflex prosthesis, the Ambicor has rear-tip fluid reservoirs and a central nondistensible chamber. The pump is moved from the distal portion of the cylinders to the scrotum, making this device easier to cycle and creating a longer central chamber for better rigidity. To our knowledge, there are no published reports of the use of this device. This device, which was introduced in 1994, is still in use.

PENILE PROSTHESIS IMPLANTATION

Indications

When the inflatable penile prosthesis was introduced in 1974, the principal treatments for men with ED consisted of sex therapy for men with psychogenic or potentially reversible ED and penile prosthesis implantation for nearly everything else. Today, the following treatment options for ED are available: sex therapy, systemic therapy, the use of vacuum erection devices, intraurethral medications, penile injection therapy, vascular surgery, and penile prosthesis implantation. Because of the attractiveness, efficacy, and safety profile of new systemic agents, many men with ED are presenting for treatment. Medications such as sildenafil citrate, and others soon to be released, are usually first-line therapy options, with sex therapy also being employed as appropriate. Men who fail these first-line treatment options are potential candidates for penile prosthesis implantation if the remaining treatment options either fail or are rejected by the patient and his partner.

The Ideal Penile Prosthesis

The ideal penile prosthesis would allow a man to control when he had an erection and would produce prosthetic flaccid and erect states resembling, as closely as possible, natural penile flaccidity and erection. To do this with an inflatable hydraulic device, a large volume of fluid must be pumped into expandable cylinders for erection and must be transferred out of the cylinders for flaccidity. This requires a device with a large abdominal fluid reservoir such as the three-piece inflatable prostheses produced by AMS and Mentor Corporation. The ideal prosthesis would provide on inflation penile rigidity, as well as girth and length expansion. Currently, there is only one device doing this and it is the 700 Ultrex Inflatable Penile Prosthesis. Should this prosthesis be offered to all potential implant recipients?

Choosing a Prosthesis

We prefer the AMS three-piece inflatable prostheses and offer nearly all patients these devices based on the following considerations. For most first-time prosthesis recipients, we offer the 700 Ultrex device, unless in addition to ED, the man has erectile deformity, for example owing to Peyronie's disease. The girth-only expanding AMS 700CX prosthesis has better straightening characteristics than the Ultrex, and thus we favor this device for these men *(25)*. We also use the AMS 700CX device for men with long penises because the CX cylinders produce better rigidity. Only rarely during primary prosthesis implantation do we encounter corpora that will not dilate sufficiently to accept 12-mm diameter cylinders. For these men, we will use the AMS 700CXM implant.

For secondary or repeat penile prosthesis implantation, we will use the girth-only expanding CX cylinders when length expansion should be avoided, for example after failed implants owing to urethral erosion or cylinder crossover. For men with small penises because of fibrotic corpora, as we see in men who have had priapism or men who have had an infected penile implant removed, we implant the small-diameter AMS 700CXM device *(18)*. For all other secondary implants, we consider the 700 Ultrex prosthesis, provided the penis is not long and it has at least 2 cm of stretch.

Patient Expectations

Following uncomplicated penile prosthesis implantation, successful healing without infection, erosion, device migration, or immediate mechanical failure should occur in about 95% of patients. If a man undergoes successful device implantation and is not satisfied, it is probably because his expectations were not met. It should be the goal of preoperative counseling to provide the patient with realistic expectations. Penile prosthesis implantation does not ordinarily interfere with penile sensation or the ability to achieve orgasm and ejaculate. However, if any of these conditions are absent or not normal, device implantation will not restore them. With today's three-piece inflatable devices, penile flaccidity is usually good and most men will feel comfortable when undressed in a locker room. Although three-piece inflatable prostheses, when inflated, resemble normal erections more than other devices, in nearly all cases, the erection will be shorter than the recipient's natural erection. This is true even with the length-expanding Ultrex prosthesis, although this disparity between prosthetic and natural erection length is less with Ultrex device than it is with other penile prostheses. The most common source of patient dissatisfaction, in our opinion, is shortness of the erection, and we try to prepare the patient for this. Although it is not possible to predict prosthetic erect length with certainty, it is usually close to the patient's preoperative stretched penile length.

Key Features of Prosthesis Implantation

Surgical Approaches

The Infrapubic Approach. With this approach, a vertical or transverse incision is made between the pubis and the penis. The sole advantage of this approach is that it permits reservoir placement under direct vision. Disadvantages include limited corporeal exposure, inability to fix the pump in its scrotal pouch, and possible damage to the dorsal nerves of the penis. Dorsal nerve damage seldom occurs during initial device implantation with this approach; however, we have seen it in men after prosthetic revisions. Possible explanations include dorsal nerve entrapment in scar or nerve damage from using the electrosurgical unit to open the corpora at the time of revision.

The Penoscrotal Approach. Penoscrotal approaches include either a vertical incision over the urethra at the penoscrotal junction or a transverse incision in the upper scrotum just below the penoscrotal junction *(26)*. Although the urethra could be damaged by the penoscrotal approach, it is easily seen and avoided. Urethral damage, which rarely occurs, is almost always confined to the corpus spongiosum and is easily repaired allowing the implant procedure to proceed. We prefer the transverse scrotal approach, which provides excellent exposure of both crura, as well as the corpora at the base of the penis. If more distal exposure is needed because of corporeal fibrosis, this incision can be extended in an inverted T fashion to the frenular area. This is the only approach that affords nearly complete corporeal exposure through a single incision.

If the cylinders and pump are implanted separately, the pump can be fixed in its sub-Dartos pouch by routing each of the three tubes through separate stab incisions in the back wall of the pouch. The principal disadvantage of the penocsrotal approach is the blind placement of the retropubic fluid reservoir.

CORPOREAL SIZING

Many implantors determine cylinder size by placing a reference suture at the midpoint of the corporotomy and then making distal and proximal measurements from this reference point. These two measurements are added to determine corporeal length and cylinder size. Using a rigid sizing instrument to determine length on the surface of the corporeal bodies over estimates the internal length of the corpora by 1 to 2 cm. If cylinders are implanted that are slightly too long for the corpora, a cylinder fold at the base of the penis occurs, which may lead to premature cylinder failure. With the Ultrex cylinders (which expand in length), using a cylinder that is too long will result in the S-shaped cylinder deformity *(27)*.

To avoid this problem, we use 2-cm corporotomies and make the distal and proximal corporeal measurements from the distal and proximal ends of the corporotomies, respectively. These two measurements are added to determine cylinder size; thus, the corporotomy is not included in this measurement. After the cylinder is placed, we make sure that it fills the entire corpus cavernosum and that it lies flat inside the corporotomy. If necessary, the cylinder size can be adjusted by adding or removing rear tip extenders until the cylinder fit is exact.

AVOIDING AUTO INFLATION

The most common cause of cylinder auto inflation is high fluid pressure in the reservoir. The prevesical or retropubic space is the best location for the reservoir. After the reservoir is placed and filled, a back-pressure test should be performed to be sure that fluid pressure in the reservoir is zero. We attach a syringe without a barrel to the reservoir tube and allow any fluid under pressure to escape into the syringe. We then apply manual pressure to the bladder area to express any additional fluid. Finally, the cylinders of the prosthesis should be kept deflated while healing is taking place so that the pseudocapsule, which forms around all parts of the prosthesis, will form around the reservoir when the device is in the deflated state.

SUMMARY

The introduction of the inflatable penile prosthesis in 1974 encouraged urologists to become more actively involved in the treatment of ED. Early models of the inflatable penile prosthesis had many mechanical problems resulting in frequent, early revisions. Numerous improvements in device design and implantation techniques over the years have resulted in today's devices, which are more reliable.

When inflatable penile prostheses and semirigid rod prostheses were first introduced, they were almost the sole treatment for organic ED. Today, a variety of treatment options, including easily used and often effective systemic therapy, have resulted in greatly increased numbers of men presenting for treatment of ED. When systemic treatments for ED fail, other treatments including vacuum erection devices, intra-urethral medications, and penile injections should be offered. If these options fail or are rejected by the patient and his partner, penile prosthesis implantation should be considered. Penile prosthesis implantation, although no longer a first-line treatment option for ED, nevertheless continues to be an important part of ED therapy.

REFERENCES

1. Scott FB, Bradley WE, Timm GW (1973) Management of erectile impotence: use of implantable inflatable prosthesis. *Urology* 2:80–82.
2. Fishman IJ, Scott FB, Light JK (1984) Experience with inflatable penile prosthesis. *Urology* 23:86–92.
3. Furlow WL (1978) The current status of the inflatable penile prosthesis in the management of impotence: Mayo Clinic experience updated. *J Urol* 119:363–364.
4. Furlow WL (1979) Inflatable penile prosthesis: Mayo Clinic experience with 175 patients. *Urology* 13:166–171.
5. Scott FB, Byrd GJ, Karacan I, Olsson P, Beutler LE, Attia SL (1979) Erectile impotence treated with an implantable, inflatable prosthesis. *JAMA* 241:2609–2612.
6. Malloy TR, Wein AJ, Carpiniello VL (1979) Further experience with the inflatable penile prosthesis. *J Urol* 122:478–480.
7. Fallon B, Rosenberg S, Culp DA (1984) Long-term followup in patients with an inflatable penile prosthesis. *J Urol* 132:270–271.

8. Montague DK (1983) Experience with semirigid rod and inflatable penile prostheses. *J Urol* 129:967–968.

13. Diokno AC (1983) Asymmetric inflation of the penile cylinders: etiology and management. *J Urol* 129:1127–1130.

14. Furlow WL, Motley RC (1988) The inflatable penile prosthesis: clinical experience with a new controlled expansion cylinder. *J Urol* 139:945–946.

15. Quesada ET, Light JK (1993) The AMS 700 inflatable penile prosthesis: long-term experience with the controlled expansion cylinders. *J Urol* 149:46–48.

16. Nickas ME, Kessler R, Kabalin JN (1994) Long-term experience with controlled expansion cylinders in the AMS 700CX inflatable penile prosthesis and comparison with earlier versions of the Scott inflatable penile prosthesis. *Urology* 44:400–403.

17. Daitch JA, Angermeier KW, Lakin MM, Ingleright BJ, Montague DK (1997) Long-term mechanical reliability of AMS 700 series inflatable penile prostheses: comparison of CX/CXM and Ultrex cylinders. *J Urol* 158:1400–1402.

18. Carbone DJ, Jr, Daitch JA, Angermeier KW, Lakin MM, Montague DK (1998) Management of severe corporeal fibrosis with implantation of prosthesis via a transverse scrotal approach. *J Urol* 159:125–127.

19. Montague DK, Lakin MM (1992) Early experience with the controlled girth and length expanding cylinder of the AMS Ultrex penile prosthesis. *J Urol* 148:1444–1446.

20. Holloway FB, Farah RN (1997) Intermediate term assessment of the reliability, function and patient satisfaction with the AMS700 Ultrex penile prosthesis [see comments]. *J Urol* 157:1687–91.

21. Mulcahy JJ (1988) The Hydroflex self-contained inflatable penile prosthesis: experience with 100 patients. *J Urol* 140:1422–1423.

22. Kabalin JN, Kessler R (1989) Experience with the Hydroflex penile prosthesis. *J Urol* 141:58–59.

23. Kabalin JN, Kuo JC (1997) Long-term followup of and patient satisfaction with the Dynaflex self-contained inflatable penile prosthesis. *J Urol* 158:456–459.

24. Anafarta K, Yaman O, Aydos K (1998) Clinical experience with Dynaflex penile prostheses in 120 patients. *Urology* 52:1098–1100.

25. Montague DK, Angermeier KW, Lakin MM, Ingleright BJ (1996) AMS 3-piece inflatable penile prosthesis implantation in men with Peyronie's disease: comparison of CX and Ultrex cylinders [see comments]. *J Urol* 156:1633–1635.

26. Scarzella GI (1989) Improved technique for implanting AMS 700CX inflatable penile prosthesis using transverse scrotal approach. *Urology* 34:388–389.

27. Wilson SK, Cleves MA, Delk II JR (1996) Ultrex cylinders: Problems with uncontrolled lengthening (the S-shaped deformity). *J Urol* 155:135–137.

12 Experience with the Mentor α-1

Ricardo M. Munarriz, MD
and Irwin Goldstein, MD

Contents

Introduction
Mentor α-1 Three-Piece Inflatable Penile
 Prosthesis
Comparison of α-1 to AMS 700 CX Mechanical
 Failure Rates
Autoinflation
Severe Corporal Fibrosis
Patient Satisfaction
Conclusion
References

INTRODUCTION

Ten years after the introduction of the Scott three-piece inflatable penile prosthesis in 1973 (American Medical Systems, Minnetonka, MN) *(1)*, Mentor Corporation introduced their first three-piece inflatable penile prosthesis, the Mentor IPP (Surgitek, Racine, WI) *(2)*. This device provided an alternative for improving the mechanical reliability of the three-piece inflatable penile prosthesis, which had been reported to be as high as 42% in some series *(3)*. The most important advance that Mentor brought to the field of penile prosthetics was the introduction of a new material, known as Bioflex. Biofelx is an aromatic polyether urea urethane elastomer that provided a tensile strength seven times higher than that of silicone without sacrificing biocompatibility and hemocompatibility *(4–6)*. The physical characteristics of this material, virtually

From: *Urologic Prostheses:*
The Complete, Practical Guide to Devices, Their Implantation and Patient Follow Up
Edited by: C. C. Carson © Humana Press Inc., Totowa, NJ

eliminated cylinder failures as a result of aneurysms or wear-induced abrasion, and provided the widest inflatable cylinder girth expansion available. As with other devices, continuous modifications of the Mentor IPP followed such as: a) modification of the pump in 1983 to improve patient identification of the deflation valve; b) use of nylon reinforced tubing in 1984 to eliminate tubing kinks; c) reinforced cylinder base in 1985 to avoid separation of the input tubing from the cylinder; d) use of a flange to the plastic clamps of the snap-on connectors in 1987 to improve stability *(7)*, yield improved clinical results *(8)*.

MENTOR α-1 THREE-PIECE INFLATABLE PENILE PROSTHESIS

The second generation of the Mentor inflatable penile prosthesis was introduced in May 1989. The Mentor α-1 was designed to improve device reliability and reduce device failure from connector leakage. This inflatable penile prosthesis (*see* Fig. 1) was the first connectorless, single pump-cylinder unit. Although continued minor modifications have occurred over the years, the basic design of the Mentor α-1 has remained the same for the last 11 yr. Some of these minor modifications to the α-1 included lengthening and reinforcement of the tubing at the exit from the pump in late 1992. The enhanced version (*see* Fig. 2) of the Mentor α-1 model increased the 5-yr survival rate from 75.3 for the original to 92.6% and lowered the failure rate of approx 5.6% for the original model to 1.3% *(9)*. Cylinder, reservoir, and pump malfunctions are rarely observed in contemporary Mentor three-piece inflatable penile prosthesis. Current data reveals device malfunction consists of tubing fluid leaks *(10–13)*.

COMPARISON OF α-1 TO AMS 700 CX MECHANICAL FAILURE RATES

In 1993, Pescatori and Goldstein reported a 16% mechanical failure rate in the AMS 700 CX as a result primarily of leaks at or near the connector site. A 4% mechanical failure rate was observed in the Mentor α-1. A common malfunction site in the AMS device was observed in the tubing from one of the cylinders as its inlet to the pump. One explanation for the difference was found to be the lower intraluminal device pressures in the Mentor device during inflation and the absence of connectors in the pump cylinder unit. This comparative paper between Bioflex (Mentor IPP and Mentor α-1) and silicon-based devices (AMS 700 CX and AMS Ultrex) revealed markedly elevated values of intraluminal

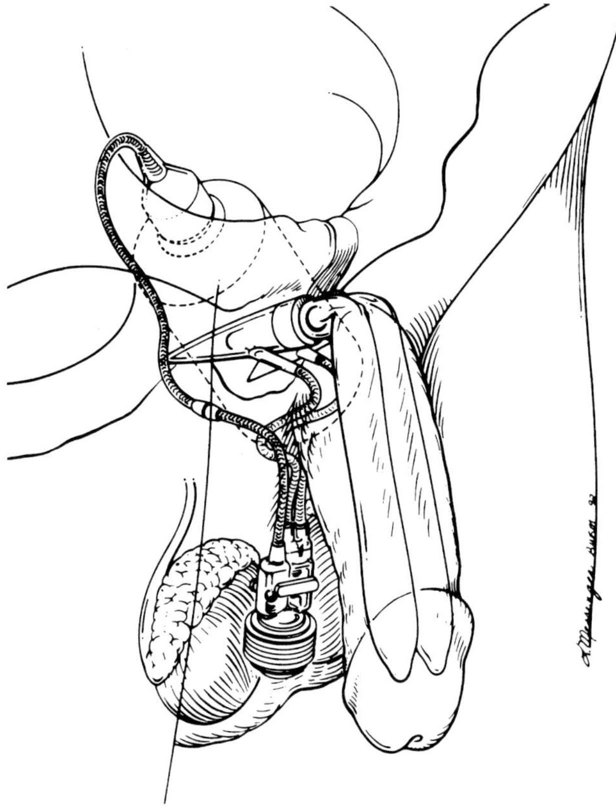

Fig. 1. Mentor α-1 inflatable penile prosthesis.

pressures in the second group (*see* Fig. 3). Such high pressures are equally transmitted to all of the communicating components, presumably causing malfunctions at the weakest locations. The difference in intraluminal pressures reflects the compliance characteristics of the wall of the cylinders. The Bioflex lining material of the Mentor cylinders has greater compliance with an ability to stretch circumferentially during inflation and increase girth to values exceeding 21 mm without deformation of the cylinders. The Dacron-Lycra sleeve surrounding the AMS 700 CX cylinder has virtually no compliance, restricting girth expansion to 18 mm *(14)*. Therefore, during inflation, fluid constraint within the AMS 700 CX will occur at lower volumes and higher intraluminal pressures than Mentor devices.

This double-digit mechanical failure rate seen in the AMS devices has not changed significantly in the last 7 yr. Carson et al. recently published the results of the AMS 700 CX study group. They found a

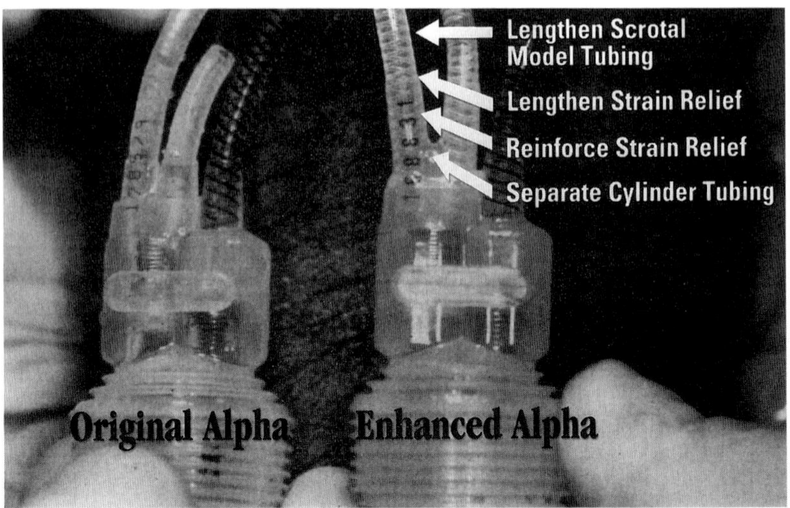

Fig. 2. Enhanced Mentor α-1 inflatable penile prosthesis. In 1992, the tubing was length and reinforced at the exit from the pump.

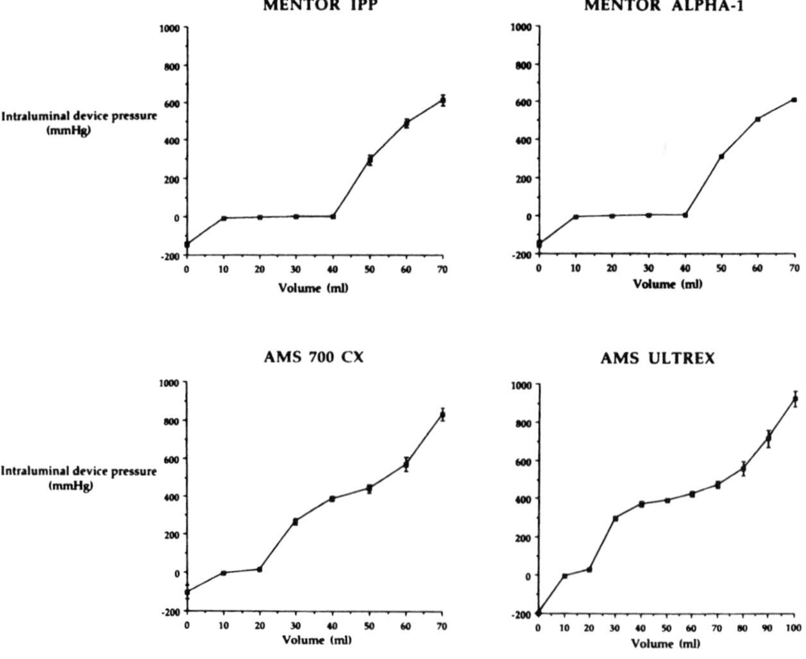

Fig. 3. Comparison between Bioflex (Mentor IPP and Mentor α-1) and silicon-based devices (AMS 700 CX and AMS Ultrex) revealed markedly elevated values of intraluminal pressures in the second group.

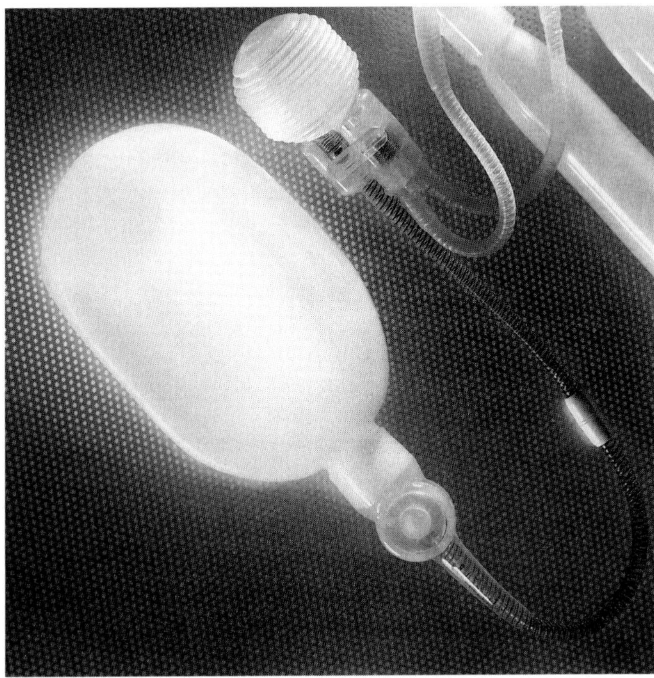

Fig. 4. Mentor α-1 inflatable penile prosthesis with the enhanced reservoir (Lock-out valve).

13.8% mechanical failure rate at 5 years with a complication rate of 45%, most commonly secondary to fluid loss or leakage *(25)*.

Based on contemporary data, the failure rate for the AMS 700 CX is therefore more than 10 times that of the Mentor α-1 inflatable penile prosthesis. The most-likely explanation for the mechanical failure rates between the two devices is the difference in the material characteristics lining the two products. Bioflex is simply a more-appropriate and reliable material when used in inflatable penile prostheses.

AUTOINFLATION

Autoinflation of the inflatable penile prosthesis is an annoying and embarrassing clinical complication, which has been reported in various degrees of severity in up to 20% of cases. Initially, both AMS and Mentor three-piece implants were reported to have spontaneous autoinflation as a complication. In 2000, Mentor Corporation introduced the enhanced reservoir with the new *"Lock-out valve"* (*see* Fig. 4). The new valve opened to allow fluid flow when the reservoir output was subjected to negative pressure. This occurred as the pump bulb recovers from a collapsed state during cylinder inflation, and when the reservoir output was subjected to positive pressure during deflation of the penile cylinders. Preliminary results reported by the Lock-out Valve Study, a group of 17 physicians of varied geographical locations and types of practices, showed 8.6% of mild autoinflation in 70 patients, with a 52-mo follow-up. All physicians reported that the lock-out valve did not affect the usual surgical procedure in any case *(15)*. Dr. Wilson also reported his experience with the Lock-out valve *(16)* at the 1999 AUA meeting in Dallas. Although, his follow-up was only 6 mo, no patients experienced autoinflation or difficult deflation.

SEVERE CORPORAL FIBROSIS

Severe bilateral corporal fibrosis because of priapism, Peyronie's disease, trauma, infection, or repeated penile placement are the most complicated penile implant insertion cases with less than satisfactory outcomes. These cases have a high incidence of complications (erosions, infections, penile shortening) and prolonged surgical time. Often, abandon of the inflatable penile prosthesis placement or placement of malleable penile prosthesis is performed as an alternative to the reinsertion of an inflatable implant. Several novel surgical techniques and instruments such as "cutting-type" dilators have been described in the past, but limited satisfactory reports of clinical outcome with inflatable penile implants are available. Controlled, sharp, corporal tissue excision with extended bilateral corporotomies has been reported to provide a 94% rate of functioning implants, and a high satisfaction rate measured by IIEF *(17)*. This technique allows the placement of a standard Mentor α-1 penile prosthesis providing the longest and widest device possible in these patients who have already lost significant length.

Mentor Corporation, recently introduced the *Mentor α-1 narrowbase inflatable prosthesis (see* Fig. 5). The α-1 NB cylinders are 3.7 mm less in diameter than the standard α-1, and have a narrower base (10 mm), with an acute tubing exit angle of 22.5°, and 9-mm rear-tip extenders, which allows easier placement within a fibrotic and scarred corpora. The use of this device in corporal fibrosis has a high rate of functioning implants (100%) with no infections or malfunctions with a 10-mo follow-up *(18)*.

PATIENT SATISFACTION

Contemporary data indicates that surgical success with inflatable penile prosthesis is 95–97% *(19,20)*, but surgical success not always represents patient satisfaction. To answer this important question, we

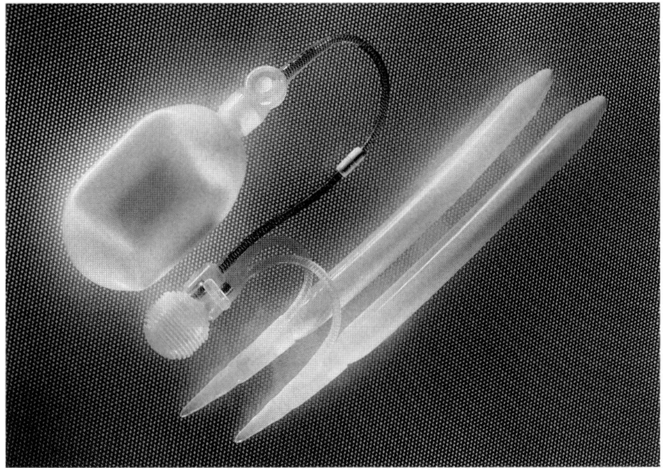

Fig. 5. Mentor α-1 narrow base inflatable prosthesis. The α-1 NB cylinders are 3.7 mm less in diameter than the standard α-1, with a narrow base (10 mm), acute tubing exit angle (22.5°), and 9-mm rear-tip extenders.

Table 1
Literature Experience with Mentor α-1 Inflatable Penile Prosthesis

	Goldstein (22)	Randrup (23)	Garber (24)	Goldstein (21)	Wilson (9) (O/E*)
Year	1993	1993	1996	1997	1999
No Pts	112	333	150	434	410/971
Mechanical failure (%)	4	2.7	0	2.5	5.6/1.3
Infection rate (%)	2	1.2	1	2.8	3.9/4.8
Follow-up (mo)	27	15.4	19	22.2	
Reoperative rate (%)	9	4.5	2	6.9	21.7/2.78
Complications	7.5	3	9.2		

*(Original/enhanced)

performed a Phase-2, multiinstitutional, large-scale retrospective study, with independently analyzed medical records and questionnaire data from consecutive eligible patients of seven physician investigators *(21)*. In those that returned the questionnaire, 89% of patients with Mentor α-1 prosthesis fulfilled expectations as a therapy for erectile dysfunction, including 28% who claimed fulfillment as expected, 31% better than expected and 30% much better than expected. Satisfaction responses of 80% or greater were noted regarding intercourse ability and confidence, device rigidity, and function. Interestingly, implantation of inflatable penile prosthesis did not result in 80% or greater satisfaction responses in partner relationship changes (as judged by the patient), partner feelings about the relationship (as judged by the patient), or increased confidence in social activities and work. Such information is important when providing preoperative counseling to patients so that postoperative expectations will be appropriate.

CONCLUSION

The introduction of penile prosthesis in 1973 revolutionized the field of sexual medicine. Urologists in conjunction with basic and clinical researchers have established the contemporary knowledge of erectile function and dysfunction allowing the development of less invasive alternatives to the penile implant. Recently, with the advent of oral therapy, the number of medical visits and urologic referrals for the sexual medical problem of erectile dysfunction has increased. Patients with erectile dysfunction are now advised to proceed first with step-care treatment for erectile dysfunction where first-line therapy (oral agents, vacuum devices, and sex therapy) and second-line therapy (intraurethral and intracavernosal pharmacologic administration of vasoactive agents) are completed prior to any consideration for surgical treatment.

Should penile prosthesis insertion be indicated, the Mentor α-1 inflatable penile prosthesis is the device that provides the widest diameter penile erection during inflation and the lowest mechanical failure rate. The Bioflex material has an increased abrasion resistance and higher tensile strength than silicone-based devices. The superior outcome data in terms of mechanical reliability have remained durable over the last 10 yr. In addition, the Mentor α-1 has a high degree of patient satisfaction.

REFERENCES

1. Scott FB, Bradley WE, Timm GW (1973) Management of erectile dysfunction: use of implantable inflatable prosthesis. *Urology* 2:80.
2. Merrill DC (1983) Mentor Inflatable penile prosthesis. *Urology* 22:504.
3. Scott FB, Byrd GJ, Karacan I, Olsson P, Beutler LE, Attia SL (1979) Erectile impotence treated with an implantable, inflatable prosthesis. *JAMA* 241:2609.
4. Pescatori ES, Goldstein I (1993) Intraluminal device pressures in 3-piece inflatable penile prosthesis: the "pathophysiology" of mechanical malfunction. *J Urol* 149:295–300.
5. Hackler RH (1986) Mentor inflatable penile prosthesis: a reliable device. *Urology* 28:489.
6. Whalen RK, Merrill DC (1991) Patient satisfaction with Mentor inflatable penile prosthesis. *Urology* 37:531.
7. Brooks MB (1988) 42 months experience with Mentor inflatable penile prosthesis. *J Urol* 139:48.

8. Merrill DC (1988) Clinical experience with the Mentor inflatable penile prosthesis in 301 patients. *J Urol* 140:1424.

9. Wilson SK, Cleves MA, Delk JR (1999) Comparison of the mechanical reliability of Original and enhanced mentor alpha I penile prosthesis. *J Urol* 162:715–718.

10. Steinkohl WB, Leach GE (1991) Mechanical complications associated with Mentor inflatable penile prosthesis. *Urology* 38:32.

11. Kabalin JN, Kessler R (1988) Five-year follow-up of the Scott inflatable penile prosthesis and comparison with semirigid penile prosthesis. *J Urol* 140:1428.

12. Earle CM, Watters GR, Tulloch AGS, Wisniewski ZS, Lord DJ, Keogh EJ (1989) Complications associated with penile implants used to treat impotence. *Aust New Zeal J Surg* 59:959.

13. Montague DK (1990) Penile prosthesis implantation: special considerations. *Int J Impot Res*, suppl, 2:3.

14. Woodworth BE, Carson CC, Webster GD (1991) Inflatable penile prosthesis: effect of device modification on functional longevity. *Urology* 38:533.

15. Goldstein I, Geffin M, and the Mentor Lock-Out Valve study Group. Prevention of auto-inflation in the Mentor Alpha-1 three piece inflatable penile prosthesis: preliminary results of the Lock-Out Valve Study. 1999 AUA Meeting.

16. Wilson SK, Delk JR, Van Buren, Dhabuwala CB. Early results with new Lock-out Valve to prevent auto inflation of Mentor Alpha 1 penile prosthesis. 1999 AUA Meeting.

17. Geffin M, LaSalle M, Patel R, Krane RJ, Goldstein I. Clinical outcome of Alpha-1 three piece inflatable penile prosthesis insertion in patients with bilateral severe corporal fibrosis. 1998 AUA Meeting.

18. Hakim LS, Pham H. Initial clinical experience with the Mentor alpha-one narrow base inflatable penile prosthesis: an effective option for the management of severe corporal fibrosis. 1999 AUA Meeting.

19. Merril DC (1989) Mentro inflatable penile prosthesis. *Urol Clin North Am* 16:51–66.

20. Furlow WL, Motley RC (1988) The inflatable penile prosthesis: clinical experience with a new controlled expansion cylinder. *J Urol* 139:945–946.

21. Goldstein I, Newman L, Baum N, Brooks M, Chaikin L, Goldberg K, et al. (1997) Safety and efficacy outcome of Mentor Alpha-1 inflatable penile prosthesis implantation for impotence treatment. *J Urol* 157(3):833–839.

22. Goldstein I, Bertero E, Kaufman JM. Witten FR, Hubbard JG, Fitch WP, et al. (1993) Early experience with the first pre-connected 3-piece inflatable penile prosthesis: The Mentor Alpha-1. *J Urol* 150:1814–1818.

23. Randrup E, Wilson S, Mobley D, Suarez G, Mekras G, Baum N (1993) Clinical experience with Mentor Alpha I inflatable penile prosthesis. *Urology* 42(3):305–308.

24. Garber BB (1996) Inflatable penile prosthesis: results of 150 cases. *Br J Urol* 78(6):933–935.

25. Carson CC, Mulkahy JJ, Govier FE, and the AMS 700 Cs study group (2000) Efficacy, safety and patient satisfaction outcomes of the AMS 700CX inflatable prosthesis: results of a long-term multicenter study. *J Urol* 164:376–380.

13 Peyronie's Disease and Penile Implants

Steven K. Wilson, MD, FACS
and Kevin L. Billips, MD

CONTENTS

INTRODUCTION
PATHOGENESIS
MEDICAL TREATMENT
SURGICAL MANAGEMENT
PROSTHESIS PLACEMENT IN PEYRONIE'S DISEASE
THE MODELING PROCEDURE
CAVEATS TO THE MODELING PROCEDURE
CONCLUSION
REFERENCES

INTRODUCTION

Peyronie's disease is a benign condition characterized by the formation of fibrotic plaques of the tunica albuginea. The French physician Francois Gigot De La Peyronie first described the condition in 1743. Dr. Peyronie suggested the etiology of the condition might be chronic irritation from sexual activity or an inflammatory (venereal) disease *(1)*. Two-hundred fifty years later, medical authorities are still puzzled over the etiology of this annoying condition.

Peyronie's first theory of continued minor sexual trauma is considered today the most likely cause of the disease. The consensus thinking is that the repeated trauma of sex is thought to injure the collagen

From: *Urologic Prostheses:*
The Complete, Practical Guide to Devices, Their Implantation and Patient Follow Up
Edited by: C. C. Carson © Humana Press Inc., Totowa, NJ

composition of the tunica albuginea. This results in induration and the formation of fibrous plaques that decrease the elasticity of the corpora and cause curvature or constriction of the penis during erection (2). Despite this widely held opinion, the majority of patients cannot give a history of injury to the penis during sexual activity

Discrete penile injuries can produce lesions indistinguishable from Peyronie's disease. Trauma must not be the only factor, however, since large series have shown inherited predisposition. In addition, there is a 20% association with Dupuytens contractures of the hand, a disease inherited via autosomal dominant gene.

The disease affects middle-aged men primarily, although reports of patients as young as 19 yr old have been recorded. The prevalence in American men is between 0.3% and 1%, but could well be higher as a result of patient embarrassment and limited reporting by physicians. In our series of more than 2000 penile implants, Peyronie's disease was the cause of implantation in between 8–12% of patients.

PATHOGENESIS

Peyronie's disease is thought to have two phases. Initially, the inflammatory phase is characterized by penile pain on erection, progressive curvature or narrowing of erection, and palpable plaque formation. The second, or chronic phase sets in after 1–1.5 yr. The patient will demonstrate a stable, painless plaque that rarely may even calcify. The plaque causes shortening of the affected side of the penis upon tumescence as the noncompliant tunica fails to stretch with erection. Clinical expression results in various appearances. The patient may complain of curvature, hourglass deformity, or portions of the penis with restricted girth when erect. Seventy percent of the curvatures are dorsal. The less-frequent downward curvatures and lateral deflections are more likely to interfere with intercourse and tend to precipitate physician consultation. The patient may have combinations of all of the aforementioned descriptions resulting in corkscrew or a flail penis.

The reported association of Peyronie's disease and erectile dysfunction (ED) is variable. In reviewing the literature, it is difficult to ascertain whether the erectile dysfunction is because of the lack of decent tumescence (proximal or distal flaccidity) or whether the reported dysfunction is owing to angulation or flail penis. Many authorities have attempted to link the condition with accelerated aging of the penile arterial vessels or associated venoocclusive disease precipitated by the noncompliant plaques. Suffice it to say, the older the Peyronie's patient, the more likely he is to report significant sexual dysfunction (3).

Clinical Diagnosis and Patient Evaluation

Patient evaluation should consist of a detailed history of symptoms including presence and duration of pain, quality of erection before and after onset of symptoms, progression of symptoms, and the degree of penile deformity. Finally, the physician should determine the degree of impairment associated with sexual intercourse because of the pain (early phase) or curvature (late). A history of trauma or instrumentation may be found in a minority of patients.

Genital examination could include a measurement of stretched penile length and girth at the time of initial evaluation because many of these men will complain of penile shortening after any surgical intervention. The hands and feet could be examined for any signs of Dupuytrens palmar fibromatosis because as many as 20% of Peyronie's patients will have this disease.

It is important to document ED for the clinical record particularly if prosthesis implantation is contemplated. An injection of vasoactive material will demonstrate the curvature, hourglass deformity, distal flaccidity, or diffuse inelasticity of the tunica. Prostaglandin E1 (PGE1) is the drug of choice for stimulating the erection and, at the same time, the physician can obtain penile duplex ultrasonography to document associated arterial disease or venous leakage. In addition, visualization of the extent of plaque formation may be possible with the ultrasound. Duplex ultrasonography is very useful for scientific documentation of Peyronie's disease and the degree of sexual impairment *(4)*. In the United States, ultrasound documentation makes it easier to obtain precertification in today's managed care environment, particularly, if prosthesis implantation is contemplated. Nocturnal penile tumescence (NPT) may be useful for the same purpose. NPT may show poor filling and a decreased number of erectile events *(3)*. In patients complaining of distal floppiness or flail penis, NPT commonly will record inequality of tumescence between the proximal and distal penis.

MEDICAL TREATMENT

Most non-surgical therapies are directed at the acute stage of the disease. Oral therapies include vitamin E (an antioxidant known to prevent fibrosis) *(5)*, aminobenzoate potassium (Potaba, used to limit collagen synthesis) *(6)*, colchicine (decreases collagen synthesis and increases collagenase activity) *(7)*, and Tamoxifen [decreases production of transforming growth factor-β (TFG-β)] *(8)*. Most investigations with these agents have been small series, not well controlled or blinded, and the results are inconclusive.

Radiation therapy had a period of popularity, but is thought by most now to cause more harm (penile fibrosis) than good *(9)*. Intralesional injections have been tried with steroids, collagenase, verapamil *(10)*, and interferon *(11)*, with limited success in small series. In our practice, we give generous doses of reassurance and rarely use any therapy for the acute phase. If the patient is insistent, we prefer vitamin E, which is cheap and well tolerated, and may alleviate the pain *(12)*.

SURGICAL MANAGEMENT

Surgery must be directed at correction of the problem after the acute inflammation stage. Several criteria have been established as guidelines for considering surgical intervention. Peyronie's disease should be past the acute inflammatory stage. Lack of pain on erection and stability of degree of impaired erection signify passage into the chronic state. Continuation of pain indicates prolongation of the acute phase and surgery should be delayed. The progression of penile curvature and associated ED should have been stable for at least 3 mo. Finally, difficulty with intercourse must be well documented in the clinical record. Some authorities believe surgery of Peyronie's disease for palpable lump or curvature without sexual limitations is meddlesome *(13)*.

Once the disease is fully stable, the surgical management consists of either correction of the penile deformity or insertion of a penile prosthesis in those patients who have significant concomitant ED. The method of correction of the penile deformity is very controversial. Surgical intervention without prosthesis implantation can be broken into two categories with numerous technical variations contained within each group. The first category includes operations, which shorten the long side by corporal plication or removing ellipses—the Nesbit procedure. The second group of operations lengthens the short side. This is accomplished by incision/excision of the plaque with grafting (natural tissue or synthetic).

In patients with associated impotence, Peyronie's disease is corrected by prosthesis implantation with modeling and/or plaque incision/excision with or without grafting (natural tissue or synthetic). The scope of this chapter does not allow for a full discussion of all the surgical options for Peyronie's disease. Discussion will focus on the appropriate use of penile implant surgery in the treatment of Peyronie's disease after a brief mention of the other two categories of operation.

Shortening the Long Side—Nesbit Procedure

Originally described in 1965, Nesbit initially reported his operation as a surgical correction of congenital penile curvature in young men *(14)*.

The technique was to shorten the long side of the penis by plication with sutures or elliptical excision and closure. Pryor reported the application of the Nesbit operation to Peyronie's disease with good results *(15)*. Unfortunately, penile shortening complaints and postoperative development of ED troubled long-term follow up of Nesbit procedures for Peyronie's disease. Pryor, in a recent publication, claims experience has diminished these drawbacks because of a combination of better patient education ("the shortening is rarely troublesome and was only more than 2 cm in 17 of 359 men") *(14)* and better preoperative assessment of associated ED (availability of penile duplex doppler).

Lengthening the Short Side—Plaque Excision and Grafting

Devine and Horton introduced this popular method of treatment of Peyronie's disease in 1974 *(16)*. The plaque is excised and the tunical defect is replaced with a dermal graft obtained from the abdominal wall, buttock, thigh, or iliac crest skin. Austoni, in a series of 481 patients, reported disturbing long-term results with the Devine operation citing the need for further corrective surgery (17%) and a high percentage of erectile impairment (20%) *(17)*. Other covering tissues have been, substituted for dermis, e.g., dura, tunica vaginalis, fascia, cadaver fascia, split thickness skin, and vein. Synthetic grafts have been fashioned from a variety of fabrics, with GoreTex and Dacron being the most popular. Currently, the method of Lue utilizing autologus saphenous vein is in vogue *(18)*.

Patients need to be informed of the risk to their erectile function with all these procedures. Some patients will have their deformity corrected, but then need pharmacological treatment to achieve an erection *(19)*. If the resulting impotence is severe enough, they may require secondary placement of penile implant. Discussion about the risks of injury to the neurovascular bundle and subsequent decreased penile sensation also needs to be emphasized. Although loss of penile sensation is rare as a complication of plaque resection, ED seems fairly common *(20)*. In our opinion, plaque excision and grafting is a formidable surgical exercise. For patients in whom a complex repair will be necessary, we suggest the option of a penile prosthesis *(21)*.

For patients without ED, we prefer simple Nesbit plication of the short side. We avoid Nesbit elliptical excision or the more-extensive surgery of plaque excision and grafting. Our feeling is that any procedure that interrupts tunical integrity by incision may lead to impairment of erections. Furthermore, because 70% of Peyronie's disease occurs on the dorsum of the penis, elliptical excision or plaque resection usually requires elevation of the neurovascular bundle. Dorsal nerve injury and consequent decreased penile sensation may be possible during dissection of the neurovascular bundle. This complication, unfortunately, has no treatment.

PROSTHESIS PLACEMENT IN PEYRONIE'S DISEASE

Men with both ED and Peyronie's disease should be considered as candidates for implant surgery. Penile prosthesis placement is most appropriate for men who have significant ED or flaccidity distal to the plaque. Because the other surgical interventions aforementioned may be associated with penile shortening and subsequent development or exacerbation of ED, the candidate pool for prosthesis placement can be expanded to include men with short penises and partially impaired erectile function. In our practice, all men over age fifty are counseled to consider prosthesis placement. Many of these older men will demonstrate poor rigidity distal to the plaque after an injection of PGE1. Additionally, penile duplex Doppler may demonstrate impairment of penile blood flow (arterial or venous) in these older subjects increasing the possibility that impotence will result as a result of any straightening procedure without prosthesis placement.

Malleable Prosthesis and Peyronie's Disease

The simple placement of a pair of semirigid rods may be enough to straighten the curvature without the need for adjunctive procedures. Insertion of the semirigid prosthesis is not difficult because the Peyronie's plaques are subtunical and usually do not obliterate the corporal space. In our view, prosthetic girth is a more important factor than prosthesis length in correction of curvature by malleable prosthesis placement. It is important to dilate to 14 mm to facilitate 13-mm prosthesis insertion. This additional girth, compared to smaller diameter rods, helps overcome the deformity because girth (i.e., axial rigidity) not length, is believed to be the most important contributing factor to penile rigidity *(22,23)*. Proper sizing of the length of the rods in a Peyronie's patient is imperative. If there is any question of intracorporal measurements, the shorter length should be chosen. In fact, Mulcahy advises 0.5-cm downsizing of rod implants in all patients to facilitate comfort and concealment *(24)*. Despite the apparent shortening of one side of the penis because the Peyronie's disease, the operating surgeon should attempt to place rods of the same length in Peyronie's patients. Failure to place equal lengths or placement of excessively long rods may lead to pain and difficulty bending (and thus concealing) the penis. In our view, sizing of malleable prostheses is more crucial than size selection of inflatable ones.

Many different styles of semirigid or malleable prosthetic devices have been successfully utilized in Peyronie's disease, even soft silicone rods without imbedded wires *(25)*.

After implantation of rods, it is necessary to judge the straightening and glandular deviation. Ghanem reported 7 of 20 *(35%)* patients not satisfied with straightening by rod implantation (Duraphase, Acuform, AMS 600) alone *(26)*. In 19–42% of Peyronie's patients, it will be necessary to perform plaque incision along with semirigid prosthesis placement *(27,25)*. If the deformity persists after insertion of the rods, it is easy to overcome by relaxing incision(s) with electrocautery on the short side. This results in lengthening of the concavity and resultant straightening. The tunical defects do not require closure—the gaping of the tunica adds the required length to the short side to accomplish straightening.

Use of subcoronal incision for placement of the malleable prosthesis in Peyronie's disease has an advantage over the traditional penoscrotal approach *(28)*. The subcoronal incision will facilitate degloving of the penis if additional straightening by incision of the short side is needed. The subcoronal incision is only useful in circumcised men or uncircumcised men who consent to circumcision in association with the implantation. Preputial edema and eventually phimosis will result from use of the incision with failure to circumcise. If circumcision is not possible, the ventral penile incision described by Mulcahy is an excellent substitute *(24)*.

Two Piece Hydraulic Prosthesis in Peyronie's Disease

There are no reported series utilizing either the Mentor Mark II or the AMS Ambicor for patients with Peyronie's disease. In our experience, these prostheses are compromised in both flaccidity and erection, and less mechanically reliable *(29)* when compared to three-piece devices. There seems to be little reason to ever implant a compromised two-piece device in anybody *(30)*, particularly a Peyronie's patient in whom maximum rigidity is needed to facilitate straightening.

Three Piece Inflatable Prosthesis in Peyronie's Disease

One of the original inventors of the AMS inflatable penile prosthesis, F. Brantley Scott, conceived the modeling procedure *(31)*. Dr. Scott had noted orthopedic surgeons molding broken bones over metal rods and postulated that the concept might be useful in correction of Peyronie's disease deformities. Unfortunately, during Dr. Scott's active clinical years, the AMS cylinder was composed entirely of silicone and did not have a fabric insert to limit distention. The limitless distensibility of the pure silicone cylinder did not provide enough rigidity against deformation to act as a fulcrum for disrupting the plaque. Knoll, in 1990, reported results with AMS inflatable penile prosthesis in 67 men with Peyronie's disease without modeling. Half of the patients also required a relaxing incision through the tunica albuginea at the point of greatest concave curvature *(32)*.

In 1985, AMS introduced the PND (nondistensible) cylinder to facilitate plaque resection over an inflatable implant. The CX (controlled expansion) cylinder was an improvement over the PND and utilized three-layer construction with a layer of woven polyurethane fabric (similar to Dacron) sandwiched between two silicone layers. This allowed limited girth expansion, but restricted aneurysmal dilatation when the cylinder was bent. These distention-controlled cylinders now had sufficient rigidity to be used in overcoming Peyronie's disease. In addition, a second inflatable implant manufacturer, Mentor, introduced a new three-piece implant with cylinders constructed of Bioflex (similar to polyurethane). These cylinders were partially distensible and also generated enough rigidity to permit modeling. Whereas Dr. Scott conceptualized the modeling procedure, Wilson and Delk reported the first large series in 1994 using AMS CX, AMS Ultrex, Mentor IPP, and Mentor Alpha cylinders *(33)*.

At the turn of the new century, the modeling procedure for treatment of Peyronie's disease has achieved worldwide acceptance *(34)*. In the *Textbook of Erectile Dysfunction* Ralph and Pryor wrote, "operative modeling of the penis over a prosthesis may look and sound horrible but gives a good result in any deformity" *(14)*. In another recent textbook, Hellstrom considered the approach effective, but, "rather simplistic" *(35)*.

THE MODELING PROCEDURE

Mentor α-1, AMS 700 CX inflatable cylinders of equal lengths are placed and the 2-cm corporotomies are closed with multiple interrupted sutures of 00 Vicryl or Dexon. Running closure of the corporotomy seems more likely to rupture during modeling and the resultant corporotomy edges are more fragmented than if interrupted suturing is used.

Mentor α NB, AMS 700 Ultrex cylinders are not recommended *(36)*. In our experience, the α NB cylinder may develop cylinder aneurysm and rupture through the suddenly gaping corporotomy, if the corporotomy sutures break (*see* Fig. 1A). The Ultrex, because it is a lengthening cylinder, does not generate enough rigidity to overcome the curve without additional tunical incision *(37)*. Montague reported corporoplasty was necessary in 10

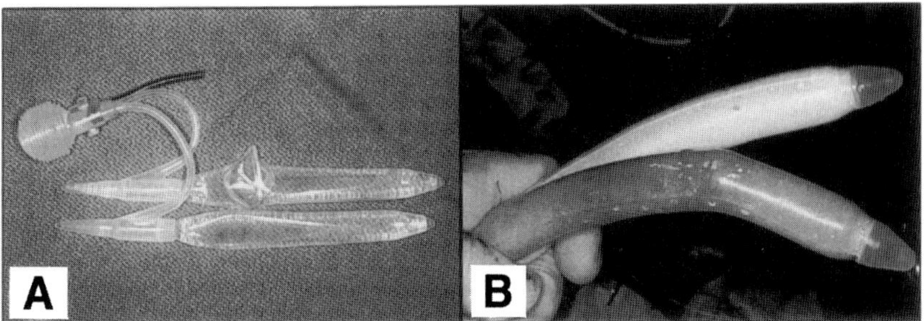

Fig. 1. (**A**) Alpha NB cylinder with aneurysm caused by modeling. (**B**) CX cylinder with abrasion of outer silicone layer caused by modeling.

of 38 patients undergoing the modeling procedure if Ultrex cylinders were utilized. This compared with none of 34 patients requiring plaque incision if the CX cylinders were implanted prior to the modeling procedure *(38)*. Fishman and the authors of this chapter had similar poor experiences using Ultrex cylinders in Peyronie's disease *(39)*.

After cylinder placement, the reservoir is placed in the prevesical space and filled with normal saline. The system is connected and the prosthesis is inflated to the absolute maximum distention. The pump is not placed in the scrotum, but remains outside the incision during the modeling manipulations. The tubing from the cylinders is crossclamped with rubber shod hemostats to prevent pump damage from excessive backpressure. During the modeling, it is also advisable to protect the corporotomies by grasping the base of the penis with thumb on one corporotomy and first two fingers on the other. This supports the corporotomies preventing suture rupture during the maximum inflation and subsequent modeling (*see* Fig. 2).

The penis is forcibly bent in a direction opposite the curvature in a maneuver similar to breaking a twig with both hands. The pressure on the penis is maintained for 90 s. The modeling probably results in splitting and rupturing of the fibrotic plaques. The operating surgeon can often hear snapping or feel movement of the cylinders as previously nonpliant tunica is expanded. After 90 s, the clamps protecting the pump are removed and additional fluid may be added to the cylinders. Addition of fluid to cylinders previously maximally distended is now possible because some expansion of restricted corporal capacity has occurred. The clamps are then reapplied, corporotomies reprotected and the modeling procedure is repeated for another 1.5 min (*see* Fig. 3). There is nothing magical about 90 s, but persistence of bending, rather than a quick fracture achieves straightening. Requiring a set amount of

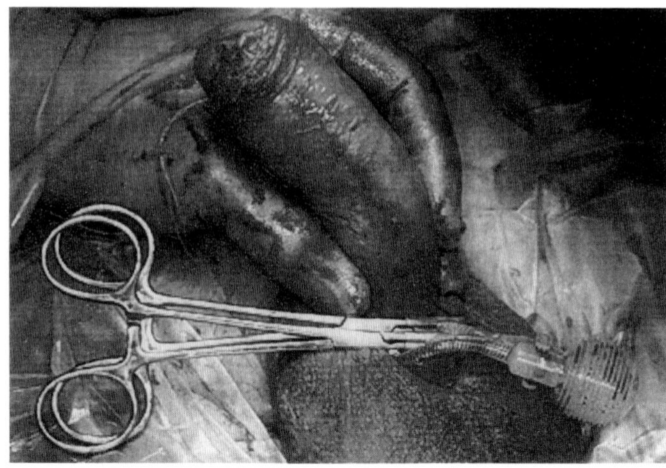

Fig. 2. Protection of corporatomies with thumb and fingers. Protection of pump with rubber shod clamps.

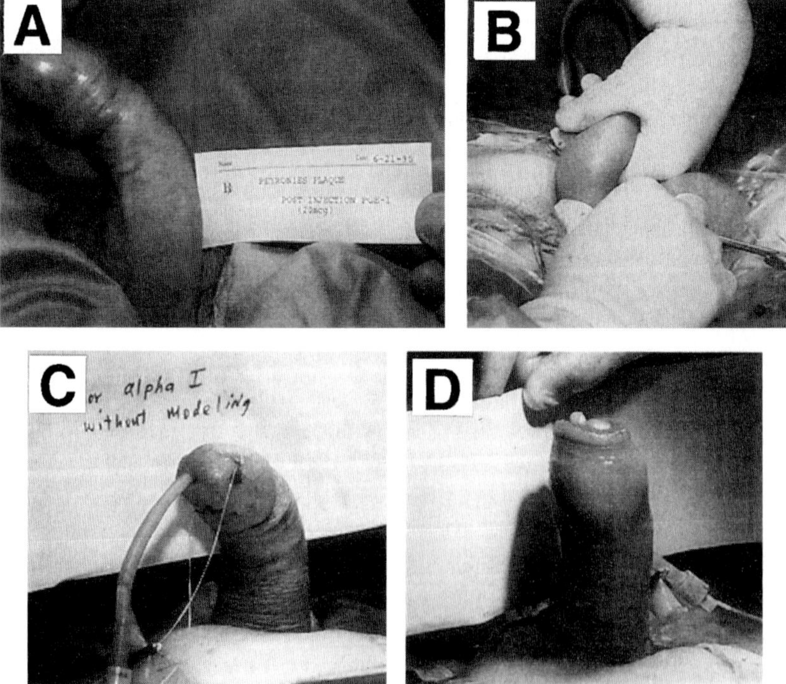

Fig. 3. The modeling procedure. (**A**) Preop appearance after PGE injection. (**B**) Modeling. (**C**) Implant alone without modeling. (**D**) After two modeling sessions.

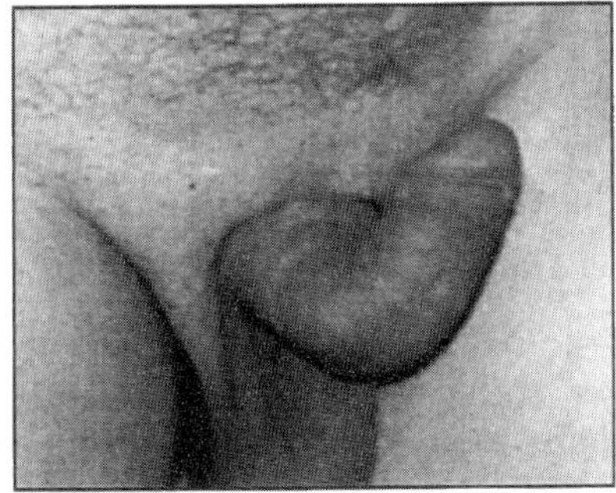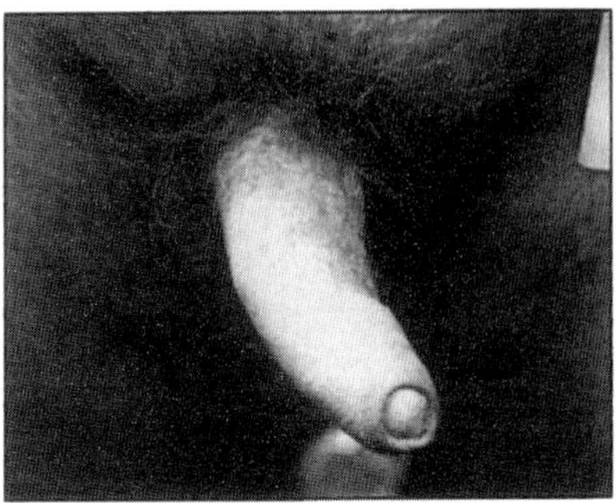

Fig. 4. Pre-op (left) and Post-op (implant and modeling).

time enforces the discipline that repeated long periods of modeling are necessary to the success of the straightening.

After two modeling sessions, the prosthesis is deflated completely. The assistant pulls on the suture guides of the cylinders and the surgeon reinflates the prosthesis only as far as necessary to achieve a rigid erection. This complete deflation and subsequent reinflation accomplishes two important features. It allows reseating of the cylinders distally improving the appearance. It also allows the surgeon to evaluate the straightening at the degree of inflation that will be used by the patient. Maximum inflation is used for correction of the curvature, but the patient will never maximally inflate. He will only inflate enough to achieve a satisfactory erection and it is at this inflation level, not maximum inflation that the results of the modeling procedure should be judged.

A wise man once said, "perfect is the enemy of good." It is not necessary to continue to repeat the modeling procedure in order to achieve an absolutely straight erection. Twenty *(37)* to thirty *(32)* degrees (*see* Fig. 4) is considered a successful operation and will be appreciated by the patient. Adequate straightening is usually achieved with two modeling sessions. Rarely is a third session necessary. Early in our experience, modeling was occasionally not sufficient to achieve satisfactory results. The original paper reported 8% of patients required additional corporplasties. In these patients, the penis was degloved and relaxing incisions were made on the short side. Gaping of the transverse incision resulted in lengthening along the concave side of the curvature and consequent penile straightening. The incision was left open or closed in a Heineke-Mikulicz fashion. Our latest experience of the last 5 yr shows incisions are not necessary *(12)*.

Tunical incision after prosthesis insertion is best accomplished with the electrocautery. If electrocautery is needed for relaxation of curva-

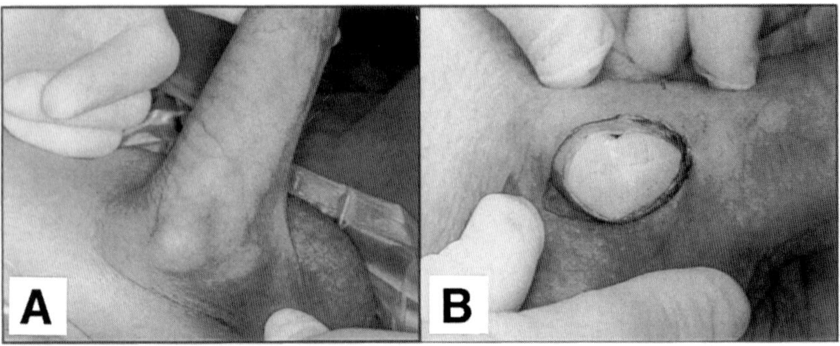

Fig. 5. (**A**) Aneurysm at site of tunical incision. (**B**) Aneurysm at surgery.

ture not overcome by the modeling procedure, cutting or coagulating current should be set below 35 W because cylinders can be injured with higher settings *(40)*. Deflation of the cylinder prior to incision gives an additional measure of safety. All but the smallest tunical defects will require closure or synthetic graft. Mentor or Ultrex cylinders having less distention control compared to CX cylinders, always require implant coverage to prevent subsequent aneurysm. The CX should be less likely to require a graft because its inside fabric wrap controls its expansion. Nevertheless, our experience has shown that coverage/closure of wide gaps is still needed with CX (*see* Fig. 5) to prevent subsequent bulging of the cylinder through the tunical defect.

There are several reasons to avoid corporoplasty if possible. Corporoplasty at penile prosthesis implantation increases operative time and usually requires mobilization of the neurovascular bundle. Simultaneous use of graft material with penile prosthetic devices has been reported to increase the risk of infection *(41)*. For these reasons, it is fortunate that corporplasty and graft coverage is only rarely necessary.

Complications of the Modeling Procedure

Review of our large database of more than 200 Peyronie's patients subjected to three-piece implant and the modeling procedure shows a consistent urethral laceration complication rate of 4%. We had hoped limiting the modeling to two or three sessions would decrease the incidence, but it has remained constant through the years. The laceration always occurs at the meatus and is heralded by blood at the meatus and visual confirmation of the cylinder tip in the fossa navicularis (*see* Fig. 6). On several occasions, we have detected (perhaps, caused) the urethral laceration upon modeling at the teaching visit (see #6 caveat later). If urethral laceration occurs, it is necessary to remove the offending cyl-

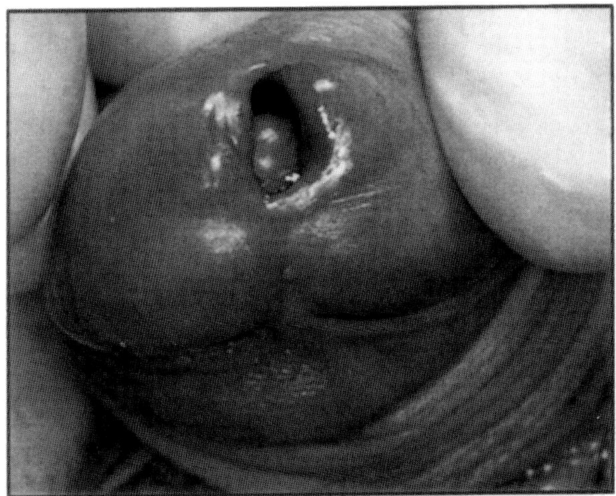

Fig. 6. Urethral rupture occurring as a complication of modeling.

inder and tie off the tubing leaving the rest of the prosthesis in place. It is not necessary (in fact, it is not possible) to close the meatal laceration and the urethral Foley catheter is only used for 2–3 d. The cylinder can be replaced after 8 wk by an additional surgery. Some patients are content with a one cylinder erection, particularly if the Mentor cylinder was utilized.

Corporal rupture at a site other than the sutured corporotomy occurs in 2% of patients. In our experience it is much more likely to occur in Asian men. It can be corrected by degloving the penile skin and repairing the defect. Increased corporal pain, edema, and petechias are common accompaniments to the modeling procedure and can be resolved with nonsteroidal antiinflammatories.

We had wondered if modeling might cause the implant to need revision more often for mechanical failure or medical cause (including reoperation for straightening) when compared to patients implanted but not modeled. We recently reported long-term follow-up of 200 patients in whom the modeling procedure was utilized for correction of the Peyronie's disease after implantation with both AMS CX and Mentor α cylinders. We compared revision free survival experience of these implants with 900 similar implants in non-Peyronie's patients. There was no significant difference in survival experiences of the two study cohorts when all reasons for revision were considered together. No significant difference in survival was observed in revision as a result of mechanical failure, patient dissatisfaction, infections, and medical/iatrogenic reasons. There was a difference in the mechanical survival

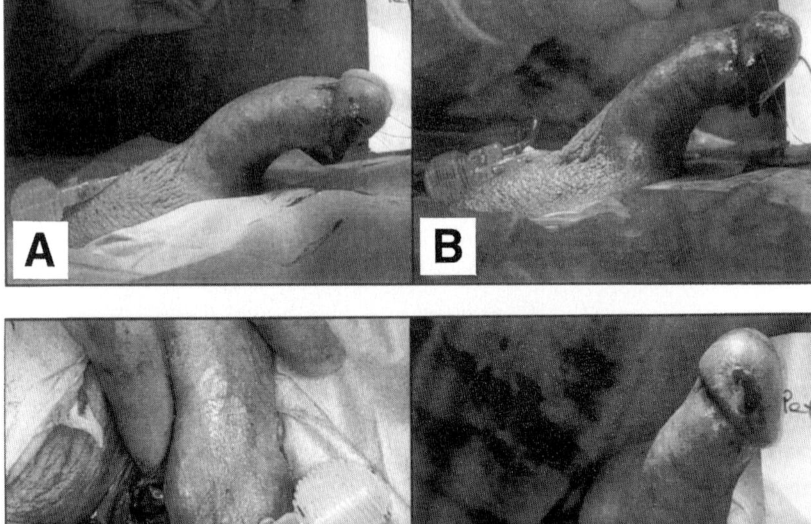

Fig. 7. (A) Implant only. **(B)** After first model. **(C)** Corporotomy rupture. **(D)** After two modeling sessions.

between the two devices used in the modeling procedure. In the Peyronie's patients, mechanical survival of the Mentor α-1 was superior to that of the AMS 700CX *(42)*. There was no difference in the mechanical reliability between the devices in the non-Peyronie's patients indicating that the trauma of modeling may predispose the AMS cylinder to future failure. We have previously reported detection of occasional abrasion of the outer layer of silicone after modeling *(see* Fig. 6B) *(24)*.

CAVEATS TO THE MODELING PROCEDURE

1. Before placement of the pump in the scrotum and closure, it is important to verify that the corporotomies have remained closed, since the modeling procedure often results in suture breakage *(see* Fig. 7).
2. Straightening continues for over 1 yr with use of the implant and the patient can be counseled to inflate and model at home if his result was less than satisfactory. The most difficult curvature to correct is in the patient with a short penis and distal upward curvature *(see* Fig. 8). It is difficult to gain enough purchase on the end of the short penis to effectively model. Fortunately, residual curvature after implantation in these patients always corrects with time and implant usage.

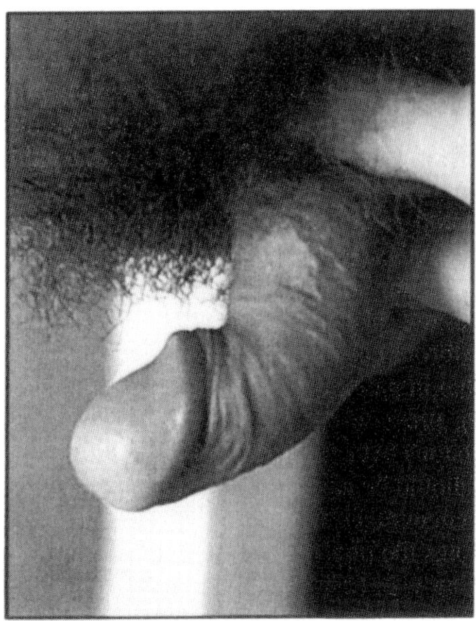

Fig. 8. The most difficult Peyronie's presentation for the Modeling Procedure—A short penis with distal curvature.

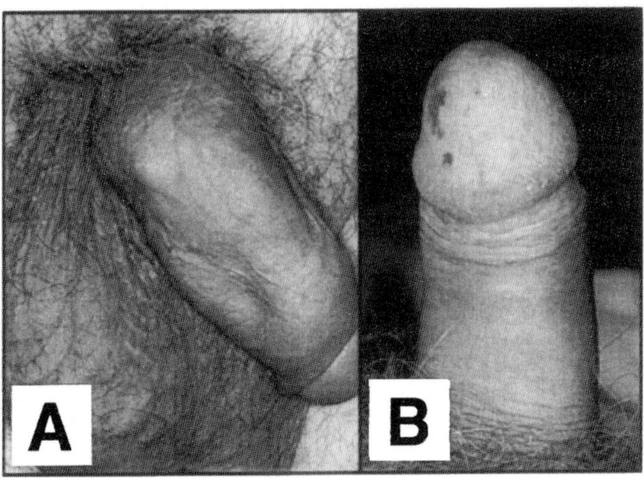

Fig. 9. After placement of prothesis and modeling, the penis is curved in flaccidity but straight in erection. (**A**) Flaccid; (**B**) Erect.

3. The patient must be warned that his penis will be curved in flaccidity, but straight in erection (*see* Fig. 9). This is exactly the opposite of his condition prior to implantation with the modeling procedure. The flaccid penis now has some rigidity because of the cylinders. The cylinders act as a stent and the penis will be carried in flaccidity with a curve to short side.

4. Early in our experience, a few patients are not satisfied with initial straightening. In these patients, we attempted another modeling under anesthesia 3–12 mo after the original implantation. The secondary procedure was not successful, probably because of the restrictive tethering of the fibrous capsule that had formed around the cylinders. We now know that in patients who are unhappy with the straightening of the modeling procedure, it is necessary to make secondary tunical relaxing incisions over the inflated prosthesis.

5. The patient should be advised to wear his penis pointed cephalad initially. This encourages capsule development around the cylinders, which promotes the physiologic cephalad extension of the erection.

6. At the teaching visit (usually 4–6 wk), the penis is modeled with the patient fully awake. Sometimes capsule development around the cylinder may have started, which would inhibit straightening. At this early stage of capsule formation, it is possible to feel reexpansion of the tunica accompanying this maneuver.

CONCLUSION

Success with surgical correction of Peyronie's disease depends upon the patient's ability to have sexual intercourse with a straightened penis. If the patient has ED after the Nesbit procedure or plaque resection and graft replacement, the operation can be considered a failure even though penile straightening has been accomplished. If any degree of tumescence problem is present before surgery, careful consideration for inflatable prosthesis placement and the modeling procedure should be discussed with the patient. In our view, this treatment has the greatest potential for trouble-free straight erections for the rest of his life. For urologic surgeons, penile prosthesis implantation with the modeling procedure is straightforward with minimal complications. More importantly, our patients receive a straightened penis useful for coitus.

REFERENCES

1. De la Peyronie F (1743) Sur quelques obstacles pui s'opposent a l'ejaculation naturelle de la semence. *Mem Acad R Chir* 1:425.
2. Ralph DJ, Mirakian R, Pryor JP, Bottazzo GF (1996) The immunological features of Peyronie's disease. *J Urol* 157:282–284.
3. Stecker JF, Devine CJ (1985) Evaluation of erectile dysfunction in patients with Peyronie's disease. *J Urol* 132:680–681.

4. Ralph DJ, Hughes T, Lees WR, Pryor JP (1992) Pre-operative assessment of Peyronie's disease using colour Doppler sonography. *Br J Urol* 69:629–632.

5. Scardino PL, Scott WW (1949) The use of tocopherols in the treatment of Peyronie's disease. *Ann NY Acad Sci* 52:390–396.

6. Shah PJR, Green NA, Adib RS, et al. (1983) A multicentre double-blind controlled clinical trial of potassium para-aminobenzoate (Potaba) in Peyronie's disease. *Prog Reprod Biol* 9:47–60.

7. Akkus E, Carrier S, Rehman J, et al. (1994) Is colchicine effective in Peyronie's disease ? A pilot study. *Urology* 44:291–295.

8. Ralph KJ, Brooks MS, Bottazo GF, Pryor JP (1992) The treatment of Peyronie's disease with tamoxifen. *Br J Urol* 70:648–651.

9. Hall SJ, Basile G, Bertero EB, et al. (1995) Extensive corporal fibrosis after penile irradiation. *J Urol* 153:372–377.

10. Levine LA, Merrick PF, Lee RC (1994) Intralesional verapamil injection for the treatment of Peyronie's disease. *J Urol* 151:1522–1524.

11. Benson RC, Knoll LD, Furlow WL (1991) Interferon alpha 2 b in the treatment of Peyronie's disease. *J Urol* (abstract); 145:1342.

12. Pryor JP, Farell CF (1983) Controlled clinical trial of vitamin E in Peyronie's disease. *Prog Reprod Biol* 9:41–45.

13. Ralph D, Pryor JP (1999) Peyronie's disease. In: Carson C, Kirby R, Goldstein I, eds., *Textbook of Erectile Dysfunction,* Oxford: Issis Med. Media, pp. 515–517.

14. Nesbit RH (1965) Congenital curvature of the phallus: report of three cases with description of corrective operation. *J Urol* 93:230–232.

15. Pryor JP, Fitzpatrick JM (1979) A new approach to the correction of the penile deformity in Peyronie's disease. *J Urol* 122:622–623.

16. Devine CJ, Horton CE (1974) Surgical treatment of Peyronie's disease with a dermal graft. *J Urol* 111:44.

17. Austoni E, Colombo F, Mantovani, et al. (1995) Chirugia radicale e conservazione dell'erezione nella malantia di La Peyronie. *Arch Ital Urol Nefrol Androl* 67:359–364.

18. Brock G, Kadioglu A, Lue TF (1993) Peyronie's disease: a modified treatment. *Urology* 42:300–304.

19. Dalkin BL, Carter MF (1991) Venogenic impotence following dermal graft repair for Peyronie's disease. *J Urol* 146:849–851.

20. Melman A, Holland TF (1979) Evaluation of the dermal graft inlay technique for the surgical treatment of Peyronie's disease. *J Urol* 120:421–422.

21. Berger RE (1995) Remodeling for Peyronie's disease with implants. *Contemp Urol* 7:45–49.

22. Udelson D, Nehra A, Hatzichristos DG, et al. (1998) Engineering analysis of penile hemodynamics and structural dynamic relationships: Part 1 clinical implications of penile tissue mechanical properties. *Int J Impot Res* 10:15–24.

23. Mulcahy JJ (1997) Overview of penile implants. In: Mulcahy JJ, ed., *Topics in Clinical Urology, Diagnosis and Management of Male Sexual Dysfunction,* New York: Igaku-Shoin, pp. 218–230.

24. Mulcahy JJ (1999) Unitary inflatable, mechanical and malleable penile implants. In: Carson C, Kirby R, Goldstein I, ed., *Textbook of Erectile Dysfunction,* Oxford: Issis Med Media, pp. 413–421.

25. Subrini L (1984) Surgical treatment of Peyronie's disease using penile implant: survey of 69 patients. *J Urol* 132:47–49.

26. Ghanem HM, Fahmy I, El Meliegy A (1998) Malleable penile implants without plaque surgery in the treatment of Peyronie's disease. *Int J Impot Res* 10:171–173.

27. Eigner EB, Kabalin, JN Kessler R (1991) Penile implants in the treatment of Peyronie's disease. *J Urol* 145:69–71.
28. Wilson S (1997) Penile prosthesis implantation: pearls pitfalls and perils. In: Helstrom WJG, ed., *Male Infertility and Sexual Dysfunction,* New York: Springer, pp. 529–549.
29. Dubocq F, Tefill EL, Gheiler HL, Dhabuwala CB (1998) Long-term mechanical reliability of multicomponent inflatable penile prosthesis: comparison of device survival. *Urology* 52:277–281.
30. Lue TF (1998) Editorial in *J Urol* 160:1728.
31. Wilson SK (1997) Management of Penile Implant Complications. In: Mulcahy JJ, ed., *Topics in Clinical Urology, Diagnosis and Management of Male Sexual Dysfunction,* New York: Igaku-Shoin, pp. 231–253.
32. Knoll LD, Furlow WL, Benson RC (1990) Management of Peyronie's disease by implantation of inflatable penile prosthesis. *Urology* 36:406–408.
33. Wilson SK, Delk JR (1994) A new treatment for Peyronie's disease: modeling the penis over an inflatable prosthesis. *J Urol* 152:1121–1123.
34. Pacik D, Kumstat P, Dolezel J, Turjanica M (1995) Implantation of an inflatable penile prosthesis as an effective alternative to surgery of impaired erection. *Rozhledy v Chirugii* 74:363–366.
35. Hellstrom WJG, Bryan WW (1997) Treatment of Peyronie's disease. In: Helstrom WJG, ed., *Male Infertility and Sexual Dysfunction,* New York: Springer, pp. 481–491.
36. Wilson SK, Cleves MA, Delk JR (1996) Ultrex cylinders: problems with uncontrolled lengthening (the "S"-shaped deformity). *J Urol* 155:135–137.
37. Kowalczyk JJ, Mulcahy JJ (1996) Penile curvatures and aneurysmal defects with the Ultrex penile prosthesis corrected with insertion of the AMS 700 CX. *J Urol* 156:398–401.
38. Montague DK, Angermeier KW, Lakin MM, Ingleright BJ (1996) AMS 3-piece inflatable penile prosthesis implantation in men with Peyronie's disease: comparison of CX and Ultrex cylinders. *J Urol* 156:1633–1635.
39. Fishman IJ (1996) Editorial comment. *J Urol* 156:1635.
40. HakimLS, Kulaksizoglu H, Hamill BK, et al. (1995) Guide to safe corporotomy incisions in presence of underlying inflatable penile cylinders: Results of in vitro and in vivo studies. *J Urol* 155:366–368.
41. Knoll LD, Furlow WL, Benson RC, et al. (1995) Management of nondilatable cavernous fibrosis with the use of a downsized inflatable penile prosthesis *J Urol* 153:366–368.
42. Wilson SK, Cleves MA, Delk JR (2001) Long term follow up a treatment for Peyronie's disease: modeling the penis over an inflatable penile prosthesis. (2001). *J Urol* 165:825–829.

14 Current Approach to Penile Prosthesis Infection

John J. Mulcahy, MD

CONTENTS

INTRODUCTION
INCIDENCE
PERIOPERATIVE PREPARATION
SIGNS AND SYMPTOMS
TREATMENT
REFERENCES

INTRODUCTION

Rapid advances in the pharmacology of erectile dysfunction (ED) have brought more patients in to inquire about alternatives and commence treatment. Viagra is now a household word with name recognition similar to Coca-Cola and Nike. Patients will more commonly choose the least-invasive effective treatment for this disorder, namely, oral medication. However, severe cases of ED may not respond to medications or, in patients with severe scarring of erectile bodies, deformed or limited erections may result. Penile implants are still a very effective therapy with the highest satisfaction rate of all ED alternatives among both patients and partners *(1)*. They are effective when medication has failed and will overcome the effects of scar tissue in the corpora cavernosa to both straighten and strengthen inadequate erections. When implants were introduced almost three decades ago, repairs were common *(2)*. Vendors have eliminated or reinforced areas that would be a source of wear or malfunction, and surgeons have developed more-reliable

From: *Urologic Prostheses:*
The Complete, Practical Guide to Devices, Their Implantation and Patient Follow Up
Edited by: C. C. Carson © Humana Press Inc., Totowa, NJ

techniques of implantation, thus reducing the incidence of reoperation. Repair rates of 15% at 5 yr and 30% at 10 yr are now realistic *(3)*.

INCIDENCE

One of the most serious problems associated with penile implant insertion is infection. The organisms usually enter the wound at the time of surgery, but there have been reports of seeding of the implant from distant sources via hematogenous spread *(4)*. The incidence of infection has been reported from 0.6% *(5)* to 8.9% *(6)*, but, in most series, averages between 1%–3%. With repairs, the reported infection rate seems to be higher at 13.3% in a series reported by Jarow *(7)*. He also noted the incidence was even higher at 21.7% when reconstructive procedures were necessary. Thomalla et al.'s series confirms this with a 37% infection rate during tertiary procedures *(6)*. In cases of reoperation for repair or reconstruction, the presence of scar tissue, reduced blood flow, longer operating time, or the introduction of foreign materials such as Gortex or Dacron to rebuild the tunica albuginea can promote bacterial growth. Patients with diabetes mellitus tend to have a higher rate of many types of infection as elevated glucose levels in tissues are a good culture medium. Jarow's series found no statistically significant increase in implant infections among diabetics *(7)*, but Fallon and Ghanem reported a threefold-greater incidence of infection in their diabetic population receiving a penile implant *(1)*. Bishop et al. suggested that glycosylated hemoglobin levels, an indicator of control of diabetes mellitus in the patient's recent past, could be used as a predictor of infection associated with penile prosthesis implantation in this group *(8)*. However, in a large series reported by Wilson et al., glycosylated hemoglobin and other parameters such as glucose level and insulin dependence could not reliably indicate the development of postoperative infection *(9)*. Patients with spinal cord injury and a neurogenic bladder tend to have a higher incidence of urinary tract infections and decubitus skin ulcers. Prosthesis infections were not more common in this group, according to Diokno and Sonda *(10)*. However, Wilson and Delk found a ninefold-greater incidence of infection among spinal cord-injured men in their series *(11)*, and Dietzen and Lloyd related a 30% incidence of infection in this patient population receiving a penile implant *(12)*. This group of patients also has diminished or absent sensation in the genital region and the incidence of erosion of a penile implant, especially the semirigid rod type, is higher than in the nonneurogenic population as a result of friction and excessive pressure against the device, which would cause pain and discomfort if sensitivity was intact. Whether an infection led to the erosion, or a primary erosion is associated with concomitant infection, is not documented in many cases. Patients with a renal transplant can undergo penile implant placement without a greater chance of device infection *(13)* and this author has placed a penile implant in three patients after cardiac transplantation without complications. The brand of prosthesis, incision site, number of components, or prior pelvic irradiation do not seem to influence the incidence of implant infection. Licht et al. found infection present on wound culture in up to 40% of penile implant cases operated on for mechanical malfunction *(14)*. There was no clinical suspicion of infection in any of these patients. Nine percent of these subsequently developed a clinical infection.

The performance of procedures such as herniorrhaphy, circumcision, or hydrocele repair in association with penile implant surgery has been implicated in an increased incidence of infection. Fallon and Ghanem *(1)*, and Thomalla et al. *(6)*, reported higher infection rates with simultaneous circumcision. If one is considering such a combined operation, the initial procedure should be insertion of the penile implant with closure of that incision. A second incision and performance of the associated procedure can then be undertaken. This reduces the duration of the open wound for penile implant placement and avoids possible contamination from manipulation of the scrotum, foreskin, or other body surface during the associated procedure. Endoscopic procedures such as transurethral prostatectomy or internal urethrotomy should not be performed simultaneously with prosthesis insertion.

PERIOPERATIVE PREPARATION

Prior to the surgery urinary tract infections should be treated. The urinary tract is usually not entered during implant surgery, but spilling of urine on the operative field during the procedure is a possibility. Sterilizing the urinary tract in neurogenic bladder patients is sometimes difficult and unpredictable, and placing a catheter in this group during surgery might be prudent to prevent leaking of urine onto the operating field. The skin of the pelvis and genital region should be inspected for infected lesions such as furuncles, sebaceous cysts, or comedomes. These should be removed prior to the antiseptic skin prep lest they be expressed during manipulations of the penile and scrotal skin during prosthesis insertion. Thoroughly washing the pelvis and perineal area with a strong antiseptic soap solution for 3 d at home prior to the surgery is recommended. The surgical site is shaved in the operating room prior to the procedure, and this is followed by a strong iodine skin prep. An alternative antiseptic prep is used if the patient is allergic to iodine.

Laminar flow systems and the surgical isolation bubble (SIBS) may reduce contamination, but are costly, cumbersome, and rarely used.

The most common organism associated with prosthesis infections in all series has been coagulase negative staphylococcus (*Staphylococcus epidermidis*). In a recent series, 58% of infections were caused by this organism *(15)*. Other bacteria less commonly seen are Pseudomonas aeruginosa, *Proteus mirabilis, Serratia marcessens, Escherichia coli, enterococcus,* and *Staphylococcus aureus. Candida albicans* and anaerobic bacteria such as bacteroides fragilis have been rarely isolated when infected implant wounds have been cultured. Most urologists use prophylactic antibiotics in association with penile implant placement. The literature has demonstrated the effectiveness of these agents in potentially contaminated procedures involving bowel, gallbladder, and uterus where bacteria may enter the wound from an open viscus *(16)*. However, no study has been reported documenting the effectiveness of use vs nonuse of prophylactic antibiotics during penile implant surgery. Infectious disease specialists have taken issue with their use in these circumstances. The operating field is sterile, numerous other precautions have been taken to prevent infection, and using such agents is expensive, may promote the development of resistant organisms, and may lead to toxic reactions or the development of allergies. If one decides to use prophylactic antibiotics, they should be started prior to the incision, usually with placement of the intravenous line. Ideally, this should occur 1 h prior to opening the wound so that tissue levels will be optimal at the start of the procedure. They should be continued for 48 h after surgery. By that time, the wound is sealed and contaminating organisms can no longer gain entry. Vancomycin and an amino glycoside are the best combination to empirically treat prosthesis infections. *S. epidermidis,* the most common pathogen, is eradicated 99% of the time by Vancomycin. The gram negative organisms, which are less commonly found, are neutralized by the amino glycoside. Excessive and prophylactic use of Vancomycin, however, is discouraged because of the potential for resistant organisms developing. Alternative prophylactic antibacterials are a quinolone or a third-generation cephalosporin, which have reasonable coverage against both *staphylococcus* and gram negative organisms. Prophylactic antibacterials for eradicating anaerobic and fungal infections are rarely used because of their infrequent occurrence. During the procedure, the wound is frequently irrigated with a solution containing antibacterials such as bacitracin and gentamicin. An Asepto syringe dispenses this cleansing solution rapidly and forcefully to wash away any organisms that might stray into the operative field.

SIGNS AND SYMPTOMS

Signs and symptoms associated with an infected penile implant may be subtle or dramatic. Fishman and Scott found that 56% of infections are manifest within 7 mo of surgery, 36% between 7 and 12 mo, and 2.6% after 5 yr *(17)*. Increasing pain, cellulitis, fever, fluctuance, and drainage from the wound, especially after squeezing on parts of the device, are signs of an acute infection. An exposed part of the prosthesis must be considered infected. Low-grade pain that never improves or increases in intensity postoperatively, persistent fixation of the pump to the scrotal wall, and increasing white blood cell count or sedimentation rate are indications of possible infection. When the diagnosis of infection is questionable, a trial of an oral quinolone antibiotic in high doses for 4–6 wk may be informative. If pain or swelling improve and then recur when the antibiotic is discontinued, then an infection is likely present.

The question sometimes arises as to when one should explore the prosthesis for a suspected infection. Certainly, an exposed part, persistent purulent drainage, cellulitis that does not recede, progressive fixation of the pump to the scrotal wall, and increasing pain are definite indications for surgical intervention. If fluctuance over a part such as the pump is present, the skin over the fluctuant area may be prepped with iodine solution and the fluid carefully aspirated and sent for culture. Not all fluctuant areas represent infection as seromas can form around prosthesis parts as well.

TREATMENT

When an infection is certain or highly suspect, removal of the implant is necessary. Oral or systemic antibacterials alone will not eradicate the organisms. With time, a sheath of fibrosis surrounds the prosthesis, as part of the body's healing process. This has relatively poor blood supply, thus limiting the inflammatory response in the area. In addition, many bacteria produce a biofilm or slime, which surrounds the implant and provides a hiding place for bacteria where antibiotics are less able to diffuse. Bacteria may also adhere to the surface of some implants. If the implant is removed, healing will occur with time. If purulent infected material is contained within the corpora cavernosa, irrigating drains should be placed within these cavities and antibacterial washes continued for 72 h *(18,19)*. Vancomycin 1 gm/L and gentamicin 80 mg/L are used as the initial irrigants and 10 cm^3 are placed through each drain and left in place for 20 min 3x/d. At 48 h, culture and sensitivity reports

Table 1
Antiseptic Irrigating Solutions

- Antibiotics (Kanamycin-Bacitracin)
- Half-strength hydrogen peroxide
- Half-strength Betadine
- Pressure irrigation (water pic) with Igm vancomycin and 80 mg gentamicin in the 5-L irrigating solution
- Half-strength Betadine
- Half-strength hydrogen peroxide
- Antibiotics (Kanamycin-Bacitracin)

are available and more appropriate antibacterials can be substituted if necessary. Closing the wounds with these drains in place has resulted in less postoperative morbidity than leaving the wound open to granulate with wet to dry dressings. After 6 mo when the wound has healed and inflammation resolved, one can return for reinsertion of a new prosthesis. However, because of the scar tissue that has now formed in the corpora cavernosa, creating cavities for the cylinders will be difficult, and the resulting erection will have a ventral bowing and be noticeably shorter (about 2-in shorter) than that created with the original implant.

A new concept has evolved in recent years termed rescue or salvage. The implant is removed completely, together with all foreign materials such as sutures, Gortex, or Dacron. The wound is thoroughly washed with a series of irrigating solutions listed in Table 1. A red rubber Robinson catheter is used to instill the solutions to the extremities of the corporal bodies and all other cavities containing foreign body parts (*see* Fig. 1). The operative field is changed including new gloves, gowns, drapes, and instruments and a new prosthesis is placed at the same procedure with closure of the wound without drains. The success rate using this technique was 82% in 55 patients with a mean follow-up of 3 yr *(15)*. The antibiotic solution is designed to neutralize bacteria, hydrogen peroxide gives superoxygenation to eradicate anaerobes, the iodine solution kills 99% of organisms, and the pressure wash loosens and washes away the slime or biofilm produced by many bacteria. Variations of salvage have been used, but the principles of the most successful techniques have involved complete removal, washing, and immediate reinsertion *(20,21)*.

The rationale and success of salvage has been demonstrated in other medical areas where the presence of prosthetic or graft material is essential for the preservation of life or limb. Bandyk et al. found that infections of aortic vascular grafts were characteristically containing

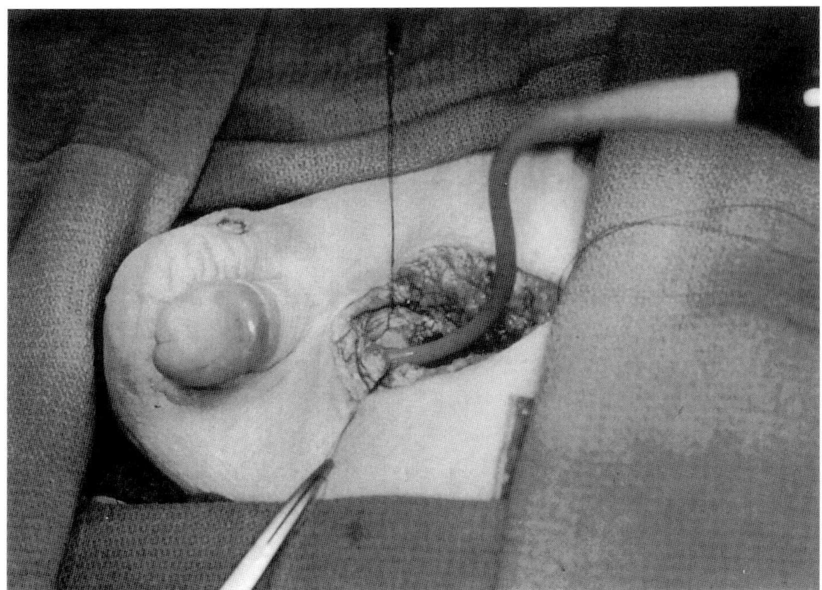

Fig. 1. A red rubber catheter is passed to all parts of the body which contained prosthesis parts. Copious amounts of irrigation are used through this catheter.

organisms of low virulence with few systemic symptoms and almost exclusively a result of *S. epidermidis (22)*. They successfully replaced 15 consecutive aortic grafts in situ with no recurrent graft infections. Hip prostheses *(23)* and prosthetic heart valves *(24)* have been salvaged with a 90% success rate. A theory for such good results in eradicating these infections involves the characteristics of *S. epidermidis*. The unique environment provided by a foreign body may enhance the ability of this organism and others to establish a foothold.

Local tissue trauma during insertion, the immediate microenvironment around the foreign body, which is acidic and hypovascular, and the appearance of a new surface with no intact cellular barrier provide opportunity for bacteria to adhere and grow *(25)*. A foreign material placed in the body usually acquires a thin fibrous tissue capsule composed of a variety of proteins *(26)*. This acellular surface coating may provide binding sites for otherwise nonpathogenic bacteria. Evidence shows that staphylococcal species adhere to foreign surfaces with much greater affinity than do other bacteria.

Parsons et al. removed penile implants that were painful and irrigated the wound with a solution of protamine and vancomycin before replacing a new prosthesis *(27)*. Systemic vancomycin was used pre- and postoperatively and a success rate of 90% in eradicating infection was achieved. Teloken et al. successfully salvaged three penile implants with a protocol using rifampin antibiotic irrigations *(28)*.

Delayed salvage has had comparable results. This involves removing the prosthesis, placing drains for wound irrigation, and returning in 72 h after the infection has been eradicated to place a new prosthesis. Cultures at the time of removal document that the appropriate antibiotics are being used and more specific antibiotics can be substituted at 48 h, if necessary. The prolonged hospitalization and second trip to the operating room are more costly, the cavities containing the cylinders have contracted, and the wound is difficult to close, especially in the thin patient, because of the inflammatory process present at this juncture, making delayed salvage less practical. Salvage procedures where parts of the device have been left behind have been less successful. Furlow and Goldwasser removed an infected pump and replaced it with a new pump in the opposite hemiscrotum leaving the cylinders in place *(29)*. Bacteria can migrate along tubing to other parts of the device and although infection may not be obvious at the time, symptoms may become evident in the future as bacterial propagation occurs. A success rate of 73% was seen with this type of procedure. Removal of a prosthesis or salvage should be performed promptly when infection is evident. To leave such a prosthesis in place, hoping infection will clear, may result in increased pressure within the penile shaft from edema and inflammation. Glans penis and distal corporal necrosis have been seen associated with infection and also in the absence of infection (*see* Fig. 2). This is usually a slowly progressive process resulting from diminished blood supply, not necessarily the infection itself. Prompt removal of the prosthesis helps take the pressure off the ischemic tissue, thus allowing more adequate tissue perfusion.

The avoidance of urethral catheters, the use of loose noncompressive dressings, and making longitudinal incisions parallel to the shaft of the penis, rather than circumferential incisions, will help avoid diminished distal blood flow, especially in high-risk patients such as those with advanced diabetes mellitus or severe peripheral vascular disease. Salvage has been successfully performed in patients with cylinder erosion to the external surface of the penis. In such cases, the entire device is removed, the wound cleansed as aforementioned, and a new device inserted. A distal corporoplasty is performed to reseat the cylinder on the previously eroded side more medially in a more secure location *(30)* (*see* Fig. 3). Consideration should also be given to using a pair of narrower cylinders in such a circumstance, because a tight girth fit may have contributed to the original erosion.

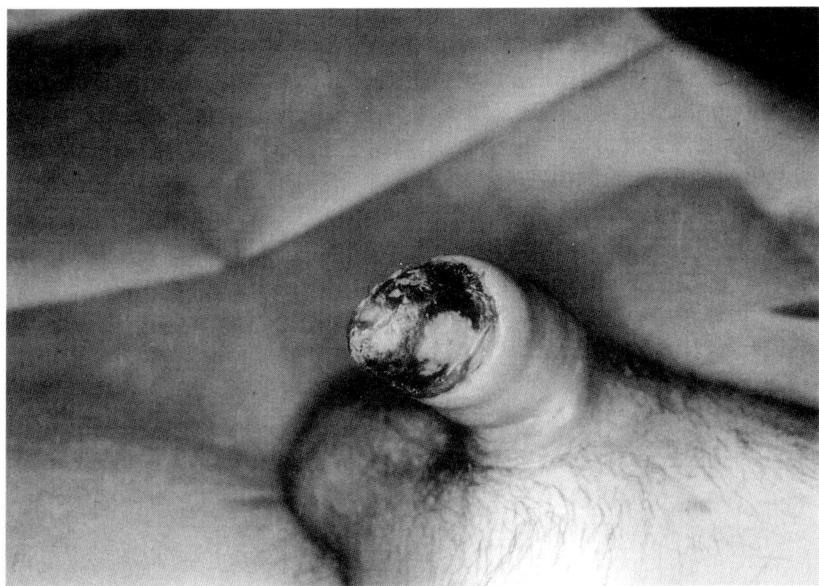

Fig. 2. Necrosis of the glans penis in a patient with Peyronie's disease and no vascular risk factors. Removal of the implant halted the progression of the necrosis. Cultures taken at the time of explant showed no growth.

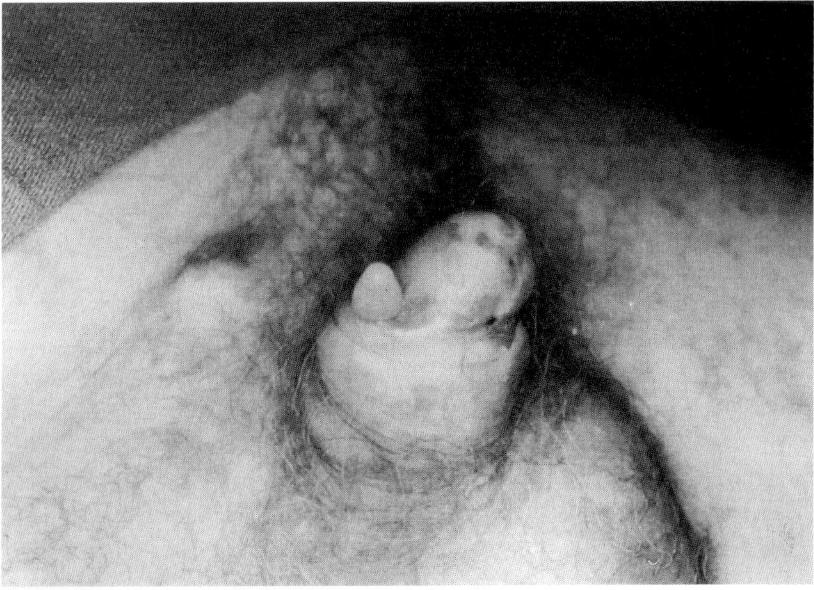

Fig. 3. Erosion of a penile implant cylinder. A successful salvage procedure combined with distal corporoplasty was performed to reseat the cylinder in its proper location.

Contraindications to salvage would include bilateral cylinder erosion into the urethra, necrotizing infections, severely toxic patients such as those in diabetic ketoacidosis or septicemia, and immunosuppressed patients. The greatest success with salvage has been in those patients in whom the infection is manifest long after surgery, is not associated with extensive cellulitis, and is caused by less-virulent organisms such as *S. epidermidis*. Salvage has been successful in those patients with extensive purulence and marked cellulitis caused by virulent organisms when preceded by abscess drainage and culture and appropriate systemic antibiotics for a number of days prior to the salvage procedure. In such cases, sterilization of the tissues with systemic antibiotics followed by sterilization of the cavity containing the prosthesis by the surgical irrigations has given a gratifying result.

Infection of a penile implant was once a catastrophic complication, which necessitated removal. Now, with salvage and reconstructive procedures, most infections can be successfully treated and patients restored to sexual function using the modality for treating erectile problems with the highest satisfaction and success rate, i.e., the penile implant.

REFERENCES

1. Fallon B, Ghanem H (1990) Sexual performance and satisfaction with penile prostheses in impotence of various etiologies. *Int J Impot Res* 2:35–42.
2. Apte SM, Gregory JG, Purcell MH (1984) The inflatable penile prosthesis, reoperation and patient satisfaction: a comparison of statistics obtained from patient record review with statistics obtained from extensive follow up research. *J Urol* 131:894–895.
3. Carson CC, Mulcahy JJ, Govier FE (1999) Efficacy and safety outcomes of the AMS 700 CX inflatable penile prosthesis: results of a long term multicenter study. *J Urol* 161 Suppl:259, Abstr 999.
4. Carson CC, Robinson CN (1988) Late hematogenous infection of penile prostheses. *J Urol* 139:50–52.
5. Montague DK (1987) Periprosthetic infections. *J Urol* 138:68–69.
6. Thomalla JV, Thompson ST, Rowland RG, Mulcahy JJ (1987) Infectious complications of penile prosthetic implants. *J Urol* 138:65–67.
7. Jarow JP (1996) Risk factors for penile prosthetic infection. *J Urol* 156:402–404.
8. Bishop JR, Moul JW, Sehelnik SA, Peppas DS, Gormley DS, McLeod DG (1992) Use of glycosylated hemoglobin to identify diabetics at high risk for penile prosthetic infections. *J Urol* 147:386–388.
9. Wilson SK, Carson CC, Cleaves MA, Delk JR (1998) Quantifying risks of penile prosthesis infection with elevated glycosylated hemoglobin. *J Urol* 159:1537–1540.
10. Diokno AC, Sonda LP (1981) Compatibility of genitourinary prostheses and intermittent self catheterization. *J Urol* 125:659–667.
11. Wilson SW, Delk JR (1995) Inflatable penile implant infection: Predisposing factors and treatment suggestions. *J Urol* 153:659–661.
12. Dietzen CJ, Lloyd LK (1992) Complications of intracavernous injections and penile prostheses in spinal cord injured men. *Arch Phys Med Rehab* 73:652–655.

13. Sidi AA, Peng W, Sanseau C, Lange PH (1987) Penile prosthesis surgery in the treatment of impotence in the immunosuppressed man. *J Urol* 137:681, 682.

14. Licht MR, Montague DK, Angermeier KW, Lakin MM (1995) Cultures from genitourinary prostheses at reoperation: Questioning the role of staphylococcus epidermidis in periprosthetic infection. *J Urol* 154:387–390.

15. Mulcahy JJ (2000) Long term experience with salvage of infected penile implants. *J Urol* 163:481, 482.

16. Nichols RL (1981) Use of prophylactic antibiotics in surgical practice. *Am J Med* 70:686–692.

17. Fishman IJ, Scott FB, Selim AM (1987) Rescue procedure: An alternative to complete removal for treatment of infected penile prosthesis. *J Urol 137:Suppl 202A:Abst* 396.

18. Maatmann TJ, Montague DK (1984) Intracorporeal drainage after removal of infected penile prosthesis. *Urology* 23:184, 185.

19. Kim JC, Lunati FP, Khan SA, Waltzer WC (1995) T-Tube drainage of infected penile corporeal chambers. *Urology* 45:514–515.

20. Kaufman JM, Kaufman JL, Borges FD (1998) Immediate salvage procedure for infected penile prosthesis. *J Urol* 159:816–818.

21. Fishman IJ, Scott FB, Selim A, Nguyen TA (1997) The rescue procedure: an alternative for managing an infected penile prosthesis. *Contemp Urol* 11:73–80.

22. Bandyk DF, Bergamine TM, Kinney EV, Seabrook GR, Towne JR (1991) In situ replcement of vascular prostheses infected by bacterial biofilms. *J Vasc Surg* 13:575–583.

23. Carlson AS, Josefsson G, Lindberg L (1978) Revision with gentamicin-impregnated cement for deep infections in total hip arthroplasties. *J Bone Joint Surg (AM)* 60A:1059–1064.

24. Slaughter L, Morris JE, Starr A (1973) Prosthetic valvular endocarditis: a 12 year review. *Circulation* 47:1319–1326.

25. Gristina AG, Giridhar G, Gabriel BL, Naylor PT, Myrvik QN (1993) Cell biology and molecular mechanisms in artificial device infections. *Int J Artif Organs* 16:755–763.

26. Ingraham FD, Alexander E Jr, Matson DD (1947) Synthetic plastic materials in surgery. *N Engl J Med* 236:362–368.

27. Parsons CL, Stein PC, Dobke MK, Virden CP, Frank DH (1993) Diagnosis and therapy of subclinically infected prostheses. *Surg Gynecol Obstet* 177:504–506.

28. Teloken C, Souto JC, Daros C, Thorell E, Souto CAV (1992) Prosthetic penile infection: Rescue procedure with rifamycin. *J Urol* 148:1905, 1906.

29. Furlow WL, Goldwasser B (1987) Salvage of the eroded inflatable penile prosthesis: A new concept. *J Urol* 138:312–314.

30. Mulcahy JJ (1999) Distal corporoplasty for lateral extrusion of penile prosthesis cylinders. *J Urol* 161:193–195.

15 Reoperation for Penile Prosthesis Implantation

Run Wang, MD and Ronald W. Lewis, MD

CONTENTS

INTRODUCTION
DIAGNOSIS
PATIENT PREPARATION
GENERAL SURGICAL PRINCIPLES
FIBROSIS
INFECTION
EROSION AND IMPENDING EROSION
POSITION PROBLEMS
MECHANICAL FAILURES
PAIN
CONCLUSION
REFERENCES

INTRODUCTION

Upon introduction to treat male erectile dysfunction (ED) in the 1970s, penile prosthesis implantation revolutionized our practice for managing ED. Even in the era of effective oral medications for ED, sales of penile prostheses have been relatively stable in the past decade *(1)*. It is possible to foresee the continuous need for penile prostheses as more and more patients are seeking treatment for ED, thanks to the recent media coverage and the improved knowledge of the general population about ED. The modifications and improvements of penile

From: *Urologic Prostheses:*
The Complete, Practical Guide to Devices, Their Implantation and Patient Follow Up
Edited by: C. C. Carson © Humana Press Inc., Totowa, NJ

prostheses have maximized the device's reliability and longevity. The 5-yr survival of some models has reached more than 92% *(2,3)*. It is our belief that the modern inflatable devices are very mechanically reliable. Reoperations for penile prosthesis implantation are now more likely for infection, patient dissatisfaction, or physician error than for mechanical breakdown. Before 1990, about 57% of the reoperations at the Mayo Clinic were for mechanical failure or device malfunction *(4)*. The mechanical failure of some current devices has been as low as 0.8%/yr for the first 3.5 yr and then 3.1% in the next 1.5 yr of observation *(2)*. However, reoperation for penile prosthesis implantation is a challenge even for the experienced prosthetic urologist. In this chapter, we discuss the techniques of reoperation for penile prosthesis implantation under different situations.

DIAGNOSIS

Establishment of diagnosis for patients who need reoperation is straightforward. A history of previous penile implantation with removal of the prosthesis and a simple physical evaluation of the patient will establish the diagnosis for penile fibrosis. The majority of patients with prosthesis infection will present with erythematous and fluctuant areas over the corporeal bodies and/or scrotal pump. Some patients may have drainage of pus from these areas, with or without fever. Erosion and impending erosion of implants can be easily identified by physical examination. For erosion of implants into the bladder and urethra, some imaging studies or cystoscopy may be needed. Mechanical failure will not be a diagnostic dilemma because the device will simply not produce a rigid penis suitable for intercourse. However, identifying the problematic parts of the device may not be established before the surgery. If the system is filled with diluted contrast material, pelvic X-ray will indicate complete loss of fluid. Pelvic X-ray may also reveal a break in the metal core in some semirigid devices, or malposition of components of a device; but this kind of conventional radiology study may not be accurate. Most prostheses are now filled with saline that will preclude evaluation by conventional radiology. As a matter of fact, some authorities do not believe that contrast medium would help the diagnosis of the cause of the device failure because the contrast would be absorbed after leaking from the device *(5)*. Aneurysms of cylinders, S-shaped deformity of cylinders, and SST deformity caused by inadequate cylinder length should easily be diagnosed by physical examination. Prolonged pain after penile implantation (more than 6 wk) can be very difficult to deal with because the etiology of this pain is not well understood. Subclinical infection, malposition of the device, and autonomic neuropathy in diabetes mellitus have all been proposed as explanations. Sometimes this prolonged pain can be caused by inappropriate sizing of the cylinders; i.e., they are too large in diameter or too long for the corporeal space. By using magnetic resonance imaging (MRI), Moncada et al. have reported that buckling of cylinders could be the cause of prolonged penile pain and reoperation to correct the buckling cylinder resolved the pain in all their cases *(6)*.

PATIENT PREPARATION

Patient education is one of the most important strategies to achieve patient and partner satisfaction for penile prosthesis implantation. This is particularly true for reoperation. It is imperative for the prosthetic urologist to ensure that the patient and partner have proper expectations and an understanding of common anticipated complications associated with a reoperation. Our previous study showed that patients who have had more than one reoperation should be prepared that they are more likely to need a third or fourth (or even more) reoperations *(7)*. The patient needs to be informed that reoperation, particularly the reoperation involving corporeal reconstruction, may have 10 to 20 times-higher infection rates *(8)*. The patients with diabetes should have their glycosylated hemoglobin (Hgb A1-C) checked, as a poorly controlled diabetic may not be suitable for a salvage procedure *(9)*. However, this is debatable because Wilson et al. did not find the association between diabetic control and prosthesis infection *(10)*. Patients with cavernosal fibrosis or scar should be informed that a replacement device will not reproduce the original cosmetic result and that penile shortening may occur. In patients who have had a prior urethral erosion or urethral tear during dilation, we warn them of the risk of reentry into the urethra and the potential need for temporary urinary diversion by means of a perineal urethrostomy or suprapubic cystotomy. Penile numbness may occur, particularly with an infrapubic approach for penile reimplantation. This numbness may be transient or permanent. Return of full sensation may take as long as 12–18 mo.

GENERAL SURGICAL PRINCIPLES

General principles are no different from those used in a primary penile implant except in certain situations, such as in a salvage operation (to be discussed later). For penile prosthetic surgery, the most common infecting organism is the opportunistic *Staphylococcus epidermidis* *(11)*. We routinely give 1 g cefazolin intravenously with the induction of anesthesia. However, if the patient is a diabetic or has a history of prior infection with the prosthetic device, the best antibiotic is a vancomycin-gentamicin regimen. We use a single dose of vancomycin (1 g intravenously) and gentamicin (5 mg/kg, intravenously) preoperatively. For a patient with multiple histories of prosthetic removal because of infection, 3 d of cephalexin preoperatively are also used to maximize the prevention of reinfection. We also suggest that these patients have a Hibiclens scrub every day for 3 d preoperatively.

The incision site is shaved after the induction of anesthesia. A 10–15 min surgical scrub with povidone-iodine is mandatory in our institute. The surgeon and all assistants will have 10 min standard surgical scrub. Povidone-iodine solution is applied to the surgeon's hands before surgical gloves are worn or povidone-iodine solution is used between the glove layers for double gloving. A Foley catheter is inserted to facilitate urethral identification. If the patient has had multiple infections and is uncircumcised, we prefer to perform a circumcision before revision of the penile prosthesis, allowing time for it to heal. We do not like to perform a circumcision at the time of surgery unless a subcoronal approach is being used for a semirigid or self-contained inflatable device. Even under those conditions, if the foreskin shows any signs of infection, placement of the prosthesis should be delayed until this infection is cleared. If a penoscrotal or infrapubic incision is to be used, we do not believe there is a need for circumcision. However, we routinely obtain the patient's consent for possible need of circumcision, particularly if reseating of the cylinder tip in the corpus cavernosum under the glans penis is needed or degloving of penile skin is necessary for complex penile implantation.

The choice of surgical approach varies according to the condition that requires reoperation. A study by Garber and Marcus demonstrated that the infection rate was not different when scrotal or infrapubic surgical approaches were used *(12)*. We recommend use of a bipolar electrode for electrocoagulation of bleeding vessels to decrease the possibility of injury to neural and arterial structures. This is not mandatory if the penile neurovascular anatomy is well understood by the surgeon and care is taken during the dissection. We like to have a handheld Doppler unit available in case there is concern about the penile arterial supply.

The vancomycin-gentamicin regimen is given for 24-h postoperatively. Oral cefazolin or ciprofloxacin is given thereafter for 2–3 wk to patients who underwent reoperations for a noninfection cause, and for 4–6 wk to patients who underwent reoperation as a result of infection or for a complex reoperation *(9,11,13)*.

FIBROSIS

The most common and difficult problem in dealing with reoperation of patients with penile implants is corporeal fibrosis. The etiologies for corporeal fibrosis are Peyronie's disease or its treatment, priapism, penile trauma, and intracavernosal injection. However, the most common corporeal fibrosis in reoperative prosthetic surgery is caused by the removal of a previously implanted device secondary to infection or erosion *(13–15)*. After removal of an infected penile prosthesis, corporeal fibrosis can be very severe and fibrosis contraction will then result in a shortened penis. Reimplantation of penile prosthesis cylinders into such a scared corporeal body becomes a technical challenge in prosthetic urology. However, successful reimplantation surgery can be obtained by keeping the following four steps in mind. These include: 1) ideal corporeal dilation; (2) appropriate choice of prosthesis; 3) complete closure of the corpora cavernosa; and 4) maximizing penile length.

Techniques to manage fibrotic corpora vary according to the fibrotic severity, the location, and the surgeon's preference and experience. We often use combination incisions, such as an infrapubic and circumcision-like incision for penile degloving for safe and accurate corporeal dilation (*see* Fig. 1). Certainly, multiple openings in the corpora allow for better access to dissect or serially dilate intracorporeal fibrotic tissue. Sometimes, a plane between the fibrous scar tissue and the tunica albuginea can be developed with sharp dissection. However, we found that in many cases, a complete bivalving of the dense fibrotic corporeal tissue is necessary with coring out of the fibrotic tissue under direct vision and sharp dissection to make a suitable space for a penile device. This technique allows us to avoid urethral injury and has been very successful in the majority of our complex cases. We also found that Carrion-Rossello cavernotomes could be very helpful in the dilatation of the scarred corpora (*see* Fig. 2). These cavernotomes are sized 9–12 mm with cutting rasp-like surfaces, which enhance passage through the fibrotic tissue. Some prosthetic urologists use careful scissor dissection to create a narrow cavity adjacent to scar tissue, which can be achieved with Metzenbaum scissors by dissecting scar away from the tunica albuginea of the corpus cavernosum or by bluntly dissecting through scar with the scissors *(15)*. After a narrow cavity is created down to or near the ischial tuberosities, the Otis urethrotome can be used for sharp incision of the tissue in a direction away from the urethra. However, great care should be taken not to cut through the tunica albuginea. This technique requires experience to know the direction of the crus, and

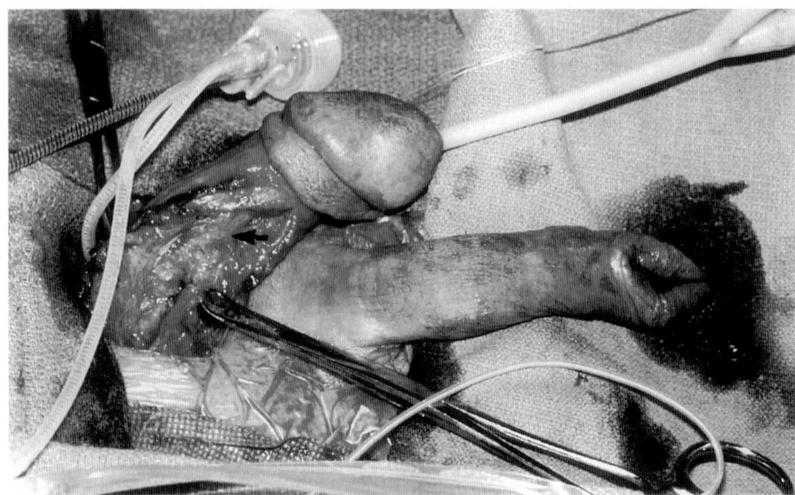

Fig. 1. Two-incision approach very often necessary to operate on the patient with severe fibrosis. The upper and lower Allis clamps are on the edge of the corpora cavernosa. The excised fibrotic tissue that has been removed by direct dissection is marked with an arrow. The two incisions that have been used in this case are an infrapubic incision and a circumcision incision allowing for full exposure of the corpora cavernosa tissue. In this particular slide, the left cylinder has been placed and this photograph is prior to placement of the right cylinder. The attached pump is shown also in the picture after placement of the left cylinder.

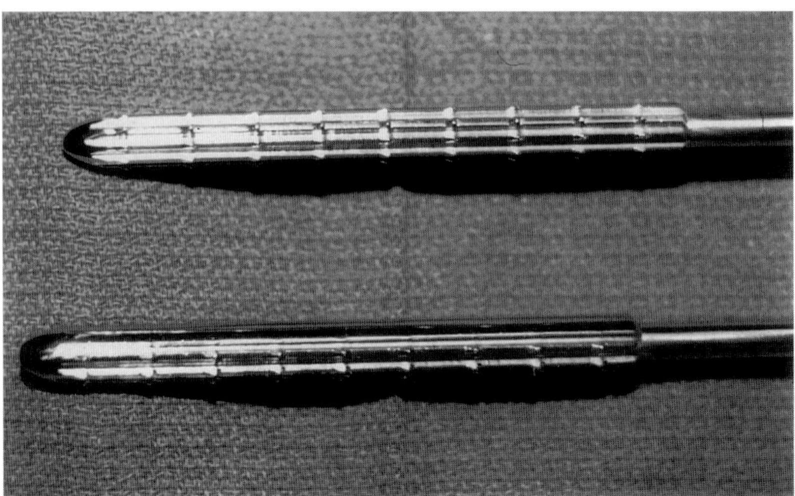

Fig. 2. The rasping end of the Carrion-Rosello cavernotomes is shown. The rasp are smooth as they are introduced in a forward direction and have a cutting, rasping surface as they are removed for dilating tissue in a corpora cavernosa that has significant fibrosis.

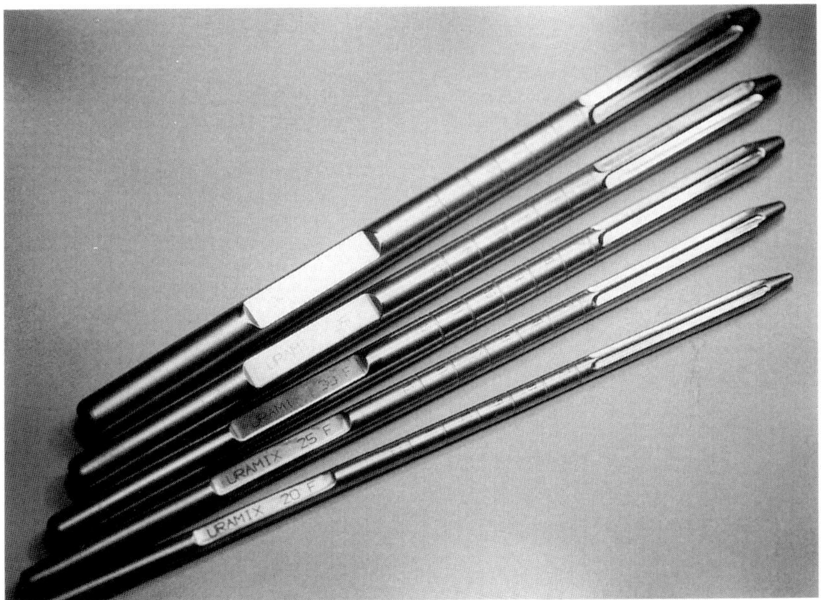

Fig. 3. A demonstration of the new penile cavernotome as proposed by Mooreville and Wilson.

what tissue can be incised and what must be avoided. When operating distally to create a cavity to the subglandular area, fibrotic tissue incision in both directions through multiple sites can be made to create the cavities with the urethrotome, cavernotome, or sharp scissors. Rajpurkar et al. reported their success with multiple incisions and minimal scar tissue excision in extensive penile fibrosis patients *(13)*. They use a midline perineal incision in all their cases. A 2-cm corporotomy is made on the corpus cavernosum and minimal scar tissue is excised at the site of corporotomy to facilitate the initiation of corporal dilation. The initial dilation is performed from the corporotomy site to the ischial tuberosity almost under direct vision starting with Metzenbaum scissors. The 7–11 gage Hegar dilators and/or Dilamezinsert were then used for further dilation. An additional subcoronal incision is made if necessary and dilation of the distal fibrotic area is carried out under direct vision through the distal corporotomy. It is exemplary, and to their credit, that they could achieve successful dilation and implantation without using any cavernotome or Otis urethrotome. No urethral perforation and only one crural perforation were reported in their study. A new penile cavernotome that allows drilling a space in fibrotic corpora was recently reported by Mooreville et al. *(15)* *(see* Fig. 3–4). This cavernotome set

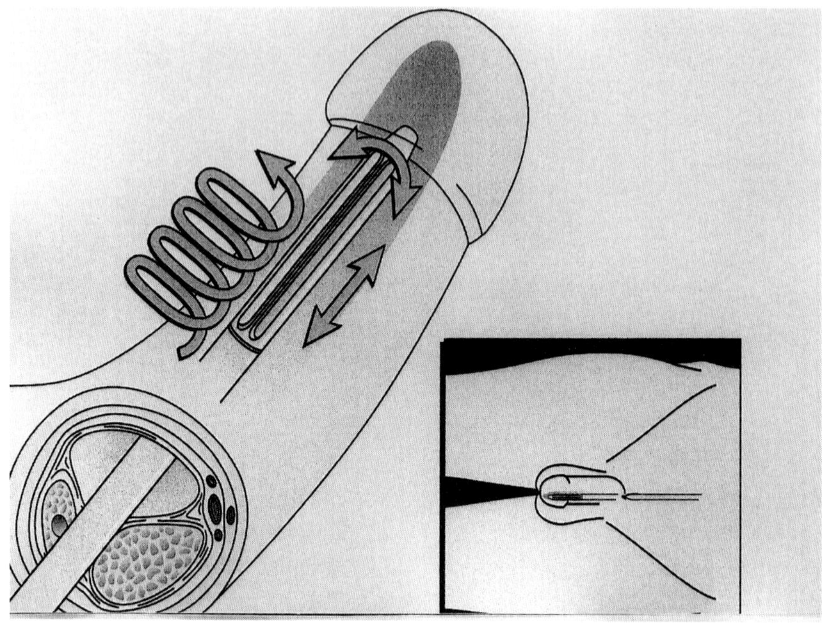

Fig. 4. The action necessary to remove fibrotic tissue with the cavernotome shown in Fig. 3.

consists of five cavernotomes with diameters from 6 to 13 mm. The head of the cavernotome is blunt and tapered for 1 cm. The height of the 6-cm-long working blade is 1 mm. This working blade rises from a beveled surface, which allows 1-mm shavings of tissue to be resected. As reported by authors, the dilation of fibrotic corpora was easier and quicker because extensive corporeal resection was not necessary. However, great care should be taken to avoid possible corporeal perforation.

Even with optimal corporal dilation, the standard penile prosthesis cylinder will be unable to be placed in the majority of cases of severe fibrosis without corporeal reconstruction. We now have more choices for penile prostheses than at any time before. As a matter of fact, we are now routinely preparing downsized versions of prostheses [Mentor α-1 (narrow base) and AMS 700 CXM] for patients with severe corporeal fibrosis. We have found the Mentor α-1 (narrow base) to be very useful because of its narrow-base feature, better girth expansion and softer tip than the AMS 700 CXM. Carbone et al. also reported their experience in the management of severe corporeal fibrosis with placement of the AMS 700 CXM prosthesis *(14)*. In all 26 men with severe corporeal fibrosis, the AMS 700 CXM prostheses were successfully implanted with primary closure of the tunica albuginea without need of corporeal reconstruction.

For tunica albuginea closure, we preplace sutures to prevent possible needle puncture to the prosthesis. This is particularly necessary in a resident-training institute. If corporeal closure is performed after the cylinder is placed, it is imperative to use a protector for cylinder protection from needle perforation. In some circumstances, even with the use of a downsized device, the edges of the tunical albuginea cannot be approximated over the cylinders. Corporeal reconstruction using synthetic material will be needed, even though there has been controversy about increased risk of infection with the use of synthetic material *(14)* (*see* Fig. 5A). We like to use a Dacron netting overlaid on either side by silastic material, which allows some elasticity (*see* Fig. 5B).

Even after successful penile prosthesis implantation in patients with extensive penile fibrosis, some patients will complain of insufficient penile length for satisfactory sexual intercourse. It is important to discuss limitations of the reoperation for penile implantation thoroughly to make sure that patients understand the penile shortening is caused by severe fibrosis and scar contraction. Use of AMS 700 Ultrex or Ultrexplus with a hope of length enhancement has been disappointing. Daitch et al. also demonstrated that Ultrex cylinders exhibited an increased mechanical failure rate *(3)*. If functional penile length will not reach more than 10 cm after implantation of a penile prosthesis, then release of the suspensory ligament, V-Y flap advancement, and/or lower abdominal tissue debulking may gain an additional penile length. Knoll et al. reported their experience in 11 patients with extensive cavernous fibrosis who underwent penile prosthesis implantation with a modified suprapubic V-Y advancement flap and lower abdominal tissue debulking *(16)*. An additional 3.5- to 6.5-cm functional penile length was obtained.

INFECTION

Infection after the insertion of a penile prosthesis is the most devastating complication. Previous dogma has advised immediate removal of the penile implant and reinsertion of a prosthesis 3–6 mo later, which almost always results in corporeal fibrosis, scaring, and penile shortening. Because more successful salvage procedures were reported, immediate replacement of the infected penile prosthesis has become possible. We previously reported our successful salvage operation in 17 out of 21 patients *(7)*. We placed a fenestrated drain along with the new prosthesis to allow for intermittent irrigation for 5–7 d with Dabs antibiotic solu-

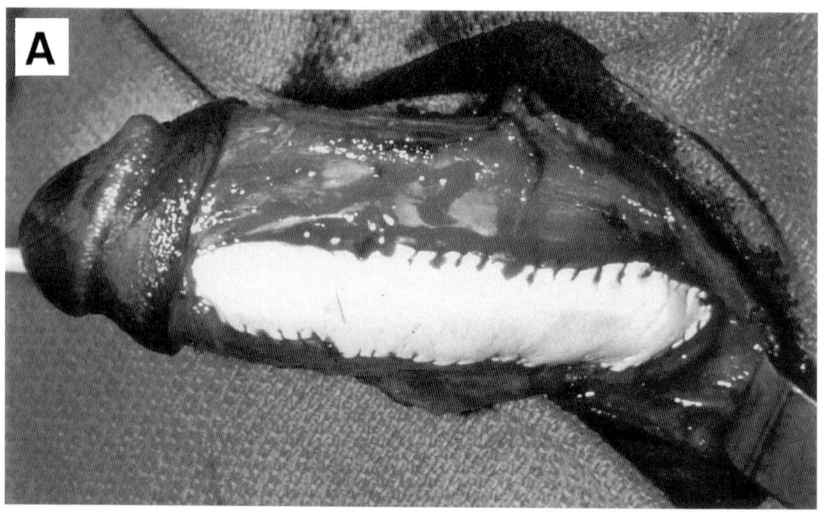

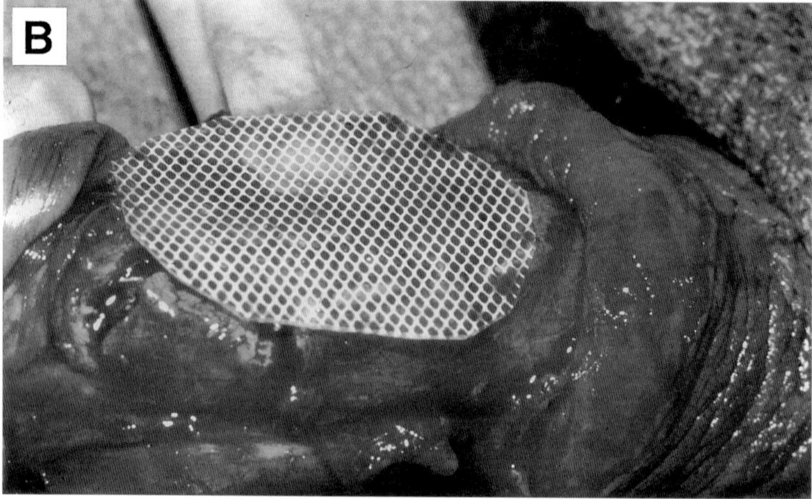

Fig. 5. (A) A closure of a defect in a corpora cavernosa with a gortex patch. **(B)** The covering of the defect in the corpora cavernosa with a patch of dacron netting that is covered with silicone (not commercially available).

tion (500 mg neomycin, 80 mg gentamicin, and 100 mg polymyxin in 1000 mL normal saline).

Brant et al. in 1996 proposed a 7-step vigorous intraoperative irrigation protocol in their immediate salvage procedure for infected penile prostheses (*see* Table 1) *(17)*. Do not use intraoperative irrigation if the reservoir site is intraperitoneal. The pump location is usually changed.

Table 1
Sequential Irrigating Solutions
for Immediate Salvage Procedure

- Kanamycin 80 mg/L, bacitracin 1 g/L
- One-half strength hydrogen peroxide
- One-half strength povidone-iodine
- Pressure irrigation with 5 L NS containing
- 1 g vancomycin and 80 mg gentamicin
- One-half strength povidone-iodine
- One-half strength hydrogen peroxide
- Kanamycin 80 mg/L, bacitracin 1 g/L

Salvage was successful in all 11 patients, even though one patient had a repeat salvage procedure. Their contraindications for immediate salvage attempt included necrotic infections, diabetic patients with purulence in the corporeal bodies, rapidly developing infections, and erosion of the device cylinders. Kaufman et al. used this 7-step irrigation protocol in their immediate salvage procedure in seven patients for infected penile prosthesis with success in six patients (9). They suggested that a salvage procedure could be successful even for patients with diabetes with visible pus in the corpora. Mulcahy recently summarized his long-term experience with this salvage protocol and 7-step sequential irrigation in managing penile prosthetic infection (18). He obtained 82% (45 of 55 patients) infection-free rate after 6–93 mo follow-up.

Knoll compared delayed and immediate salvage techniques in managing penile prosthetic infection (11). A delayed salvage procedure (3 d) included complete removal of all prosthesis, intraoperative antibiotic irrigation with Dabs solution of all locations where a component of the device was placed, and placement of drains in these locations. This was followed by postoperative intermittent drain irrigation with Dabs solution every 8 h clamped for 20 min for 3 d and subsequent reimplantation of a new three-piece device. An immediate salvage procedure was performed by following the same kind of protocol as aforementioned by Brant et al. Knoll found that an immediate salvage appears as successful as a delayed salvage procedure.

EROSION AND IMPENDING EROSION

Erosion of a penile prosthesis is uncommon, but it can be calamitous. The most common sites of erosion are the distal cylinder and scrotal pump (see Fig. 6). The etiology of cylinder erosion is mostly because of loss of distal penile sensation in the patient with spinal cord injury,

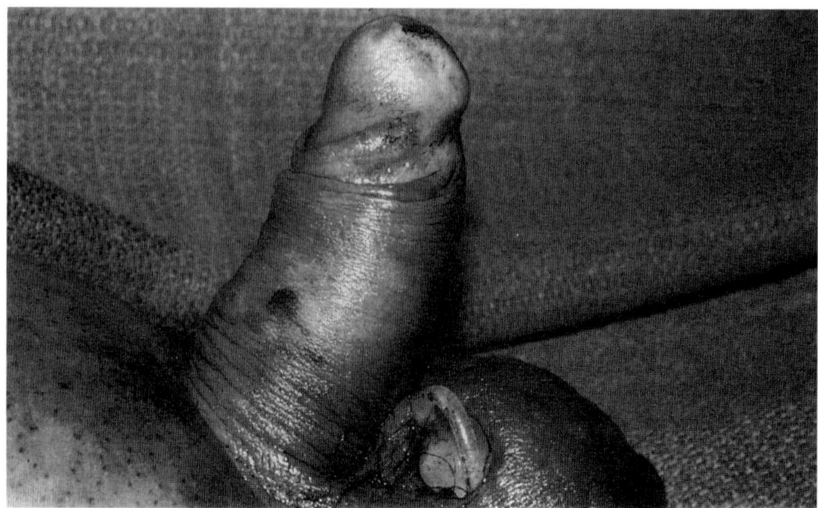

Fig. 6. A patient who presents with scrotal erosion of pump and tubing attached to the pump without purulent discharge. This case was successfully salvaged by removing the old pump and placing the new pump on the opposite side of the scrotum after thorough antibiotic irrigation.

diabetes, or postradiation. Erosion can also result from oversizing of the prosthesis, or failure to keep the prosthesis deflated when not in use. Management of erosion associated with obvious infection should follow the principles for treating infection as aforementioned. We attempt to perform salvage surgery for every patient with erosion without frank purulent material.

Erosion of the reservoir into the bladder or into the bowel is a rare occurrence. This is often owing to the tension on the tubing leading from the reservoir or a small reservoir cavity that exerts pressure on the balloon, pushing it into the viscus. This will need to have the affected bowel segment resected or bladder closed, and the reservoir replaced into a new site with an adequate cavity without tension on the tubing *(19)*.

Scrotal erosion may be salvaged by transferring the pump or pump/reservoir combinations to the opposite scrotum. Impending erosion of the proximal cylinders or the rear-tip extenders in the perineum can often be repaired through a perineal incision.

Distal erosion or impending erosion of the penile prosthesis can be repaired with a variety of methods. Mulcahy described a distal corporoplasty to repair lateral impending erosion *(1)*. He reseats the cylinder in a more medial and secure position under the glans penis by creating a new cavity for the cylinder behind the back wall of the fibrotic sheath containing it. One of the authors has used this technique for more than 10 yr and has always found normal appearing corporeal tissue after making an incision into the dorsal medial wall of the old cylinder sheath. This corporeal tissue can easily be dilated to make a space for inserting the cylinder in the appropriate subglanular position. In Mulcahy's report, all 14 patients who underwent corporoplasty using this technique had satisfactory results after 2-yr follow-up *(1)*. Alter et al. reported their successful two-stage procedure with prefabricated tunica vaginalis fascia flaps to repair recurrent penile prosthesis extrusion in two patients *(20)*. A variety of synthetic and natural substitutes has also been used for corporeal reconstruction to repair the distal erosion. These include polyester, polypropylene mesh, polytetrafluoroethylene (PTFE), rectus fascia, and fascia lata. Recently, there was a report of the use of human cadaveric allograft skin for reconstruction of the corpus cavernosum in the repair of distal erosion of a penile prosthesis *(21)*. Smith et al. treated five patients with impending erosion of penile prosthesis with PTFE distal wind sock graft *(22)*. All patients had satisfactory and functional erections after 32 mo follow-up. Again, as aforementioned, use of synthetic material has been controversial as a result of a possible increased risk of penile prosthesis infection. We agree with Smith et al. that the simple addition of a synthetic graft will not increase the rate of penile prosthesis infection.

Urethral erosion is a more difficult problem to manage. As a preventive measure, it is recommended that a temporary proximal urinary diversion be performed in patients who are undergoing self-intermittent catheterization and desire a penile implant. We prefer perineal urethrostomy. When urethral erosion is diagnosed, the eroded cylinder should be removed and inserted at a later date after the urethra heals completely. It is important to determine whether there is a communication with the cylinder on the opposite side during the surgery. If this cylinder is not involved, it can be left in place to help maintain the length of the penis; otherwise this cylinder should be removed also if it is communicating with the erosive process. Whether the remainder of the prosthesis should be kept or removed depends on the duration of the erosion and the associated infection. Should any question about the infection of a multicomponent exist, the device should be removed and a salvage procedure performed.

POSITION PROBLEMS

The two most common position problems include inappropriate cylinder length and a high-riding pump or reservoir/pump combination in the scrotum. We have also seen a case in which the pump was located behind the testis possibly because of migration as the patient complained of gradual difficulty finding the pump for inflation. The malpositioned pump or reservoir/pump combination can be easily corrected by simple open surgery. If there is difficulty in replacing a pump or reservoir/pump combination into the ipsilateral scrotum, the contralateral scrotum often can be used. If the original tubing appears to be too short to allow adequate placement, we recommend placing a new pump.

A difference in length between two cylinders can sometimes be addressed by Yachia corporeal plasty on the convex side of the curvature. However, erectile deformities after placement of AMS 700 Ultrex are best corrected by replacement with AMS 700 CX cylinders *(23)*.

An inappropriate cylinder length can cause glans bowing or SST deformity. The effective way to correct this type of deformity is with the Ball procedure *(24)*. In this procedure, a circumcising or hemicircumcising incision is made and the plane between the glans and the distal portion of the tunica albuginea of the corpora cavernosa is developed by sharp dissection. Place a nonabsorbable soft suture through the glans substance and through the tunica albuginea adjacent to the cylinder head. When all sutures are in position, securely tie the sutures dorsally, ventrally, or laterally, wherever the glans needs to be secured over the cylinder head. Sometimes, the cylinders are too short, which should be corrected by adding rear-tip extenders to the cylinders or replacing them with longer cylinders. Improper placement of the cylinders, such as crossover into the other corpora, can be corrected through a circumcision incision for the distal penile crossover or a perineal incision for crossover in the crural corpora.

MECHANICAL FAILURES

True mechanical failure for inflatable penile prostheses includes tubing leak, pump leak, reservoir leak, and cylinder aneurysm. When mechanical failure occurs, as a rule of thumb, every effort should be made to replace a three-piece prosthesis with a similar prosthesis if possible. Patients are usually dissatisfied if this is not done. Some authors suggested that AMS 700 prostheses over 3 yr old should be totally explanted and replaced with a new multicomponent prosthesis *(5)*. Others suggested replacing all parts after 5–6 yr if a three-piece inflatable device develops a mechanical problem *(19)*.

Replacement of involved components can be done by isolating the connecting tubing to observe for tubing fracture; particularly where excessive angulation of the tubing is present as it joins to the connector.

Kim et al. has found that the input tube exited through a separate stab wound has higher incidence of tubing fracture than when the input tubing runs alongside the cylinder within the corpus and exits through the corporotomy *(25)*. If fracture is observed, bypass it by connecting intact parts of the tubing. Sometimes it may be difficult to identify the defective part or parts. Some authors suggested using an ohmmeter; others used pressure testing to locate the defect *(19)*. We like to replace any part, if not all, when there is doubt about the integrity of any component of the device. Modern reservoirs are usually not a source of mechanical failure. Encapsulation of the reservoir can be managed by hydrodilation and rupture of the restricting capsule using a hand-held syringe through a scrotal incision. An aneurysmal defective cylinder should be replaced and corporoplasty should be performed to maintain the tunical strength and prevent replacement cylinder aneurysm *(23)*. When there are mechanical problems in a unitary hydraulic device or rod-type penile prosthesis, both cylinders should be replaced. This is also true for two-piece prostheses and three-piece devices without connectors as both the cylinders and pump are part of one continuous system. A two- or three-piece IPP is recommended replacement of unitary hydraulic devices.

PAIN

Persistent pain beyond 4–6 wk in the absence of fever, elevated white count, erythema, or purulent drainage should be carefully evaluated. Even though we may not be able to identify the etiology in many cases, the penile pain, as aforementioned, can be caused by inappropriate sizing of the cylinders. As reported by Moncada et al., buckling of cylinders could cause prolonged penile pain after prosthesis implantation. This pain can be resolved by reoperation to correct the buckling cylinder *(6)*.

CONCLUSION

Reoperation after insertion of a penile prosthesis continues to be a challenge for prosthetic urologists. However, if the surgery is well planned, it can be very successful.

REFERENCES

1. Mulcahy JJ (1999) Distal corporoplasty for lateral extrusion of penile prosthesis cylinders. *J Urol* 161:193.
2. Wilson SK, Cleves MA, Delk JR II (1999) Comparison of mechanical reliability of original and enhanced Mentor Alpha I penile prosthesis. *J Urol* 162:715.
3. Daitch JA, Angermeier KW, Lakin MM, et al. (1997) Long-term mechanical reliability of AMS 700 series inflatable penile prostheses: comparison of CX/CXM and Ultrex cylinders. *J Urol* 158:1400.

4. Lewis RW, Morgan WR (1995) Failure of the penile prosthesis. In: Cohen MS, Resnick MI, eds., *Reoperative Urology*, Boston: Little, Brown and Company, pp. 235–243.

5. Wilson SK (1997) Penile prosthesis implantation: pearls, pitfalls, and perils. In: Hellstrom WJG, ed., *Male Infertility and Sexual Dysfunction*, New York: Springer, pp. 529–548.

6. Moncada I, Hernandez C, Jara J, et al. (1998) Buckling of cylinders may cause prolonged penile pain after prosthesis implantation: a case control study using magnetic resonance imaging of the penis. *J Urol* 160:67.

7. Lewis RW, Mclaren R (1993) Reoperation for penile prosthesis implantation. *Problems Urol* 7:381.

8. Jarow JP (1996) Risk factors for penile prosthetic infection. *J Urol* 156:402.

9. Kaufman JM, Kaufman JL, Borges FD (1998) Immediate salvage procedure for infected penile prosthesis. *J Urol* 159:816.

10. Wilson Sk, Cleves MA, Delk JR II (1996) Glycosylated hemoglobin and the risk of infection among penile implant patients. *Int J Impot* Res 8:120.

11. Knoll LD (1998) Penile prosthetic infection: management by delayed and immediate salvage techniques. *Urology* 52:287.

12. Garber BB, Marcus SM (1998) Does surgical approach affect the incidence of inflatable penile prosthesis infection? *Urology* 52:291.

13. Rajpurkar A, Li H, Dhabuwala CB (1999) Penile implant success in patients with corporal fibrosis using multiple incisions and minimal scar tissue excision. *Urology* 54:145.

14. Carbone DJ Jr, Daitch JA, Angermeier KW, et al. (1998) Management of severe corporeal fibrosis with implantation of prosthesis via a transverse scrotal approach. *J Urol* 159:125.

15. Mooreville M, Adrian S, Delk II JR, Wilson SK (1999) Implantation of inflatable penile prosthesis in patients with severe corporeal fibrosis: introduction of a new penile cavernotome. *J Urol* 162:2054.

16. Knoll LD, Fisher J, Benson RC Jr, et al. (1996) Treatment of penile fibrosis with prosthetic implantation and flap advancement with tissue debulking. *J Urol* 156:394.

17. Brant MD, Ludlow JK, Mulcahy JJ (1996) The prosthesis salvage operation: immediate replacement of the infected penile prosthesis. *J Urol* 155:155.

18. Mulcahy JJ (2000) Long-term experience with salvage of infected penile implants. *J Urol 163:* 481.

19. Mulcahy JJ (1997) The complex penile prosthesis. In: Hellstrom WJG, ed., *Male Infertility and Sexual Dysfunction*, New York: Springer, pp. 549–562.

20. Alter GJ, Greisman J, Werthman PE, et al. (1998) Use of a prefabricated tunica vaginalis fascia flap to reconstruct the tunica albuginea after recurrent penile prosthesis extrusion. *J Urol* 159:128.

21. Landman J, Bar-Chama N (1999) Initial experience with processed human cadaveric allograft skin for reconstruction of the corpus cavernosum in repair of distal extrusion of a penile prosthesis. *Urology* 53:1222.

22. Smith CP, Kraus SR, Boone TB (1998) Management of impending penile prosthesis erosion with a polytetrafluoroethylene distal wind sock graft. *J Urol* 160:2037.

23. Kowalczyk JJ, Mulcahy JJ (1996) Penile curvatures and aneurysmal defects with the Ultrex penile prosthesis corrected with insertion of the AMS700CX. *J Urol* 156:398.

24. Ball TP (1980) Surgical repair of penile "SST" deformity. *Urology* 15:603.
25. Kim SC, Seo KK, Yoon SH (1999) Fracture at the input tube-cylinder junction of AMS 700 inflatable penile prostheses as a complication of a modified implantation technique in a series of 99 patients. *Urology* 54:148.

16 Corporeal Fibrosis

*Penile Prosthesis Implantation
and Corporeal Reconstruction*

Kenneth W. Angermeier, MD
and Drogo K. Montague, MD

CONTENTS

INTRODUCTION
PATIENT EVALUATION
PROSTHESIS IMPLANTATION
POSTOPERATIVE CARE
COMPLICATIONS
REFERENCES

INTRODUCTION

Implantation of a penile prosthesis in the setting of corporeal fibrosis can be a significant challenge. This condition occurs most commonly following removal of a previously implanted penile prosthesis for infection or erosion *(1,2)*. Additional etiologies of corporeal fibrosis include priapism *(3)*, penile trauma *(4)*, Peyronie's disease *(5,6)*, intracavernosal injection therapy *(7)*, and idiopathic *(8)*. The extent of fibrosis within the corporeal bodies may vary, and it may occur unilaterally or bilaterally. The primary problem presented by the fibrosis during penile prosthesis implantation is interference with satisfactory dilation of the corporeal bodies and subsequent corporotomy closure. Following surgery, the main problem encountered is often patient dissatisfaction regarding

From: *Urologic Prostheses:*
The Complete, Practical Guide to Devices, Their Implantation and Patient Follow Up
Edited by: C. C. Carson © Humana Press Inc., Totowa, NJ

functional erectile length. This can be a significant issue that must be extensively reviewed with the patient preoperatively to ensure that he understands the inherent difficulties of the surgical procedure and has realistic expectations.

PATIENT EVALUATION

History

As in any patient, a careful history is important. The presence of corporeal fibrosis may be suspected based upon a history of any of the conditions aforementioned. The premorbid status of the erect penis should be elucidated, as well as the timing of the onset of erectile dysfunction (ED). If the patient has a history of intracavernosal injection, the duration of treatment and agents used should be recorded. A history of erectile curvature or erectile discomfort should be documented if present. Although rare, a patient with idiopathic corporeal fibrosis may present with primary ED. A review of previous surgical procedures on the penis is also important in operative planning.

Physical Examination

Careful palpation of the stretched penis should be carried out to identify areas of tunical or intracorporeal fibrosis. These are generally documented with a drawing. We also assess penile extensibility and corporeal compliance. It should be noted whether the patient is circumcised, and the possibility of circumcision at the time of the implant needs to be discussed if one feels that adjunctive distal penile incisions might be required.

Additional Studies

In patients who have not undergone previous evaluation and treatment for ED, a nocturnal penile tumescence study is obtained. This would primarily include those with a history of priapism, penile trauma, or previous treatment for Peyronie's disease. We have also used biothesiometry in these situations to document vibratory thresholds preoperatively. The index finger, penile shaft, and glans penis are assessed bilaterally *(9,10)*. The thresholds detected by the patient during both increasing and decreasing amplitude of vibration are recorded. This is primarily useful for comparison to postoperative biothesiometry in patients complaining of changes in penile sensation. Except in unusual circumstances, we have not found penile imaging studies to be very helpful in the surgical treatment of patients with corporeal fibrosis.

PROSTHESIS IMPLANTATION

Implantation of a penile prosthesis in the setting of corporeal fibrosis is one of those cases during which the surgeon must be familiar with a variety of techniques to aid with corporeal dilation and closure. There do not seem to be any highly reliable preoperative predictors of surgical difficulty and the patient needs to be aware of this. In our standard implant procedure *(11)*, we make an upper transverse scrotal incision and dilate the corporal bodies through 2-cm corporotomies using Hegar dilators. If corporeal fibrosis does not allow this, there are adjunctive procedures and devices that can help to accomplish a successful implant.

Dilators

When fibrosis impedes corporeal dilation, the most common initial maneuver is the use of Metzenbaum scissors to create a channel through the fibrosis. The scissors are advanced and intermittently spread, using the opposite hand to palpate the tips of the scissors and monitor their location. The tips are directed dorsolaterally to decrease the risk of urethral injury. Once the distal or proximal corporal body has been reached, the scissors are spread and then withdrawn. Hegar dilators are then used to fully dilate the corpora. If it remains difficult to pass Hegar dilators, the Dilamezinsert[1] may be used to aid sequential dilation. Some authors have advocated the use of the Otis urethrotome as another option for corporeal dilation *(10,12)*. The instrument should be positioned away from the urethra, and multiple cuts may be needed at different locations to allow subsequent passage of Hegar dilators. We have not used the Otis urethrotome in this setting.

In addition to the aforementioned, two special dilators or cavern-otomes have been manufactured for use in the presence of corporeal fibrosis. The Carrion-Rosello cavernotome[2] has a smooth surface along one aspect of its circumference while the other is covered with rows of small pointed edges that provide a rasping action (*see* Fig. 1). The smooth aspect is oriented toward the urethra as the dilator is inserted to the distal or proximal end of each corporeal body. They are available in sets of 4, with diameters of 9, 10, 11, and 12 mm. Our experience is that these devices can aid dilation in difficult situations, however, they are at times a bit difficult to withdraw following insertion through dense fibrosis. A more recently developed penile cavernotome[3] is designed as a cutting

---

[1]Lone Star Medical Products, Houston, TX.
[2]UROAN - XXI, Electromedicina, Spain.
[3]Uramix, Inc., Landsdowne, PA.

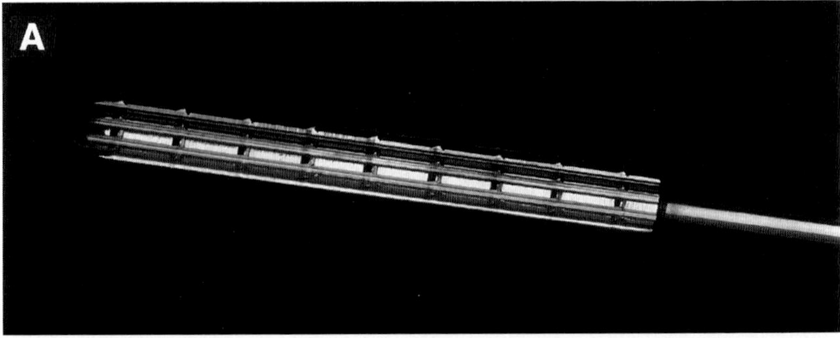

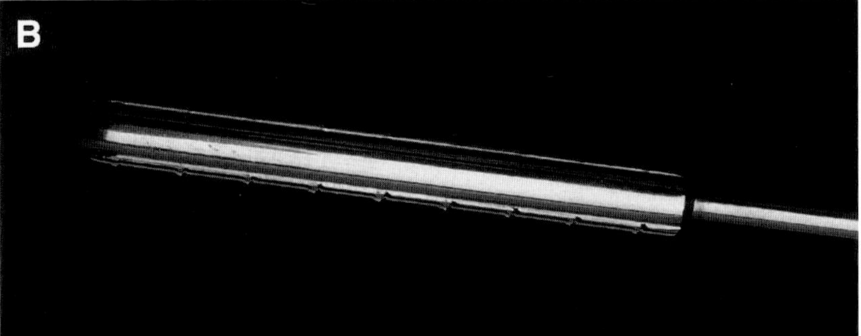

Fig. 1. Carrion-Rosello cavernotome.

dilator, with a blunt distal tip and a 6-cm-long working blade with a height of 1 mm (*see* Fig. 2). The blade does not extend beyond the diameter of the dilator, and arises from a beveled surface that allows the actual resection of small shavings of tissue if necessary. The dilator is advanced slowly with an oscillating motion or by rotation. It is available in sets of 5, with diameter ranging from 6–13 mm. Use of this device in 16 patients with severe corporeal fibrosis has been reported *(13)*, with successful implantation of an inflatable penile prosthesis in all cases. Operative time was reduced and no patient required a synthetic graft. Four patients required a secondary procedure to correct impending distal corporeal erosion of a cylinder tip. These new dilators seem to have the potential for easier dilation of fibrotic corpora, and it will be interesting to monitor future results as experience increases.

Downsized Penile Prosthesis

A major advance in the management of patients with corporeal fibrosis occurred with the introduction of the downsized inflatable penile prosthesis. Our experience has been primarily with the AMS

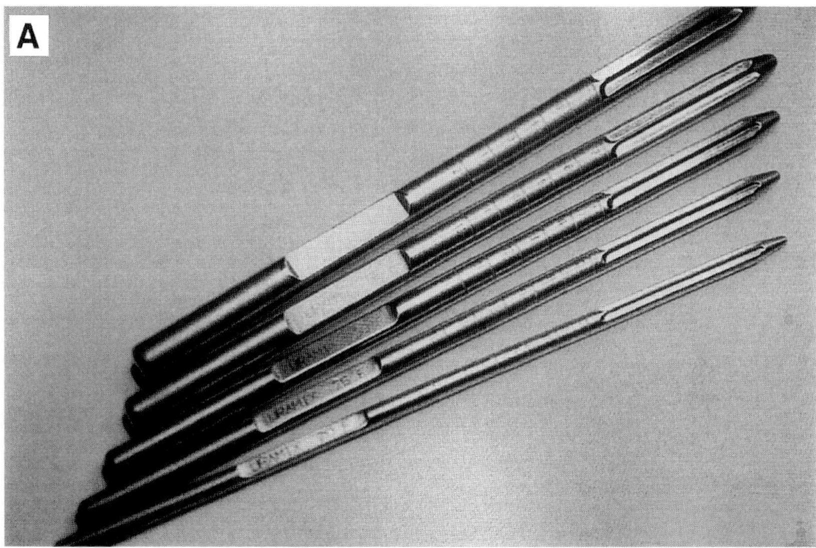

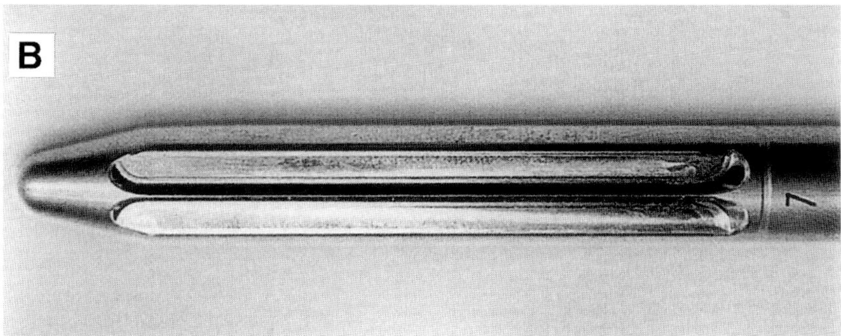

Fig. 2. Cutting penile cavernotome. (From Mooreville M, Adrian S, Delk JR, II, Wilson SK (1999) Implantation of inflatable penile prosthesis in patients with severe corporeal fibrosis: introcuction of a new penile cavernotome. *J Urol* 162:2005. With permisison, and courtesy of Michael Mooreville, MD.)

700 CXM[4] (*see* Fig. 3), which was introduced in 1990. Originally developed for men with smaller penises, it is now used primarily in patients with corporeal fibrosis. The deflated cylinder diameter is 9.5 mm and inflated diameter 14.2 mm, which is a significant advantage when corporeal dilation is difficult. The addition of rear-tip extenders allows the cylinder input tubing to exit almost directly out of the corporotomy, and may therefore lessen the degree of dilation required for proximal

---

[4]American Medical Systems, Inc., Minnetonka, MN.

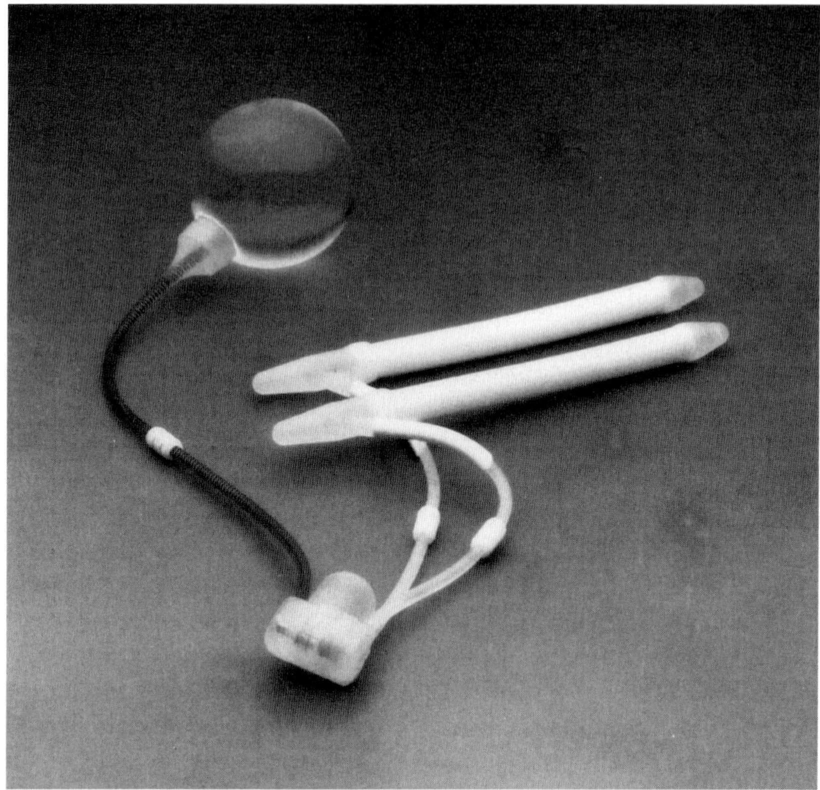

Fig. 3. AMS 700 CXM inflatable penile prosthesis. (Courtesy of American Medical Systems, Inc., Minnetonka, MN.)

insertion. Studies have shown that this device can often obviate the need for corporeal reconstruction with synthetic grafts in patients in whom it would have been otherwise necessary *(14,15)*. In addition, the rate of infection was decreased to 4–5% and the majority of patients have had a satisfactory functional outcome.

Corporotomies

When dense corporeal fibrosis precludes adequate dilation using the aforementioned techniques, or when it is difficult to localize the dilator within the distal corpus, additional corporotomy is often helpful. In order to aid distal dilation, exposure to the corporeal body is gained via a subcoronal skin incision or by extending the transverse scrotal incision distally in the midline (*see* Fig. 4). A dilator or scissors can then be advanced as far as possible, followed by a secondary corporotomy over

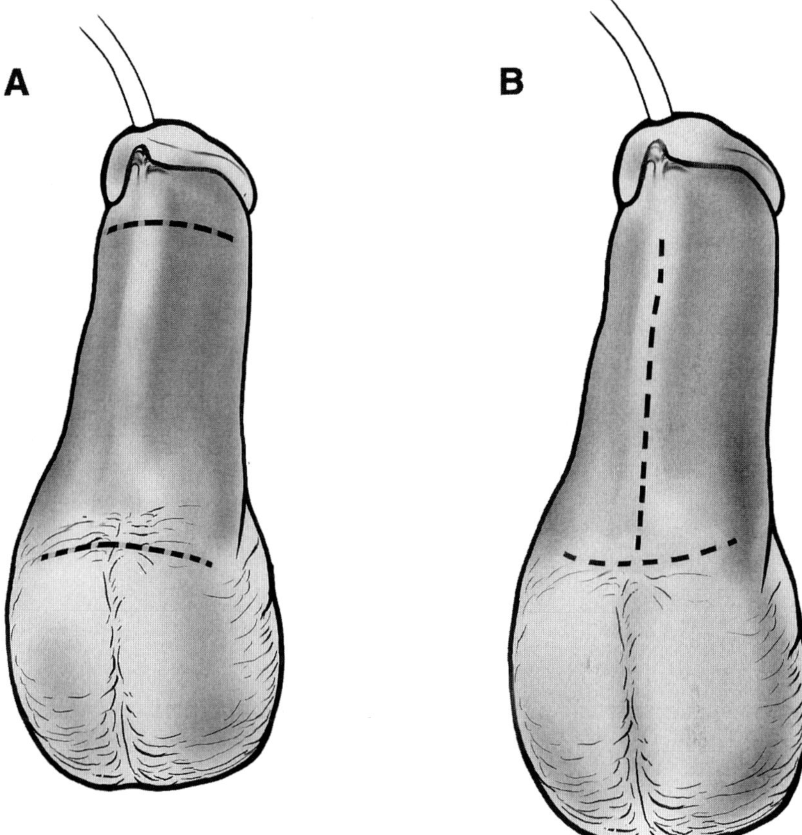

Fig. 4. Skin incisions for exposure of distal corpora. (**A**) Subcoronal incision. (**B**) Transverse scrotal incision extended distally in midline.

the tip (*see* Fig. 5). Alternatively, initial advancement of a dilator is not an absolute requirement and the tunical incision can merely be made along the distal corpus *(16)*. Distal dissection and dilation with Metzenbaum scissors can then be accomplished virtually under direct vision (*see* Fig. 6). The area between the corporotomies is then dilated from both directions until a satisfactory diameter has been reached.

If this maneuver fails, extended corporotomies may be required. The initial corporotomy incision is lengthened and often includes the majority of the shaft of the penis back to the proximal corpus (*see* Fig. 7). This allows dilation proximal and distal to the tunical incision, and nay be accompanied when necessary by excision of a sufficient amount of the intervening fibrotic tissue to allow prosthesis insertion *(17,18)*. With the emergence of special dilators and the downsized inflatable penile

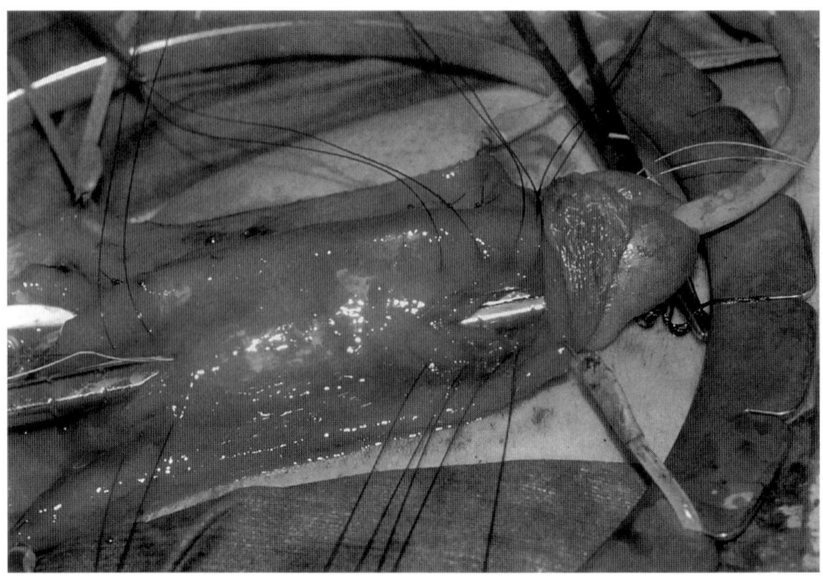

Fig. 5. Secondary corporotomy: tunical incision over tip of dilator.

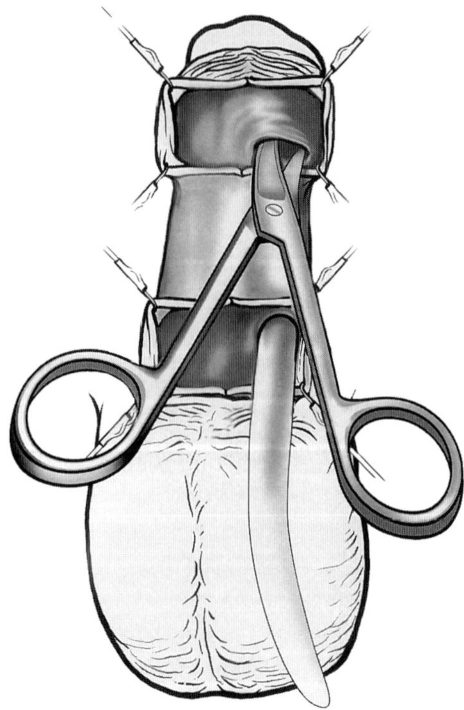

Fig. 6. Secondary corporotomy: scissors dissection and dilation of distal corpus.

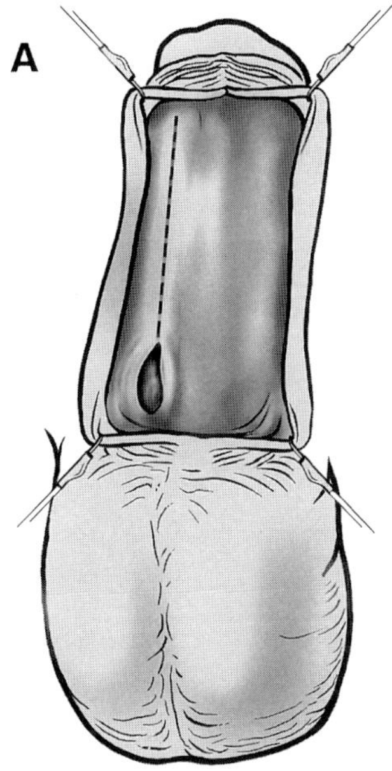

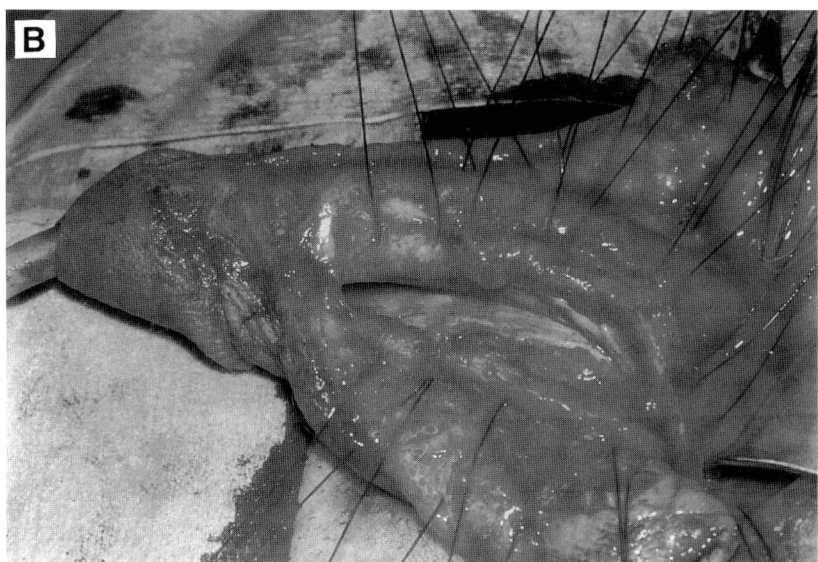

Fig. 7. Extended corporotomy. (**A**) Proposed tunical incision. (**B**) Extended corporotomy with stay sutures in place.

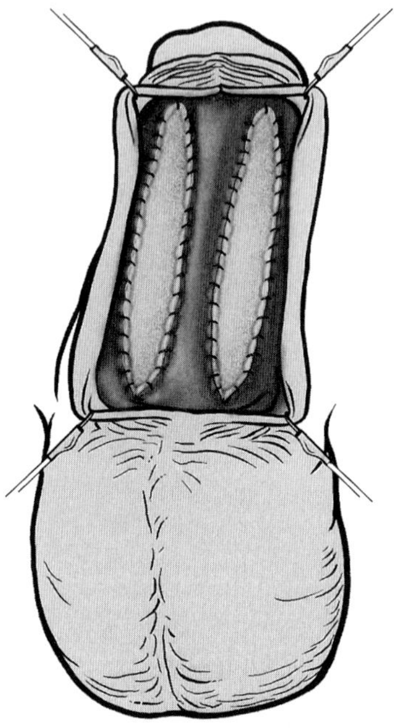

Fig. 8. Extended corporotomy: closure with PTFE patch.

prosthesis, extended corporotomy was required in only 8% of men with corporeal fibrosis in a recent study *(15)*.

Corporeal Reconstruction—Synthetic Grafts

Although increasingly uncommon, there may be situations where the tunica albuginea cannot be closed over a prosthetic cylinder following secondary or extended corporotomy. Corporeal reconstruction with a synthetic graft is therefore required, most commonly using a polytetrafluoroethylene (PTFE) patch. The patch is tailored to the tunical defect allowing full coverage of the prosthetic cylinder, and sutured in place with a running 3-0 polypropylene or PTFE suture (*see* Fig. 8). An early report of experience with this technique in 30 men with corporeal fibrosis demonstrated an infection rate of 30% *(19)*. However, there have been several smaller series using a similar approach with no infectious complications *(20–22)*. In general, however, most surgeons seem to agree that it is preferable to avoid corporeal reconstruction with synthetic grafts when possible, in order to minimize the potential risk of infection and distal cylinder migration.

POSTOPERATIVE CARE

The postoperative care following penile prosthesis implantation in the setting of corporeal fibrosis is similar to that following a standard implant *(11)*. A Foley catheter is left indwelling overnight. Based upon surgeon preference, a small suction drain may be placed in the subdartos space and brought out through a stab incision in the inguinal region opposite the reservoir. Most patients are discharged after a 23-hr hospital stay, although an occasional patient may stay longer for pain control following an extensive reconstructive procedure. Patients with corporeal fibrosis are treated with ciprofloxacin or a cephalosporin for 1 wk postoperatively. An attempt is made to maintain the penis in an upward orientation during the first month to prevent ventral tethering. Patients can generally resume intercourse 6–8 wk postoperatively.

COMPLICATIONS

Injury to the urethra may occur during difficult corporeal dilation. In these complex cases, if such an injury is recognized intraoperatively the implant procedure should probably be aborted. Orienting scissor tips and dilators laterally, with localization of the distal aspect of the device by palpation as it is advanced can minimize the risk of urethral injury. The appropriate use of a secondary or extended corporotomy can also help in this way. A second complication of dilation is tunical perforation, which is most common within the proximal crura during the implant procedure. Distal perforations may present postoperatively as impending lateral or distal erosion in the region of the glans penis. A proximal crural perforation can, at times, be bypassed with larger dilators, precluding the need for formal repair. Several techniques for managing this problem have been described, and primarily involve placement of synthetic material such as PTFE or a rear-tip extender as a windsock into the proximal crus *(23)*. A plug and patch technique has also been reported *(24)*. Late distal erosion laterally may be managed with a procedure described by Mulcahy *(25)*, in which the distal cylinder tip is relocated using natural tissues. A windsock technique has also been reported *(26)*.

With current techniques, infection rates in the setting of corporeal fibrosis are similar to those associated with standard prosthesis insertion *(13–15)*. This may be related to a decreasing need for corporeal reconstruction and facilitation of the implant procedure with decreased operative time *(27)*. Periprosthetic infection may be managed with a salvage procedure *(28)* when feasible. Prosthesis removal may result in further shortening of an already fibrotic penis, but will be required in some individuals.

REFERENCES

1. Gasser TC, Larsen EH, Bruskewitz RG (1987) Penile prosthesis reimplantation. *J Urol* 137:46.
2. Montague DK (1987) Periprosthetic infection. *J Urol* 138:68.
3. Macaluso JN, Sullivan JW (1985) Priapism: review of 34 cases. *Urology* 25:233.
4. Orvis BR, McAninch JW (1989) Penile rupture. *Urol Clin North Am* 16:369.
5. Furlow WL, Swenson HE, Lee RE (1975) Peyronie's disease: a study of its natural history and treatment with orthovoltage radiotherapy. *J Urol* 114:69.
6. Devine CJ, Horton CE (1987) Bent penis. *Semin Urol* 5:251.
7. Larsen EH, Gasser TC, Bruskewitz RG (1987) Fibrosis of corpus cavernosum after intracavernous injection of phentolamine/papaverine. *J Urol* 137:292.
8. Fishman IJ (1987) Complicated implantation of inflatable penile prostheses. *Urol Clin North Am* 14:217.
9. Padma-Nathan H (1988) Neurological evaluation of erectile dysfunction. *Urol Clin North Am* 15:77.
10. Knoll LD (1995) Use of penile prosthetic implants in patients with penile fibrosis. *Urol Clin North Am* 22:857.
11. Montague DK, Angermeier KW, Lakin MM (1996) Penile prosthesis implantation. In: Marshall FF, ed., *Textbook of Operative Urology,* Philadelphia: WB Saunders, ch. 85, pp. 712–719.
12. Carson, CC (1989) Infections in genitourinary prostheses. *Urol Clin North Am* 16:139.
13. Mooreville M, Adrian S, Delk JR II, Wilson SK (1999) Implantation of inflatable penile prosthesis in patients with severe corporeal fibrosis: introduction of a new penile cavernotome. *J Urol* 162:2054.
14. Knoll LD, Furlow WL, Benson RC, Bilhartz DL (1995) Management of nondilatable cavernous fibrosis with the use of a downsized inflatable penile prosthesis. *J Urol* 153:366.
15. Carbone DJ, Daitch JA, Angermeier KW, Lakin MM, Montague DK (1998) Management of severe corporeal fibrosis with implantation of prosthesis via a transverse scrotal approach. *J Urol* 159:125.
16. Herschorn S, Barkin M, Comisarow R (1986) New technique for difficult penile implants. *Urology* 27:463.
17. O'Donnell PD (1986) Operative approach for secondary placement of penile prosthesis. *Urology* 28:108.
18. Fishman IJ (1989) Corporeal reconstruction procedures for complicated penile implants. *Urol Clin North Am* 16:73.
19. Knoll LD, Furlow WL (1992) Corporeal reconstruction and prosthetic implantation for impotence associated with non-dilatable corporeal cavernosal fibrosis. *Acta Urol Belg* 60:15.
20. Herschorn S, Ordorica RC (1995) Penile prosthesis insertion with corporeal reconstruction with synthetic vascular graft material. *J Urol* 154:80.
21. George VK, Shah GS, Mills R, Dhabuwala CB (1996) The management of extensive penile fibrosis: a new technique of minimal scar-tissue excision. *Brit J Urol* 77:282.
22. Seftel AD, Oates RD, Goldstein I (1992) Use of a polytetrafluoroethylene tube graft as a circumferential neotunica during placement of a penile prosthesis. *J Urol* 148:1531.
23. Mulcahy JJ (1987) A technique of maintaining penile prosthesis position to prevent proximal migration. *J Urol* 137:294.

24. Szostak MJ, DelPizzo JJ, Sklar GN (2000) The plug and patch: a new technique for repair of corporal perforation during placement of penile prostheses. *J Urol* 163:1203.

25. Mulcahy JJ (1999) Distal corporoplasty for lateral extrusion of penile prosthesis cylinders. *J Urol* 161:193.

26. Smith CP, Kraus SR, Boone TB (1998) Management of impending penile prosthesis erosion with a polytetrafluoroethylene distal wind sock graft. *J Urol* 160:2037.

27. Jarow JP (1996) Risk factors for penile prosthetic infection. *J Urol* 156:402.

28. Mulcahy JJ (2000) Long-term experience with salvage of infected penile implants. *J Urol* 163:481.

17

Artificial Urinary Sphincter for Treatment of Male Urinary Incontinence

Ananias C. Diokno, MD

and Kenneth M. Peters, MD

CONTENTS

INTRODUCTION

INDICATIONS AND PATIENT SELECTION FOR ARTIFICIAL
  URINARY SPHINCTER IMPLANTATION

SURGICAL TECHNIQUES

POSTOPERATIVE FOLLOW-UP

POTENTIAL PROBLEMS

RESULTS WITH THE AMS800 ARTIFICIAL
  URINARY SPHINCTER

CONCLUSIONS

REFERENCES

INTRODUCTION

Insertion of the artificial urinary sphincter (AUS) in the male is presently still the most effective treatment for stress incontinence secondary to sphincter dysfunction. The AUS was one of the initial successful applications of a prosthetic implant in management of the genitourinary system. Historically, Foley is credited for introducing the first artificial urinary sphincter in 1947 *(1)*. The device consisted of an inflatable cuff, made of latex, that was placed around the corpus spongiosum just distal

From: *Urologic Prostheses:*
The Complete, Practical Guide to Devices, Their Implantation and Patient Follow Up
Edited by: C. C. Carson © Humana Press Inc., Totowa, NJ

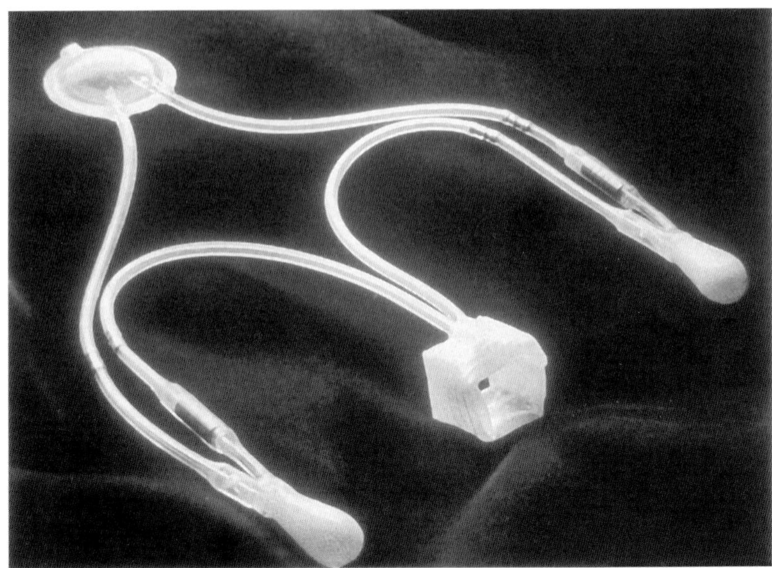

Fig. 1. The original artificial sphincter introduced in 1973 named AS 721.

to the penoscrotal junction. It was connected by tubing to a valve and syringe that were kept by the patient in his trouser pocket. The cuff was inflated to prevent incontinence and deflated to empty the bladder. Unfortunately, pressure necrosis and infections occurred, which led to fistulas and other unmanageable complications.

The modern AUS was introduced by Scott et al. in 1973 *(2)*. This device was made of silicone rubber and consisted of three major components: the reservoir, an occlusive cuff, and two pumps. The reservoir contained fluid used to activate the device and was implanted in the prevesical space. The cuff encircled the bulbous urethra or the vesical neck and the inflate and deflate pumps were placed in each hemiscrotum or labium (*see* Fig. 1).

Experience with this initial prosthesis was favorable with an overall success rate of 60%–70% *(3)*. Most of the complications and failures encountered with this device were attributable to urethral erosion and infection. Other problems that could be repaired included mechanical failures such as tube kinks, valvular failure, and device leakage.

Although the device was fairly successful, there were clearly areas for improvement. Over the next 10 yr, through the efforts of American Medical Systems (Minnetonka, MN) and several urologists active in implanting the AUSs, the device was constantly modified in an effort to simplify the design, improve reliability, and reduce the complication

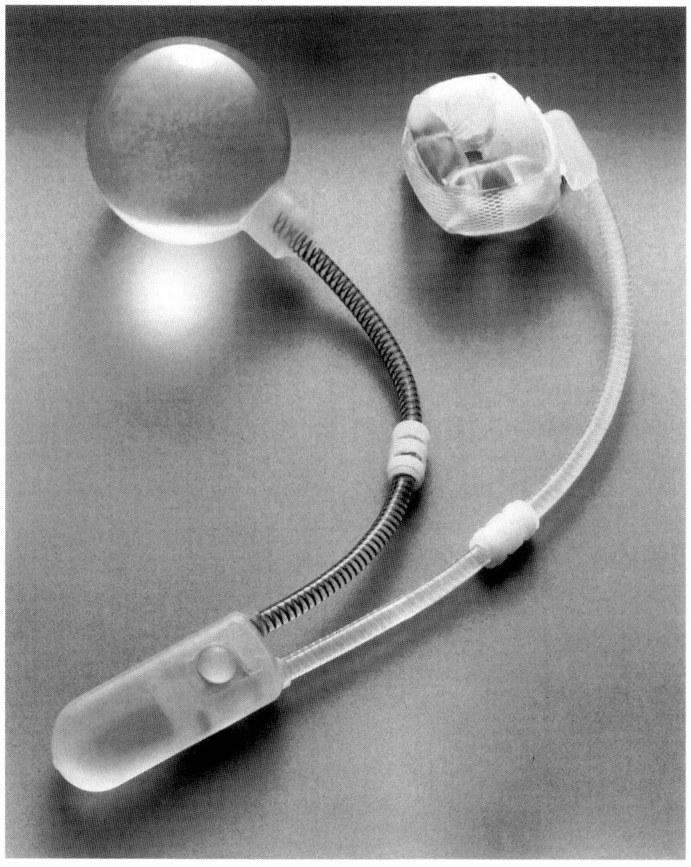

Fig. 2. AMS 800 Artificial Urinary Sphincter.

and reoperative rates. In 1983, American Medical Systems (AMS) introduced the latest AUS model, the AMS800 (*see* Fig. 2). This model has been very successful and has changed very little since then. The modifications that occurred appear to have significantly improved the durability and reliability of this AUS. The current device is constructed of a wear-resistant, biocompatible silicone elastomer and consists of three components all connected by special kink-resistant color-coded silicone tubing: a soft, pliable, dip-coated silicone cuff that is placed around the urethra or bladder neck, a seamless pressure-regulating balloon placed in the prevesical space of Retzius and a pump placed in the scrotum or labia majora with a flow resistor that acts to slow cuff refill, allowing adequate voiding time, and a deactivation button that, when engaged, prevents cuff refill altogether. This button is located on the cephalad portion of the pump mechanism (easily palpated through the skin). By squeezing it, one can move a poppet valve to a position such that fluid cannot be transferred. Reactivation is accomplished with a sharp squeeze on the pump that releases the poppet. An important point in sphincter deactivation is that some fluid in the pump is necessary to unseat the poppet valve. To accomplish this, we generally allow the pump to refill to the point where only a shallow dimple is palpable before deactivating the device. This feature was an important addition to the AUS in that Furlow showed that deactivation for 6–8 wk after implantation (to allow for periurethral swelling to decrease and tissue healing) decreased the incidence of infection and erosion with artificial urinary sphincters *(4)*. The ability to deactivate a sphincter is also an important feature when the patient requires Foley catheter drainage or undergoes instrumentation, events that increase the risk for cuff erosion or infection. In these situations, the cuff should always be emptied and then the device be deactivated (as aforementioned).

The AMS800 system is fluid filled and works hydraulically. The occlusive force of the cuff is determined by the pressure of a regulating balloon, and the balloon is manufactured so that precalibrated reservoirs are available in different pressure ranges: 51–60, 61–70, 71–80, and 81–90 cm H_2O. The intraabdominal prevesical location of the reservoir also permits the transmission of abdominal pressure changes to the cuff, helping reduce leakage with straining maneuvers *(5)*. The patient squeezes the pump to empty the cuff, transferring fluid to the regulating balloon. As the cuff empties, the occlusive force on the urethra is removed, and the patient can void. Resistors in the pump mechanism delay cuff refill for approx 2–3 min, allowing the patient adequate time to empty his bladder (*see* Fig. 3A, 3B).

INDICATIONS AND PATIENT SELECTION
FOR ARTIFICIAL URINARY SPHINCTER IMPLANTATION

Male patients who are considered for implantation of an AUS fall into one of four groups: neuropathic bladder dysfunction (mainly congenital), postprostatectomy incontinence, congenital anomalies, and trauma. A recent surge in radical prostatectomy surgery has led to more men with significant urinary incontinence as a result of sphincter dysfunction. This group consists of the most common indication for insertion of AUS in adult men.

Before considering an incontinent patient for AUS implantation, one must realize that an AUS is a treatment for incontinence because of sphincteric incompetence only *(5,6)*. Thus, the importance of preopera-

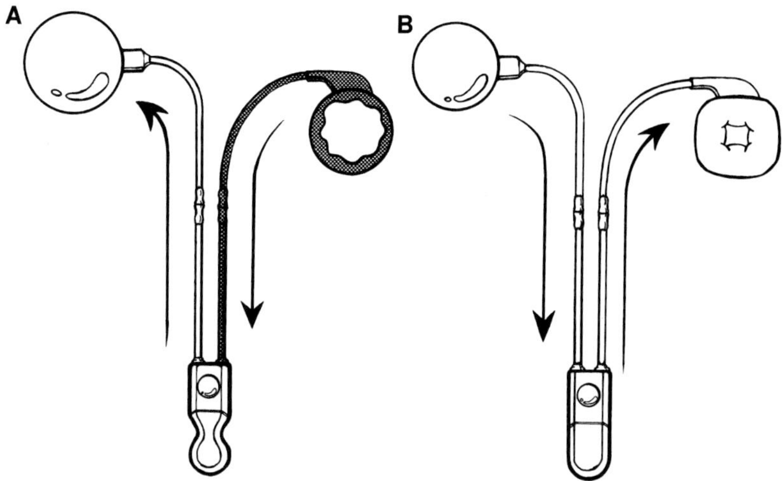

Fig. 3. Hydraulic cycling mechanism for the AUS. (**A**) Squeezing the pump will transfer fluid from the cuff to the balloon (see arrow). (**B**) The pressurized balloon will transfer the fluid from the balloon to cuff gradually (takes 1-2 minutes) because of the resistor in the pump.

tive evaluation cannot be overemphasized. Patients must be screened to ensure they are mentally and physically capable of using an AUS. In this manner, it is helpful to show the patient the actual device in vitro and observe his skills at cycling the device. Dementia or physical inability to squeeze the pump is a contraindication to placing the device, which would put the patient in retention if he were not able to use it properly.

The history of urinary incontinence should be delineated to determine its cause. Physical examination should include a neurologic examination to identify neuropathologic disturbances. During this evaluation, particular attention should be paid to the patient's upper extremity motor skills. Physical examination should define or confirm the clinical impression as to the type of incontinence present. Urinary tract infection should be ruled out and eradicated. In addition, the cause of such infection should be elucidated, because recurrent infection in the presence of prosthesis may lead to prosthesis infection. Appropriate urodynamic testing should be done to document not only the mechanism of incontinence, but also the state of detrusor function. Ideal candidates for the AUS are patients with irreversible sphincteric dysfunction and normal detrusor function. Extensive experience with this device has shown that areflexia and hyperreflexia are not absolute contraindications. However, before any implantation, appropriate provisions should be made to ensure that the bladder can be emptied regularly to avoid chronic reten-

tion and that hyperreflexia can be suppressed to avoid urge incontinence. Ideal bladder capacity should be ≥400 mL with pressures of
<40 cm H_2O, although capacity of >150 mL have been implanted
successfully. Failure to identify bladder function problems could lead to
elevated bladder storage pressures and upper tract and renal deterioration in the presence of an AUS. One can treat incomplete bladder emptying by performing a flap urethroplasty at the time of sphincter
implantation as advocated by Scott et al. *(7)* to ensure complete bladder
emptying or with intermittent self-catheterization *(8,9)*, both of which
have been shown to be compatible with the AUS implant. Hyperreflexic
or hypertonic bladder may be managed with anticholinergics, and if this
is not effective, bladder augmentation with bowel segments has been
successful with the AUS *(10)*. If hyperreflexia can be controlled with
drugs or by other means, implantation of a sphincter is feasible. Otherwise, urge incontinence will persist and upper tract deterioration
could occur.

Recently, a new mode of therapy has been added to the urologist's
armamentarium in the management of urge incontinence unresponsive
the behavioral techniques and bladder relaxant pharmacological
therapy. We have now limited experience of using the Medtronic Corporation (Minneapolis, MN) Interstim™ neuromodulation program in
combination with an AUS implant. This device consisting of a wire
electrode inserted into the sacral foramen and connected into a generator
implanted subcutaneously into the superior aspect of the buttocks, provides programmed electrical pulses to the bladder and sphincters via the
sacral reflex arc *(11)*. It is theorized that such electrical pulses will
modulate the bladder function to normality. It is therefore feasible that
a patient with stress incontinence secondary to intrinsic sphincter deficiency, but with concommitant intractable urge incontinence or even
chronic nonobstructive retention may be screened and if appropriate,
receive the Interstim implant and if stress incontinence persists, receive
the AUS. Likewise, patients with AUS and associated intractable urge
incontinence may be evaluated for Interstim implant and if found appropriate, be implanted with Interstim.

Currently our workup includes a detailed history and physical examination including neurologic with postvoid residual urine determination.
If intrinsic sphincter deficiency is suspected, patients then undergo further evaluation. All patients undergo flexible cystoscopy with particular
attention paid to bladder neck and sphincteric function during provocative maneuvers. In males, endoscopic evaluation can also identify not
only bladder neck with sphincteric incompetence but also potential
urethral disorders (contracture, stricture, and so forth). Special attention

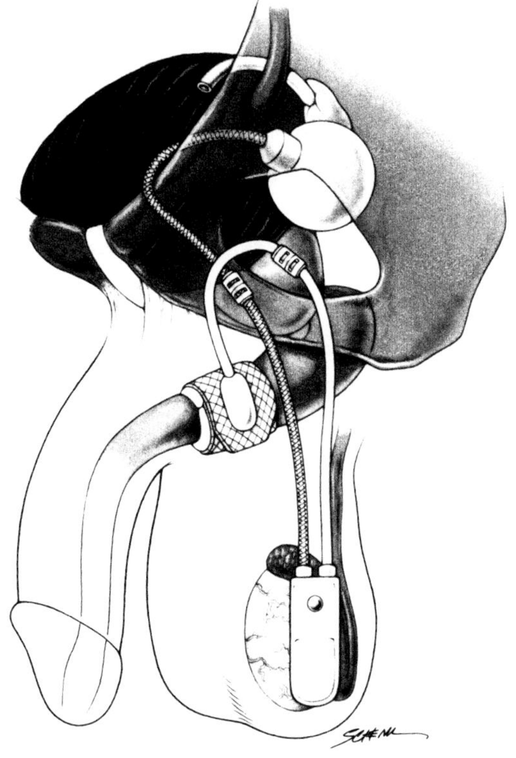

Fig. 4. Placement of the AUS at the bulbous urethra.

should be directed to the bulbous urethra, the area in the urethra where the cuff is usually implanted to assure that there are no signs of scarring, false passage, or strictures. Patients also undergo urodynamic testing, including a cystometrogram, for evaluation of bladder instability or hyperreflexia, bladder capacity, and sensation. At the completion of cystometry with the bladder full, cough stress test is performed to provoke stress incontinence. Leaking of fluid at the instant of cough confirms the presence of stress incontinence. Urethral profilometry and leak point pressure measurements are not essential when provocative cough stress test is positive.

The most common reason for insertion of an artificial urinary sphincter in adult males is for postprostatectomy incontinence. It is recommended that AUS implantation be delayed for at least 6 mo after the prostatectomy to allow time for possible spontaneous resolution. Insertion of the AUS in males can be performed at essentially two sites: the vesical neck and the bulbous urethra. For postprostatectomy incontinence, however, we recommend placement of AUS only at the bulbous urethra site primarily because of the significant postoperative changes at the bladder neck in these patients (*see* Fig. 4). In male children, the indication is generally for incontinence secondary to neurogenic dysfunction, most commonly caused by myelomeningocele. Generally in these patients, the sphincter should be placed at the bladder neck. These patients may need to receive intermittent self-catheterization and may be non-ambulatory, they will be in seated positions for long periods of time. A bulbar urethral position is of concern in this situation because it would theoretically expose the cuff to extended periods of pressure increasing the risk for erosion and infection. Potential problems with bladder neck placement in prepubertal males and subsequent prostate growth disrupting AUS function have not been reported. When one is implanting sphincters in children, it is advised to use conservative measures for management of incontinence initially and delay AUS insertion until at least 6 yr of age to allow for anatomic, emotional, and social maturation *(12)*.

SURGICAL TECHNIQUES

Patients are given antibiotics preoperatively on a prophylactic basis parenterally at least 2 h before surgery. The urine should be proved free of infection prior to hospitalization. In patients whose incontinence is managed with external devices, careful examination preoperatively is necessary to rule out cutaneous inflammation or erosion of the external genitalia. If any is present, surgery should be deferred until the skin is healed and uninflammed. All Foley catheters should be removed, if possible, 7 d prior to surgery and the urine sterilized. For those who are on clean intermittent catheterization, a urine culture is obtained 1 wk earlier and appropriate antibiotic coverage started 3 d preoperatively.

The procedure is performed under spinal anesthesia in the lithotomy position. In elderly men, care is taken when positioning the legs. Artificial hips, arthritic joints, and diminished thigh abduction ability may require special attention.

The entire lower abdomen, external genitalia, and perineum are shaved and a careful wide surgical scrub is performed and draped for access to the bulbous urethra and suprapubic area. A drape is sutured or stapled to cover the anus to isolate it from the perineal exposure. A 16-F Foley urethral catheter is passed into the bladder and the bladder is drained.

For bladder neck insertion in men, a suprapubic transverse or vertical incision is performed followed by the usual entry into the perivesical

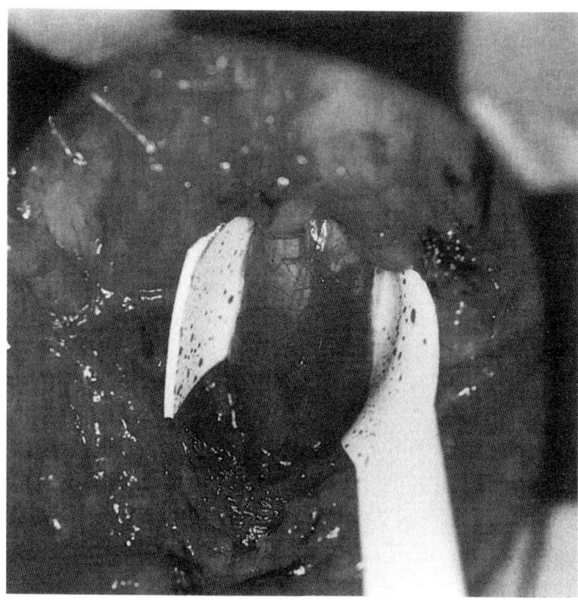

Fig. 5. Circumferential dissection of 2 cm. length bulbous urethra at the distal edge of the bulbocavernosus muscle. Note the 2 cm. wide sizer around the urethra.

space followed by exposure of the endopelvic fascia and the prostate and bladder neck area. The endopelvic fascia is then incised and the prostate and bladder neck are dissected free anteriorly and laterally. The dorsal complex of vessels and nerves are not transsected in most cases unless there is not enough space at the region of the prostatic bladder neck area. Using a right-angle clamp, blunt dissection is carried out to separate the posterior aspect of the prostate and bladder neck from the anterior rectal wall similar to the maneuver in the bulbous urethra. A 2-cm-wide space is created so that the tape measure can be passed between the bladder neck and rectal wall space to measure the circumference of the bladder neck/prostate area that will be enclosed by the cuff.

Once the cuff is inserted around the bladder neck, which is usually a 6–7-cm cuff, the cuff tubing is then brought up anteriorly. The balloon is placed in the superior prevesical space. Pressurization of the cuff is identical to the bulbous urethra technique. The tubings of the balloon (same choice as the bulbous urethral technique) and of the cuff are brought out of the prevesical space at the midline. The rectus muscles are approximated loosely at the midline and the rectus fascia closed by heavy absorbable sutures. The pump is then inserted, usually into the

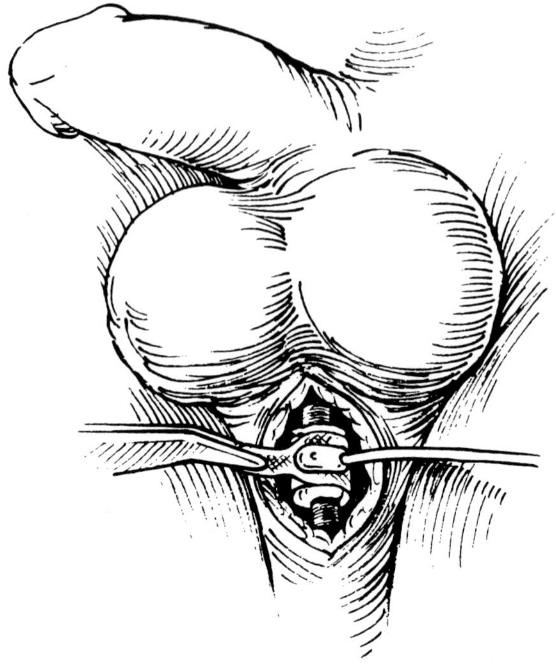

Fig. 6. Placement of the cuff around the bulbous urethra.

right hemiscrotum (same technique as the bulbous urethral insertion) and connections made over the rectus fascia avoiding any redundancy of the tubing.

For a bulbous urethral placement, a midline perineal incision is made over the bulbous urethra, which is dissected just distal to the bulbocavernosus muscle (*see* Fig. 5). The cuff is not positioned at the bulbocavernosus muscle for several reasons. First, the muscle atrophies over time causing the cuff to loosen. Second, if the muscle is divided and the cuff placed beneath the bulbocavernosus muscle, contraction of the bulbocavernosus muscle may cause the cuff to act erratically. Third, the more distal position of the cuff will prevent compression of the device while the patient is sitting, thereby reducing inadvertent opening of the cuff, and theoretically, decreasing the likelihood of atrophy and erosion. A 2-cm length of urethra must be dissected so that the cuff passes easily around the urethra (*see* Fig. 6). Care must be taken to prevent entering the tunica of the corpora spongiosum during the dissection to prevent significant bleeding and urethral injury. Once the urethra is dissected circumferentially, the proper size cuff needs to be determined. A measuring device is included in the AUS kit, which allows one to determine cuff size. The

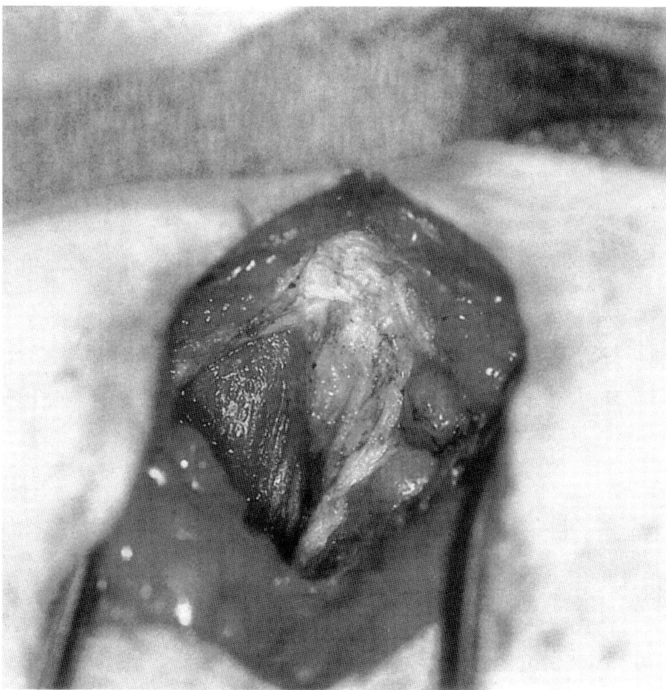

Fig. 7. Suprapubic incision to create a space for the balloon in the prevesical space behind the rectus muscle.

cuff should not be too snug, especially if the patient has had previous radiation therapy. The most common cuff size used in the male urethra is 4.5 cm. An antibiotic-soaked gauze is placed in this perineal incision while the abdominal incision is made.

Next, a pocket is created for the balloon reservoir by making a small transverse skin incision approx two-finger breadths above the pubic symphysis. The rectus fascia is incised and the rectus muscle is open at its midline. A space is created behind the rectus muscle in the perivesical area (*see* Figs. 7 and 8). Many of these men have had previous radical prostatectomies and this area may be scarred. Creating the space more cephalad along the rectus muscle will often lead to easier dissection of the perivesical space. The pocket created should be of sufficient size to prevent undo pressure on the balloon reservoir. The most common balloon size is 61–70 cm H_2O. In patients who have had radiation therapy or advanced diabetes, we use a 51–60 cm H_2O balloon. An antibiotic-soaked gauze is placed in this space while the sphincter is prepared.

The pump along with the proper size cuff and balloon is opened and placed in antibiotic solution. It is imperative to remove all air from the

Table 1
Filling Solutions

- Hypaque 25%: dilute 50 cm^3 with 60 cm^3 sterile water
- Cysto-Conray-II: dilute 60 cm^3 with 15 cm^3 sterile water
- Urovist cysto: dilute 50 cm^3 with 50 cm^3 sterile water
- Normal saline (for iodine sensitive patients)

system to prevent an airlock. This is accomplished by instilling an isotonic contrast solution composed of 50 cm^3 of 25% hypaque mixed with 60 cm^3 of sterile water. Other filling solutions can be used in the artificial sphincter (*see* Table 1). Patients with an iodine allergy should have the device filled with normal saline. The solution is instilled into the cuff and balloon using a syringe fitted with adapters designed to insert into the prosthesis tubing. With gentle tapping and aspiration, the air is removed. After removal of the air, the tubing to each device is clamped with rubber shod hemostats to prevent damage and leakage. The balloon is instilled with 22 cm^3 of contrast solution and the tubing clamped. The cuff is left empty and free of air. The pump is filled with fluid by squeezing it with both the inflow and outflow tubing in the solution. Once full and free of air, both tubes are clamped with rubber shod hemostats.

Next, the balloon is placed in the previously created pocket in the perivesical space. The pocket should be of sufficient size to be certain no pressure is placed upon the balloon. The rectus muscle and rectus fascia are closed and the tubing is brought out the midportion of the suture line.

A right-angle clamp is then passed around the previously dissected urethra. The cuff, empty of fluid or air is passed around the urethra and the tab is secured over the cuff button. The tab at the end of the cuff is trimmed so as not to protrude. The cuff is placed so that the tubing from the cuff is positioned to the left side (*see* Figs. 6 and 8). Next, a hemostat or tubing passer is passed anterior to the rectus fascia in the subcutaneous tissue, along the left inguinal region, and punctures through the tissue along the left side of the bulbous urethra at the level of the cuff. The tubing from the cuff is brought through this tunnel and externalized above the rectus fascia. A rubber shod is once again placed on the end of the tubing (*see* Fig. 8). Next, the cuff must be calibrated. To do this, the bladder is filled with irrigating fluid and the Foley catheter is removed. A temporary connection is made between the balloon filled with 22 cm^3 of isotonic fluid and the empty cuff. Prior to making any connection, fluid should be instilled in the end of each tubing to remove

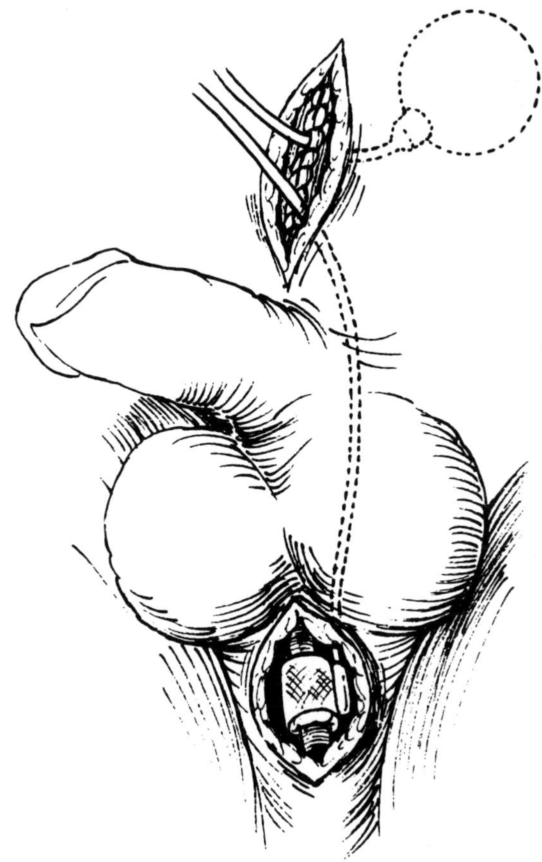

Fig. 8. Cuff tubing is routed to the left side to meet the tubing from the right-sided pump placement for easy non-angulated connection.

the small amount of air that accumulates in this region. The rubber shods are removed and fluid is allowed to flow into the cuff. The cuff is visualized to inflate and compress the urethra. Continence may be tested at this point by manually compressing the bladder with the cuff full and empty. The tubing is once again clamped and a syringe is used to aspirate and measure the amount of fluid in the cuff. The Foley catheter is then replaced. The fluid in the balloon reservoir is then adjusted for a final volume that equals 20 cm^3 plus the volume held by the cuff.

The pump is then placed by passing a large clamp anterior to the rectus fascia on the right and into the scrotum (*see* Fig. 9A). The jaws of the clamp are opened and the clamp withdrawn. The pump is then placed within this space and "milked" down into a dependent anterior scrotal position, just beneath the dartos fascia (*see* Fig. 9B). Once the pump is in

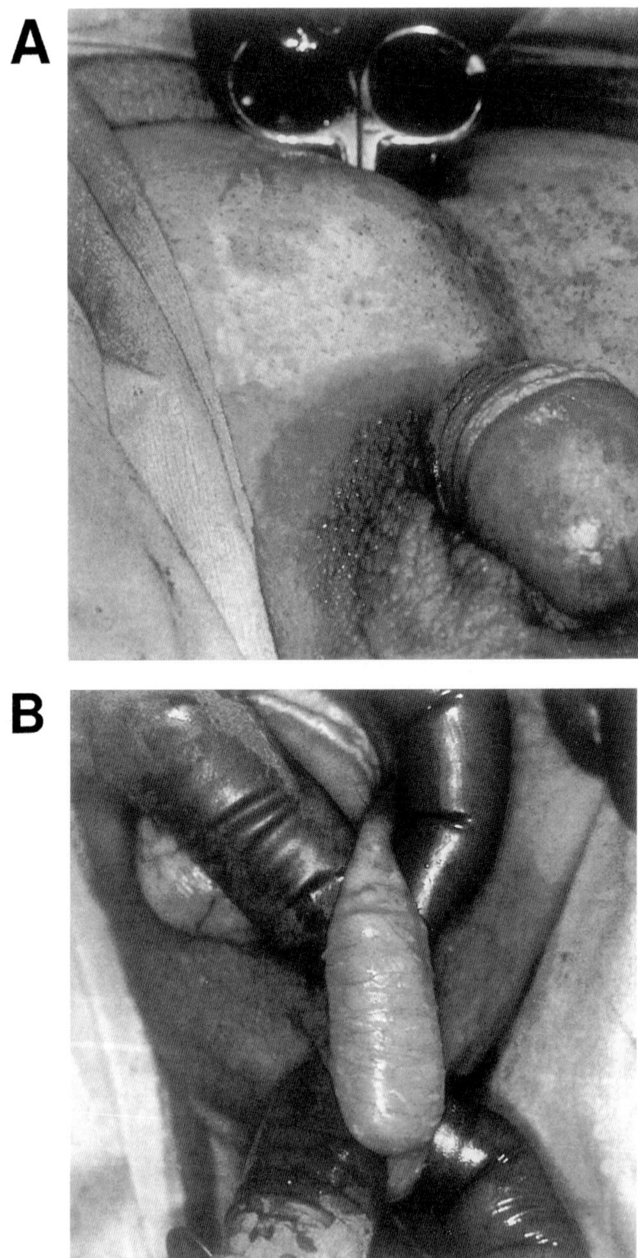

Fig. 9. (A) Clamp into the right anterior hemiscrotum. **(B)** Pump "milked" down into the anterior compartment of the right hemiscrotum.

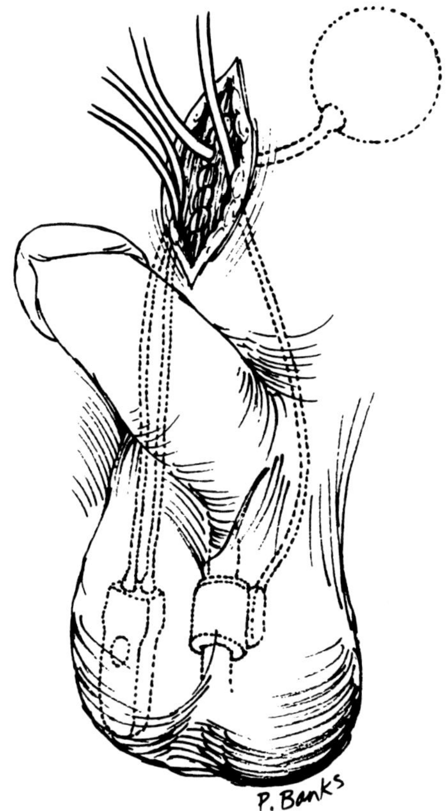

Fig. 10. Positions of AUS components prior to connections.

position, it is held in place by placing a babcock clamp on the scrotum, around the tubing.

The next goal is to complete the connections. The pump has two tubes distinct from each other but similar to the reservoir and cuff tubing (Fig. 10). Similar tubes connect to each other. Straight connectors along with a crimping tool are used to complete the connection. It is important to trim the tubing so that there is minimal redundancy, decreasing the likelihood of kinking. It is necessary to keep the tubing clamped with a rubber shod proximal to the area to be trimmed. Connections are made after removing the air at the end of the tubing by instilling isotonic solution. The integrity of the connection should be determined by gently pulling on the tubing after making the connections. The tubing is covered with tissue by approximating Scarpa's facia over the tubing.

Once the connections are complete, the rubber shod clamps are removed and the system is allowed to cycle. The system is tested by compressing the pump several times forcing fluid from the cuff to the reservoir. The cuff can be observed to deflate and fill. After the system is tested, one must lock the sphincter in the open position with the cuff deflated. By deactivating the sphincter with the cuff open, the urethra heals as vascularity is not compressed by the cuff. The deactivation period is 6 wk. The technique for deactivating the sphincter is important to prevent malfunction of the sphincter. When the pump is compressed, fluid is first forced out of the pump and then out of the cuff. When the system cycles, fluid returns to the pump first followed by the cuff. A button is on the side of the pump, which deactivates the sphincter. This button should be compressed when fluid returns to the pump, but prior to filling of the cuff. If the sphincter is deactivated with the pump empty of fluid, it will make reactivation difficult because it relies on forcing fluid through the valve lock to activate the sphincter. Next, the incisions are closed in the usual fashion and sterile dressings are applied.

POSTOPERATIVE FOLLOW-UP

Because the artificial sphincter is a prosthetic device, the patient who receives an AUS and the physician who implants it must be committed postoperatively to regular follow-up and care. Both must also be willing to deal with potential infections and mechanical problems that can arise and accept the possibility that reoperations may be required.

Our postoperative care routine begins in the operating room soon after the device is implanted. The device is tested while the patient is still under the anesthetic. Once successful cycling has been accomplished, the cuff is opened. The pump is allowed to refill until a slight dimpling is palpable, and then the device is deactivated. If the device is deactivated immediately after opening, the cuff reactivation may be extremely difficult, in that some fluid is needed in the pump to unseat the poppet used to deactivate the cuff. The patient is then taken from the operating room with a Foley catheter that remains for 24 h.

After removal of the Foley catheter, the patient is again incontinent because the sphincter is deactivated in the open position. All patients are aware of this preoperatively. Our patients remain in the hospital overnight to receive intravenous antibiotics and on discharge are orally maintained on 7 d of antibiotics. During the patient's stay, the abdominal (and perineal) wounds are inspected and the pump position is checked. Patients are instructed as to pump position and encouraged to check position at least once daily and apply light traction as needed. We believe that this may help maintain pump position during scarring and healing and also help get the patient familiar with manipulating the device.

At 6 wk postoperatively, the patient returns for a follow-up exam and pump activation. At this time, the patient is re-instructed on the use of the device and given a trial run. If a patient can successfully use the device, he or she is followed regularly (or more frequently if problems arise) at least once a year.

POTENTIAL PROBLEMS

1. Cannot activate sphincter: The most common cause preventing sphincter activation is the sphincter being deactivated with insufficient fluid in the pump. We generally allow the pump to refill to a point where a shallow dimple is palpable before deactivating the device. This will assure sufficient fluid in the pump to release the poppet valve and allow free flow through the system. Engaging the poppet valve with insufficient fluid in the pump can be a difficult problem because the sphincter relies on forcing the fluid within the pump past the poppet valve by sharply squeezing the pump. One can feel a "pop" when the valve opens. The first maneuver to overcome this problem is to stabilize the pump and squeeze forcibly over the entire surface of the pump. This may create enough pressure in the system to open the valve. If this is not successful, the following maneuver can be performed: Above the actual pump mechanism is a hardened silicone case in which the deactivation button is located. One can squeeze forcibly on the narrow sides of this silicone case 90° from the button. Squeezing this area will distort the control valve allowing fluid to flow into the pump facilitating activation. In rare instances, operative intervention is needed to replace the pump mechanism.

2. Inability to squeeze pump: Pump failure is most often caused by obstruction of fluid flow by debris, airlock, blood, or crystals from the contrast solution or antibiotics. Another cause is kinking of the tubing. Prevention is the best treatment for this problem. It is imperative to be certain that the system is free of air and that blood or tissue debris are not introduced within the system. To prevent kinking, the tubing should be trimmed so that there is minimal redundancy. The likelihood of kinking has been decreased with the introduction of kink-resistant tubing by the manufacturer This complication is rare and treated by replacement of the affected parts.

3. Urinary retention: When urinary retention in the immediate postoperative period occurs, one must immediately rule out an activated system caused by an inflated cuff. Thus, one should cycle the sphincter and deactivate the device with the cuff empty. Immediate bladder emptying should occur. If urinary retention persists, a pelvic X-ray should be performed to assess the cuff. If contrast is found to be filling the cuff, this may suggest a malfunction of the sphincter. If the sphincter is

cycled and the cuff remains inflated, in spite of being deactivated in the open position, the pump needs to be replaced as the pump mechanism is probably defective. Second, the cuff may be too tight or there may be significant postoperative edema in the periurethral area causing retention. This can be assessed with flexible urethroscopy to assess the area compressed by the cuff. In the female, retention can be managed with intermittent catheterization with the device deactivated to allow time for the edema to resolve. In our experience, male retention rarely resolves and is usually secondary to a small cuff. Thus in the male, we recommend immediate replacement of the cuff with a larger size to prevent urethral damage from compression. Urinary retention occurring as a late complication may be due to inadvertent deactivation with the cuff closed, inflammation and edema from infection or erosion, or in men with recurrent bladder neck contracture. The patient must be seen immediately and evaluated. If an indwelling Foley must be inserted, the cuff must be deactivated in an open position.

4. Urinary incontinence: Incontinence immediately after the sphincter is activated may be secondary to a large cuff, low cuff filling pressure, leak in system, detrusor instability, or malfunction of sphincter. A pelvic X-ray should be performed with the cuff in the activated and deactivated state to be certain that the cuff fills and empties appropriately. The film can also demonstrate an empty or partially filled balloon suggesting a leak within the system. If a leak is demonstrated or suspected, surgical repair should be undertaken. Only the affected component needs replaced and the revised sphincter should be tested prior to leaving the operating room. Another source of error can occur when filling the balloon reservoir and calibrating the system. The reservoir for a 61–70 cm H_2O balloon should have 20 cm^3 of fluid, plus the amount of fluid held by the cuff.

Leakage occurring after continence was achieved may be secondary to mechanical failure, erosion, urethral atrophy, or detrusor instability. Urodynamics can be performed to rule out detrusor instability. If detrusor instability is identified, this can be treated with anticholinergic medication. A retrograde urethral pressure profile can be performed to ascertain the resistance at the level of the sphincter. The maximum pressure to break through the urethra at the level of the cuff should be equal to the balloon pressure. When the cuff pressure is inadequate as in leakage or atrophy, the maximum breakthrough pressure is lower than the balloon pressure. Cystoscopy with the cuff empty can identify erosion and ischemia. If secondary to erosion, the cuff should be removed and a catheter placed until the urethra heals. If secondary to atrophy, several options exist. One can increase the balloon pressure to 71–80 cm of water. However, this maneuver does not consistently improve continence and may lead to erosion. A smaller cuff can be placed, and this may be a reasonable option in the female, but in the male the smallest cuff size is 4.0 cm and this may not resolve the incontinence. The two best options in the male are to place a new cuff in a more proximal position, at the level of the bulbocavernosus muscle *(13)*. This has been shown to be effective. Second, two cuffs can be placed along the urethra doubling the surface area compressed, increasing resistance, without diminishing tissue perfusion *(14)*.

5. Infection: Infection is a devastating complication of the AUS and most often leads to removal of the device. The infection rate has been reported to be as high as 16%; however, 1–3% is currently the most common incidence *(15)*, except in patients who had radiation therapy preimplant, where the reported infection rate is 10% *(16)*. The infection is usually in the early postoperative period and is thought to occur secondary to seeding of the prosthesis at the time of surgery. The most common organism is *Staphylococcus epidermidis.* Delayed infection may be secondary to hematogenous spread from other sources such as genitourinary or dental infections. Infection usually presents as erythema or induration at the prosthetic site. The scrotum or labia is the most common site of infection. The overlying skin can become thinned and the pump can erode through. Urethroscopy should be performed to rule out cuff erosion. Early infections may not be associated with fever or leukocytosis and patients should be made aware of subtle signs of infection. A patient found to have an infection should be admitted to the hospital and receive broad spectrum antibiotics with good gram positive coverage. On occasion, a sphincter can be salvaged with antibiotics, however, most often the device needs to be removed. A new sphincter can be placed 3–6 mo after removal of the device and resolution of the infection. Prevention is the most important defense against infections. Diabetics should have their blood sugar well controlled. The incidence of prosthetic infections have been reported to be higher if the sphincter was placed concomitantly with bowel reconstruction of the bladder. Thus, a staged procedure should be performed. Appropriate preoperative and postoperative antibiotics need to be administered. Identification and eradication of bacterial infections 1–2 wk prior to sphincter placement must occur in patients on intermittent catheterization. An aggressive surgical scrub needs to be performed and the device should be soaked in antibiotic solution and the incisions aggressively irrigated with antibiotic solution prior to inserting the prosthesis.

6. Erosion: Erosion of the cuff through the urethra has a reported incidence of 0–19%. Since the introduction of delayed activation, the current erosion rate is 1–3% (15,17). Erosion may be caused by infection, decreased vascularity secondary to radiation changes, increased cuff pressure, undersized cuff, and catheterization through a closed sphincter. Erosions manifest as perineal pain, urethral discharge or bleeding,

hematuria, irritative voiding symptoms or new onset incontinence. A common cause of erosion is a result of placement of a Foley catheter with the sphincter in the closed position. This leads to compression of the urethra between the catheter and the cuff, which may lead to erosion. It is imperative that a urologist knowledgeable in artificial sphincters cycle and lock the sphincter in the open position when an indwelling Foley is placed. Patients are encouraged to carry a medical card stating they have an AUS or to wear an Medic-alert bracelet in the event of an emergency. Diagnosis of erosion is made by urethroscopy. Treatment involves removal of the cuff and placement of a urethral catheter for approx 3 wk. A retrograde urethrogram is performed prior to catheter removal to be certain that the urethra is healed. A new cuff can be placed at a different site usually after 3 mo. Once again, prevention is important. The cuff size should be appropriate. If the patient has had previous radiation therapy a 51–60 cm H_2O balloon should be placed to decrease the pressure on the urethra. In addition, delaying activation of the sphincter for 6 wk can decrease the likelihood of erosion. Patients who are at risk or who have a history of erosion should be instructed to deactivate the sphincter at night and wear a pad for leakage. This diminishes the amount of time the urethra is compressed, allowing for increased blood flow to the urethra. In addition, if a catheter needs to be placed (i.e., for other surgical procedures), the sphincter needs to be deactivated to prevent compression of the urethra between the cuff and catheter.

RESULTS WITH THE AMS800 ARTIFICIAL URINARY SPHINCTER

Since the development of the AMS sphincter in 1973, numerous modifications of the device and insertion techniques have gradually improved the effectiveness of the AUS and reduced the reoperation and complication rates.

By far and away, most experience has been accumulated on adult males in whom the AUS has been implanted for the problem of intrinsic sphincter deficiency. Generally, male type III stress urinary incontinence occurs after prostatectomy, and results with the AUS in this group have been very successful. In 1988, Marks and Light reported on 37 patients, 95% of whom achieved socially acceptable levels of incontinence and 81% of whom were completely dry (17). This group suffered three erosions (9%) and two infections (5%) and required four revisions (11%) (20). Gundian et al. from the Mayo Clinic reported on their experience with 96 patients, 83% of whom had incontinence requiring ≥2 pads/day. This group of patients also reported a 90% satisfaction rate (15). Finally,

Malloy et al. reported a 76% complete continence rate in 42 males in whom the AMS800 device was implanted *(18)*. We have met with similar success upon review of our long-term data (>2 yr) with insertion of the AMS800 AUS.

CONCLUSION

Clearly the use of the AUS should be part of the armamentarium in the management of refractory incontinence caused by intrinsic sphincter deficiency for every urologist. The current device, the AMS800, has proved successful and effective in the short and long term. Meticulous care in the patient workup preoperatively and during insertion is necessary, however, if maximum success is to be met. Proper indications for insertion are type III urinary incontinence caused by intrinsic sphincter deficiency. This should be well documented with endoscopic, urodynamic, or video fluoroscopic evaluation. All patients and their families should be well educated about potential outcomes and problems, particularly given that the device is a prosthesis. Before implantation, the patient's ability to use the sphincter from a physical and motivational standpoint should be thoroughly assessed.

Because of the risks for infection, erosion and mechanical malfunction, extreme attention to detail and meticulous surgical technique are required during insertion. Finally, to meet with continued success after insertion, the patients must be monitored closely as long as the device is in place. Patients and physicians should be aware of signs of potential problems, changes in voiding habits, or signs of voiding dysfunction or infection. We also recommend that they carry a medical identification card to identify them as having an AUS in case of an emergency. If a catheter is to be placed, the device should first be deactivated, and if the patient undergoes any abdominal surgery, a urologist with knowledge of AUS insertion and function should be available to assist in patient circumoperative management. With careful preoperative evaluation, intraoperative technique, and postoperative follow-up, problems can be dealt with effectively if they arise, and incontinent patients can achieve a significant improvement in their quality of life.

REFERENCES

1. Foley FB (1947) An artificial urinary sphincter. *J Urol* 50:250.
2. Scott FB, Bradley WE, Timm GW (1973) Treatment of urinary incontinence by implantable prosthetic sphincter. *Urology* 1:252.
3. Diokno AC, Taub ME (1976) Experience with the artificial urinary sphincter at Michigan. *J Urol* 116:496.
4. Furlow WL (1981) Implantation of a new semiautomatic artificial genitourinary sphincter: experience with primary activation and deactivation in 47 patients. *J Urol* 126:741.

5. Light JK (1985) The artificial urinary sphincter in children. *Urol Clin North Am* 12:103.
6. Mundy AR (1991) Artificial urinary sphincters. *Br J Urol* 67:225.
7. Scott FB, et al. (1981) Implantation of an artificial urinary sphincter for urinary incontinence. *Contemp Surg* 18:11.
8. Diokno AC, Sonda LP (1981) Compatibility of genitourinary prostheses and intermittent self-catheterization. *J Urol* 125:659.
9. Barrett DM, Furlow WL (1984) Incontinence, intermittent self-catheterization and the artificial genitourinary sphincter. *J Urol* 132:268.
10. Gonzalez R, Nguyen DH, Kolielat N, Sidi AA (1989) Compatibility of enterocystoplasty and the artificial urinary sphincter. *J Urol* 142:502.
11. Schmidt RA, Jonas U, Oleson KA, et al (1999) Sacral nerve stimulation for treatment of refractory urinary urge incontinence. *J Urol* 162:352–357.
12. Belloli G, Campobasso P, Mercurella A (1992) Neuropathic urinary incontinence in pediatric patients: management with artificial sphincters. *J Pediatr Surg* 27:1461.
13. Couillard DR, Vapnek JM, Stone AR (1994) Proximal artificial sphincter cuff repositioning for urethral atrophy. *Urology* 45:653–656.
14. Brito CG, Mulcahy JJ, Mitchell ME, et al. (1993) Use of a double cuff AMS 800 urinary sphincter for severe stress incontinence. *J Urol* 149:283–285.
15. Gundian JC, Barrett DM, Parulkar BG (1989) Mayo Clinic experience with use of the AMS800 artificial urinary sphincter for urinary incontinence following radical prostatectomy. *J Urol* 142:1459.
16. Martins FE, Boyd SD (1995) Artificial urinary sphincter in patients following major pelvic surgery and/or radiotherapy: are they less favorable candidates. *J Urol* 153:1188–1193.
17. Marks JL, Light JK (1989) Management of urinary incontinence after prostatectomy with the artificial urinary sphincter. *J Urol* 142:302.
18. Malloy TR, Wein AJ, Carpiniello VL (1989) Surgical success with AMS M800 GU sphincter for male incontinence. *Urology* 33:274.

18 Female Incontinence and the Artificial Urinary Sphincter

Irving J. Fishman, MD
and F. Brantley Scott, MD

CONTENTS

INTRODUCTION
ARTIFICIAL URINARY SPHINCTER
PATIENT CANDIDATES
IMPLANTATION TECHNIQUES
RESULTS
CONCLUSION
REFERENCES

INTRODUCTION

Urinary incontinence (UI), defined as the involuntary leakage of urine sufficient to be a problem, afflicts approx 13 to 14 million Americans and, according to the National Institute of Diabetes and Digestive and Kidney Diseases (NIDDK), 11 million of them are women. One half of the residents of nursing homes are incontinent. In 1995, Americans spent approx $27.8 billion on the management of UI. Based on NIDDK statistics, the average patient with UI spent $3941 annually on the problem.

Among the various therapies available for management of UI, are use of pharmacological agents, bladder retraining, and surgical procedures, such as cystourethropexies, sling procedures, or injection of bulking

From: *Urologic Prostheses:*
The Complete, Practical Guide to Devices, Their Implantation and Patient Follow Up
Edited by: C. C. Carson © Humana Press Inc., Totowa, NJ

agents. In patients who have failed conventional treatments, the artificial urinary sphincter (AUS) is a reasonable alternative.

In 1973, F. Brantley Scott, along with Dr. Bradley and Dr. Timm, developed and implanted the first AUS. Since then, approx 3000 AUS devices have been implanted. American Medical Systems, the corporation that manufactures the device has made many improvements in its components and quality. The 800 model was first introduced in 1979, has undergone several modifications including introduction of kink-proof tubing and a more efficient and resilient narrow back cuff. Two-hundred and thirty-nine females have undergone implantation of the AUS by the authors since 1973. Of these, 108 received the earlier models (AUS 791/792) and 68 received the AS 800. The majority of these patients suffered from urethral sphincter incompetence of varying etiologies including myelomeningocoele, pelvic floor weakness with stress incontinence, and neurogenic bladders. In all of them, more conservative attempts at restoring continence had failed. Many other centers have used the AUS for treatment of urinary incontinence in females. In this chapter, the authors will review their and other's experience with this device.

ARTIFICIAL URINARY SPHINCTER

The basic objective of the AUS is to provide patients with dynamic control of the resistance to the bladder outflow as opposed to simply obstructing the outlet as with a sling procedure or with collagen injection. The latest device is the American Medical System AS 800 (*see* Fig. 1), which consists of three components made of medical-grade silicon: an occlusive cuff of variable length positioned around the bladder neck, a pump with a locking mechanism placed inside the labia majora, as well as a dip coated pressure control balloon implanted in the paravesical space (*see* Fig. 2). All of these components are interconnected with nylon-reinforced nonkinking silicon tubing. The system is filled with either normal saline or, preferably, an isotonic contrast solution that allows visualization of the device on X-ray. Normally, the device is in a closed position with the cuff inflated and uniformly compressing the bladder neck and proximal urethra. When the patient needs to urinate, she compresses the labial pump, which transfers fluid from the cuff to the balloon thereby permitting urine outflow.

The 2.0-cm-wide occlusive cuff is a longitudinal silicon balloon that incorporates a narrower (1.7 cm) outside Dacron layer with a snap-like closure. It is available in various lengths from 4.0 cm to 11.0 cm. The narrower backing improves the efficiency of the cuff and decreases the incidence of tissue pressure atrophy. An additional internal coating

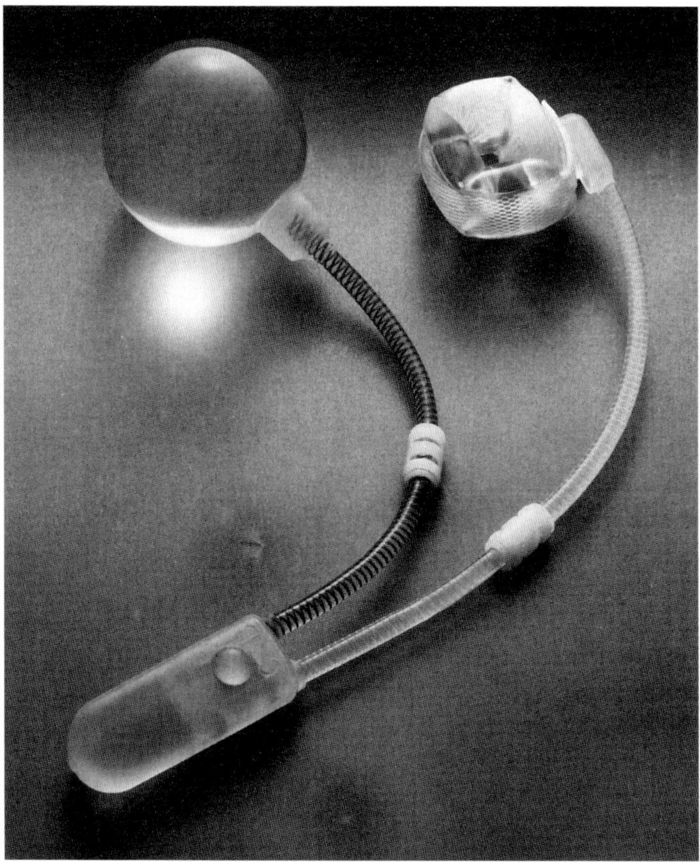

Fig. 1. American Medical System AS 800 (used with permission from American Medical Systems, Inc., Minnetonka, MN).

of a silicon material improves the pliability and the decreases the wear at the fold sites of the cuff.

The pressure-regulating balloon is available in variable pressure spectrums, ranging from 51–60 cm H_2O to 81–90 H_2O, allowing the surgeon to determine the most appropriate pressure for the individual patient. It is implanted intraabdominally, adjacent to the bladder, so that the same abdominal pressures that are exerted on the bladder are also impacting on the balloon and thereby transferred to the cuff, preventing stress leakage. The balloon is connected to the pump via reinforced silicon tubing.

The pump, which is positioned in the labia majora, consists of the pumping chamber and an ingenious control assembly that has a unique resistor and valve systems that assure delayed refill of the cuff as well

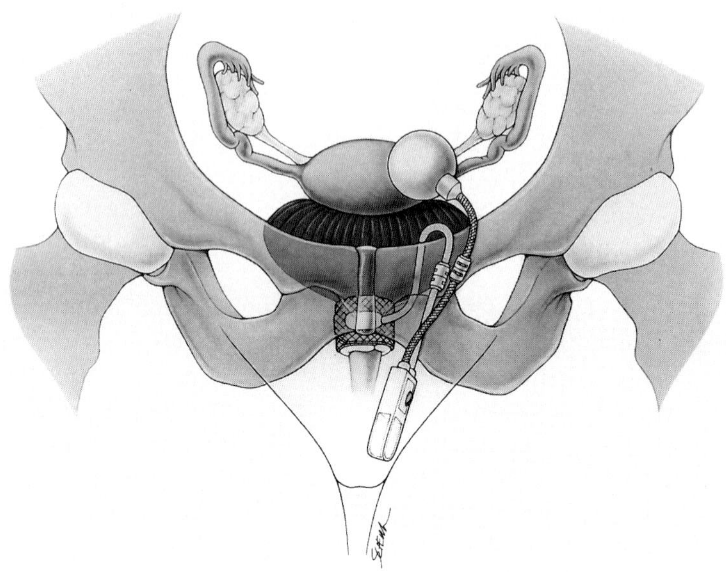

Fig. 2. Appearance of Implanted AUS 800 in female.

as instantaneous transfer of pressures from the balloon to the cuff. In addition, the control assembly pump has a button that allows the cuff to be locked in either an open or closed position. Locking the cuff in an open position minimizes the risk of injury to the urethra during catheterization or other manipulations. These new features of the AUS have improved the reliability of the device.

PATIENT CANDIDATES

Females with UI of multiple etiologies are potential candidates for the AUS implant. Among these are women (or young girls) with neurogenic bladders caused by myelomeningocoele, sacral agenesis, spinal trauma, or peripheral neuropathies and women with stress incontinence that has not responded to more conservative measures. The typical patient is a woman who has adequate bladder compliance and capacity, but whose bladder neck and urethral sphincter are nonocclusive as in Type III stress incontinence.

Potential candidates for the AUS are evaluated with a comprehensive history and physical exam, as well as with extensive urodynamic testing, which includes simultaneous pressure flow and EMG studies, voiding cystourethrography, and cystoscopy. The physician should seek out evidence for bladder instability or urgency, previous urological and/or gynecological surgery, symptoms of neurological disorders (e.g., multiple sclerosis or peripheral neuropathies), and history of recurrent urinary tract infections. Bladder compliance and associated capacity should be adequate to make the patient socially continent with the bladder neck closed. In some women with small bladder capacity or poor compliance despite anticholinergic medication, implantation of the AUS has resulted in increased bladder capacity. However, if there is persistent elevated intravesical pressure with small bladder capacity, augmentation cystoplasty should be seriously considered. Patients with evidence of outflow obstruction as a result of detrusor sphincter dyssynergia or anatomical obstruction are treated with a bladder flap urethroplasty at the time of AUS implantation or are managed with intermittent self-catheterization postoperatively. If intermittent catheterization will be required postoperatively, then the patient should be properly prepared preoperatively with instruction in the proper technique for clean intermittent self-catheterization.

In addition, a careful evaluation of the patient's past surgical or pelvic trauma is essential so that any scarring may be anticipated, especially in the area of the urethral vaginal septum. Pretreatment of postmenopausal women with estrogen cream will usually make the vaginal tissues more supple and resilient. The patient is apprised of the risk of the surgery and the possibility of device failure at any time subsequent to the surgery. Patients must be highly motivated to have the surgery, and they must have the manual dexterity as well as the mental competence and initiative to operate the device. Young girls who refuse to pump the device in order to urinate may cause significant deterioration of their renal function. The surgeon and patient must accept the fact that the patient will have to be followed regularly (at least annually) to assure stability of renal function. In addition, should the patient require abdominal or pelvic surgery in the future, she should apprise her urologist so that accidental injury to the device can be avoided.

IMPLANTATION TECHNIQUES

Two surgical approaches have evolved for implantation of the AUS. The main difference concerns the implantation of the cuff. The original technique described by Scott was a retropubic approach (1). The alternative approach is transvaginal dissection of a track around the urethra for cuff placement in combination with a suprapubic inguinal incision for placement of the other components (2).

In either case, the patient's urine must be sterile and she must be properly prepared. The patient is shaved in the operating room immediately prior to the 10-min preparation of both the abdomen and the vagina. Surgery should not proceed if there are any open lesions in the surgical field. The patient is usually given a loading dose of a broad-spectrum antibiotic 1 h before surgery. Traffic in the operating room is minimized, and the surgical team wear surgical hoods to decrease possibility of shedding into the wound.

The positioning of the sphincter cuff is the most challenging part of the operation. The plane between the bladder neck and the vagina is not very distinct, even in females who previously have not had surgery in that area. Patients who have undergone multiple conventional anti-incontinence procedures and young girls who have had bladder neck reconstruction offer the surgeon very few anatomic landmarks to work with. Two basic approaches have been advocated for implantation of the cuff. The original approach, as described by Scott was retropubic. More recently, a transvaginal perineal approach has been advocated.

The patient is placed in a lithotomy position with thighs parallel to her abdomen in order to maximize working area for the surgeon and the assistants. In addition, this position makes feasible an intraoperative cystoscopy to evaluate urethral patency. A 10-min surgical scrub of both the abdomen and the vagina is performed.

In the abdominal approach, the retropubic space is entered via a Cherney incision that transects both rectus muscles and optimizes pelvic exposure (*see* Fig. 3). The pelvic fascia is incised on either side of the bladder neck. The latter is usually well defined with the help of an intravesical Foley catheter balloon, but if there is any doubt about the anatomy because of extensive local scarring, the bladder is opened from above to facilitate visualization of the bladder neck and the ureteral orifices. Bilateral blunt and careful sharp dissection with angled scissors with simultaneous transvaginal palpation allows one to develop a space through the proximal urethrovaginal septum. An instrument that was developed specifically to expedite this portion of the operation is the Cutter clamp, which consists of two hollow detachable arms that fit together at the level of a clamp proximally and at the distal curved ends. The latter are configured into male and female tips that fit together. Once the endopelvic fascia is incised and the bladder neck is identified, the clamp is positioned in the area of the proposed cuff site (*see* Fig. 4). The arms are tightened in the clamp, and cystoscopy as well as vaginal examination allows the surgeon to rule out entrapment of excess tissue of either the bladder or vagina. Appropriate adjustments can then be made. Once it is determined that the correct plane has been chosen a cutting blade is advanced from the male clamp into the hollow of the female end, thereby cutting through the urethral vaginal plane (*see* Fig. 5).

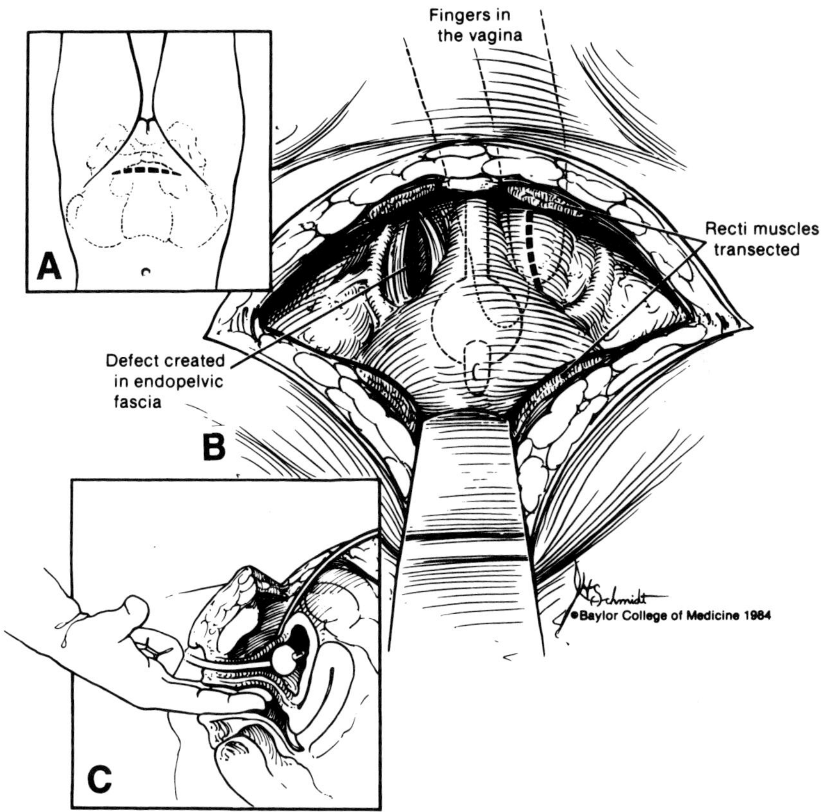

Fig. 3. Trans-abdominal approach for implantation of AUS 800.

The female arm is then unclamped and removed to expose the cutting blade. A 1-0 polypropylene suture is advanced through a hole in the blade and the latter is then gently removed, pulling the attached suture through this newly created space. A right-angle clamp is then attached to the suture and is gently guided along the new track. The space is carefully stretched to approx 2 cm to accommodate a cuff.

The cuff length is determined by measuring the loose circumference around the bladder neck with a cuff sizer. The cuff is then positioned in this space and snapped closed. Care must be exercised to avoid twisting of the cuff in the course of positioning it around the bladder neck. The length of the BN cuff ranges from 6–10 cm. The pressure-regulating balloon is then implanted in a paravesical space, assuring that there is no contact between it and the cuff. Rubbing of two silicon components can ultimately lead to thinning of the silicon and leakage. The pressure range of the balloon that is selected is determined on the basis of a

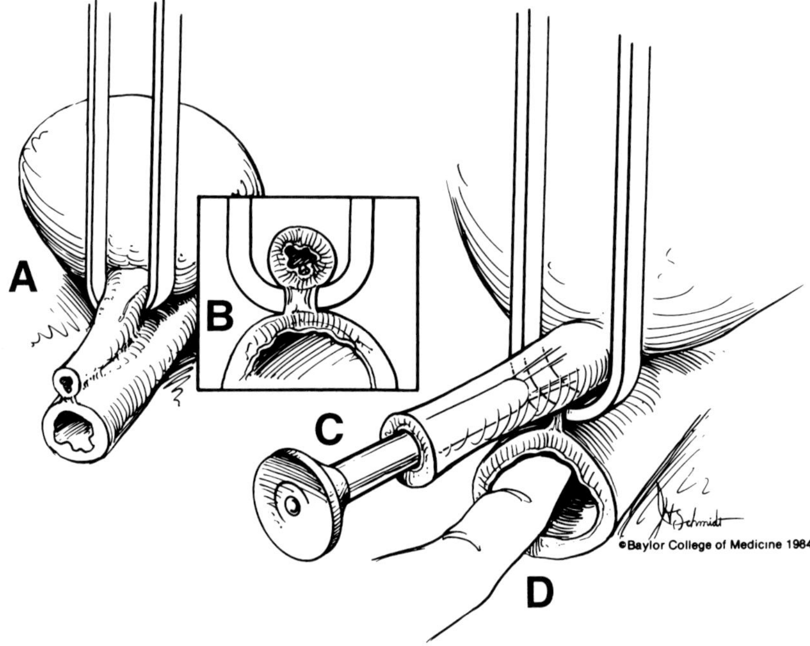

Fig. 4. Use of Cutter Clamp for implantation of AUS cuff.

variety of factors including the quality and vascular supply of the bladder neck, the intravesical pressures, and whether there was a past history of pelvic radiation. If there is evidence of poor tissue quality, then a lower pressure balloon is selected (51–60 cm H_2O). Otherwise, higher pressure balloons can be used. The balloon is filled with a volume of either saline or isotonic contrast material equal to 16 cm^3 plus the volume in the cuff, usually a minimal volume of 21 cm^3. The balloon and cuff tubings are brought through the abdominal muscles and fascia in order to help fix them in place. The deactivation pump is advanced into a space created in one of the labia majora with the help of an extended nasal speculum. The latter minimizes local trauma by bluntly dissecting a pouch for the pump. After the balloon is filled with an appropriate amount of saline or contrast-plus-water solution, the redundant tubing is amputated and Quick connectors are used to connect the appropriate tubes. Great care must be taken to keep any blood products from getting into the system because the resultant fibrinoid material will clog the valves or resistors resulting in a malfunction. The wounds are then checked for hemostasis, irrigated with copious amounts of antibiotic solution, and closed securely in multiple layers. Drains are avoided to

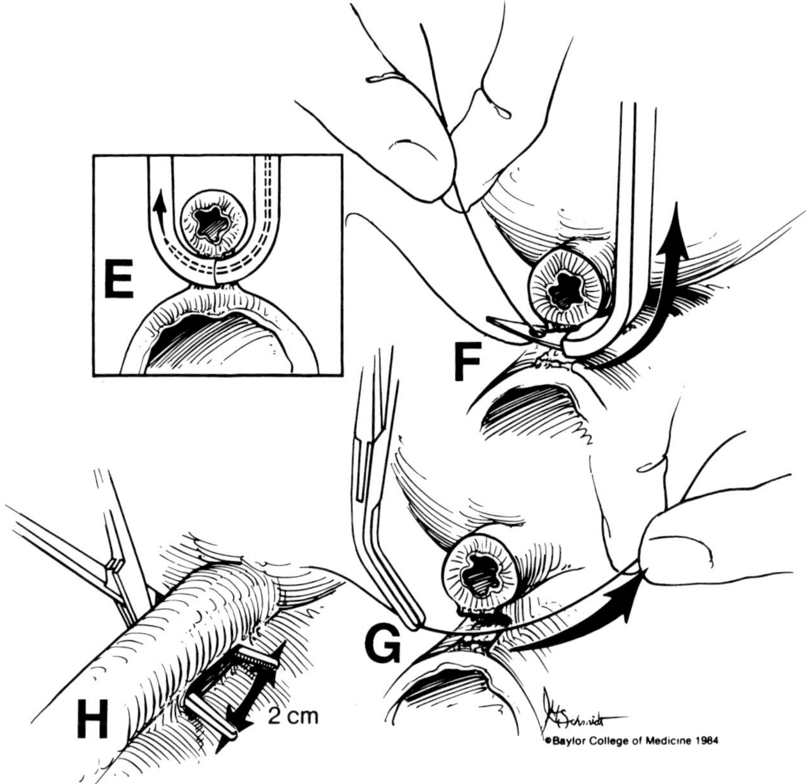

Fig. 5. Use of Cutter Clamp for implantation of AUS cuff.

minimize the risk of infection. The cuff is left deactivated for approx 4–6 wk. An X-ray of the lower abdomen is taken on the first post-operative day in order to document the location of the various components and their size. If, in the course of the cuff placement, the urethra or bladder was entered, the longer deactivation period may better allow for adequate healing. The patient is prescribed broad-spectrum antibiotics for approximately 10 d post-op. An icepack to the perineum minimizes local pain and decreases swelling.

Appell *(2)* and Hadley *(3)* popularized the transvaginal placement of the cuff around the bladder neck using a technique similar to that described by McGuire for the sling procedure. The advantage of this approach is that the dissection of the plane between the bladder neck and vagina can be performed under direct vision. The patient is prepared in a fashion similar to that aforementioned. A Foley catheter is inserted and the balloon inflated to 10 cm^3. The latter facilitates identification and

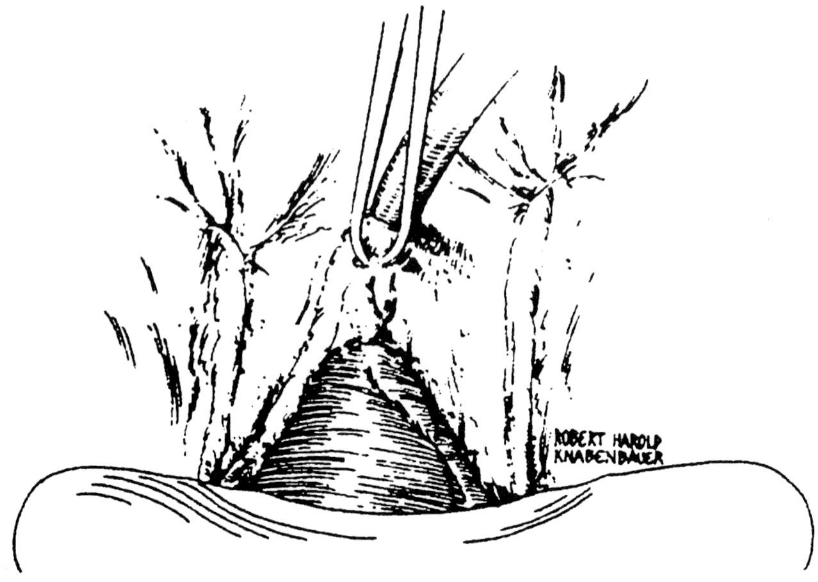

Fig. 6. Vaginal incision.

palpation of the bladder neck. A weighted speculum is placed in the
vagina and an inverted U-shaped incision is made in the anterior vaginal
wall extending from a point lateral and proximal to the bladder neck to
a point midway between the bladder neck and the urethral meatus (*see*
Fig. 6). This proximally-based vaginal flap is carefully dissected off the
urethra and bladder neck assuring adequate thickness of the flap to cover
the cuff. The proximal dissection is then extended through the
endopelvic fascia sweeping from lateral to medial, thereby creating an
opening into the retropubic space (*see* Fig. 7). Dissection of this type is
done on both sides of the bladder neck. The urethra must then be freed
from its anterior attachments to the pubis. This usually can be be done
with blunt dissection but may require sharp dissection, which adds the
risk of an accidental cystotomy. Alternatively, one may free the urethra
from the symphysis by a supra-urethral crescent-shaped incision (*see*
Fig. 8), which permits sharp dissection in the midline immediately below
the symphysis pubis (*see* Fig. 9). The dissection can then be completed
with blunt dissection, creating a circumferential space around the bladder neck and proximal urethra (*see* Fig. 10). The circumference of the
bladder neck is measured by pulling a cuff measuring tape through the
newly created space with the help of a broken back curved vascular
clamp (*see* Fig. 11). Once the measurement is obtained, a cuff, which is

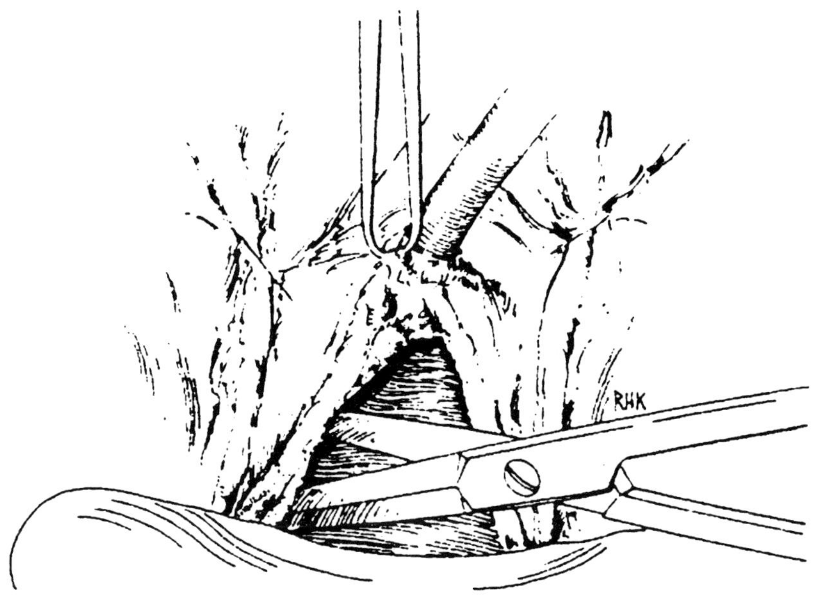

Fig. 7. Para-urethral vaginal dissection.

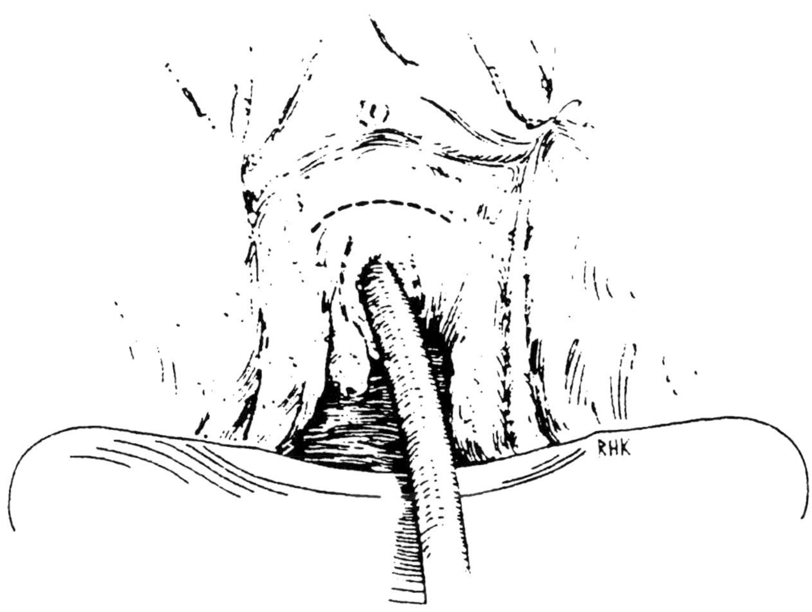

Fig. 8. Supra-urethral vaginal incision for release of scarred tissue between symphysis and urethra.

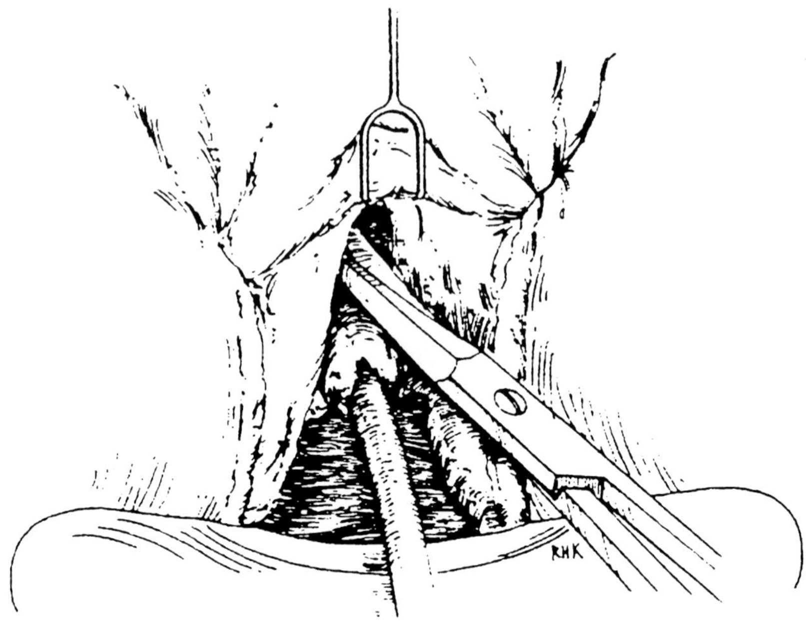

Fig. 9. Dissection of scarred supra-urethral space.

approx 0.5-cm longer, is selected and positioned around the bladder neck
(*see* Fig. 11). The direction of insertion of the cuff is determined by the
proposed location of the pump. If the pump is to be placed in the left
labia, then the cuff should be advanced tab first from the left to the right,
and vice versa if the pump is to be positioned in the right labia majora
Once the tab is snapped around the button, the whole cuff is rotated 180°
so that the button is in the infrapubic position, on the anterior portion of
the urethra or bladder neck (*see* Fig. 12). The pump and reservoir balloon are then inserted via a small transverse suprapubic incision. It is
important to position the reservoir in a paravesical space to assure
adequate pressure transfer. The cuff tubing is then passed into the suprapubic incision using a tubing passer. Once the pump is properly positioned in the labia majorum and the system has been filled with the
appropriate amount of fluid, the redundant tubing is amputated and
connections are made using Quick connectors. Usually, a right-angle
Quick connector is used between the tubing of the cuff and pump. The
vaginal flap is carefully closed over the cuff and urethra with a running
2–0 Vicryl suture. A vaginal pack is inserted and left in place until the end
of the first postoperative day. The Foley is left in place for approx 1 wk. The
AUS is deactivated for approx 6 wk to allow for adequate healing.

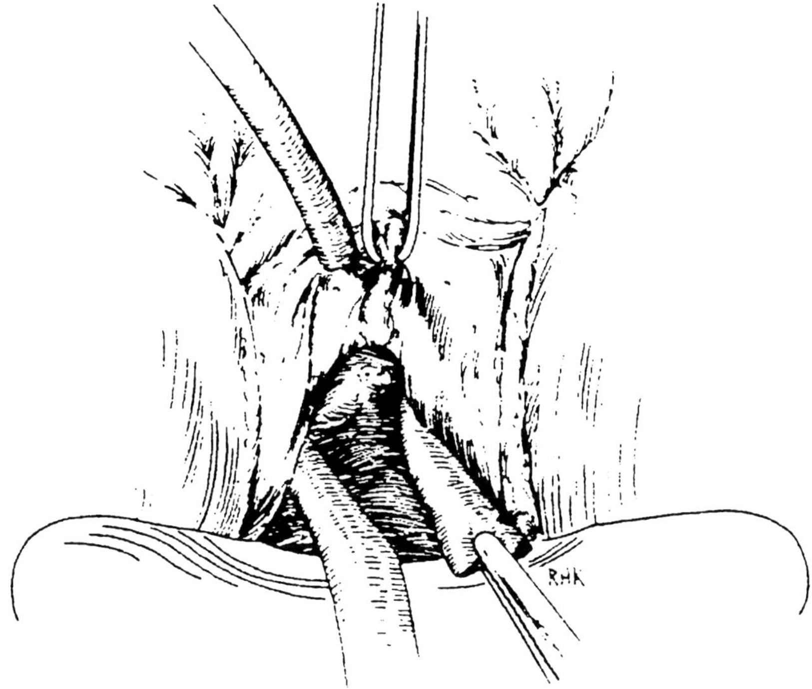

Fig. 10. Penrose drain in the space around the urethra and bladder neck.

A major concern among urologists who used the infrapubic approach preferentially was that the vaginal approach would increase the risk of infection. Surprisingly, infection has not been a major problem. In Appell's series of 34 women with type III stress urinary incontinence, no infections, erosions, or bladder instabilities were noted. Nineteen of these women had been followed for at least 3 yr. Four were emptying their bladders with intermittent self-catheterization.

RESULTS

Review of the urologic literature suggests that there has been an increase in the use of the AUS for the treatment of urinary incontinence in the female. Most reports describe implants done via an abdominal approach. In our series, 239 females underwent implantation of a variety of models of the AUS between 1973 and 1999 (*see* Table 1). Of these, 108 received the AUS 791/792 model and another 68 received the AS 800 device. The age range of patients was 5–84 yr. The 68 female patients who received the AS 800 devices were followed for as long as

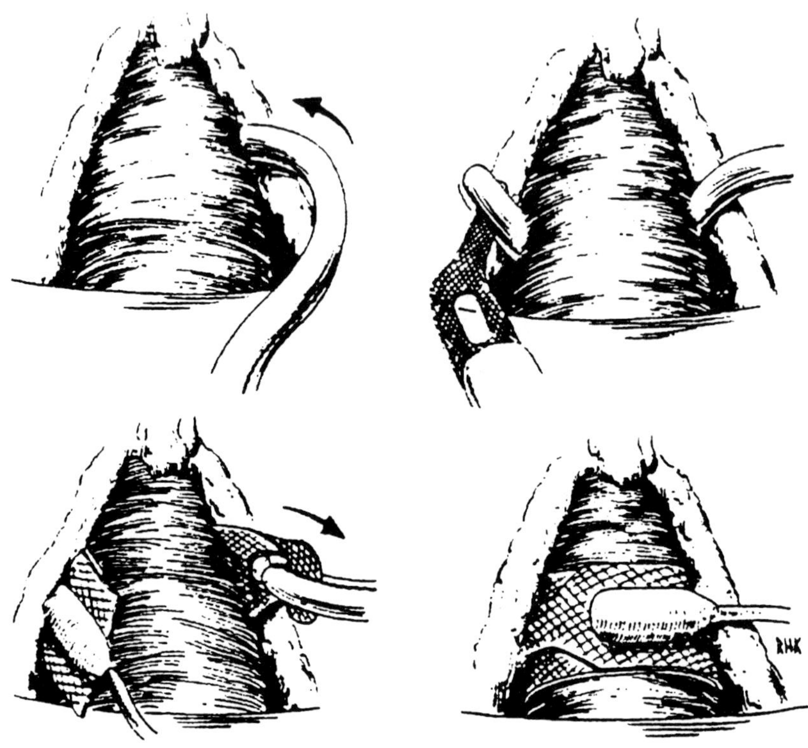

Fig. 11. A "broken back" curved vascular clamp is passed around the urethra and the cuff is grasped and positioned around the bladder neck and proximal urethra. The snap closure is secured.

12 yr. A total of 12 patients required revisions—three because of mechanical failures and nine because of surgical problems. Five devices (7%) were lost because of infections. Ten devices (14%) were total failures because of infection and erosion of the cuff. Of the remaining patients, 86% continue to be socially continent. This compares favorably with similar results obtained by Schreiter *(4)* who reported an 86% continence rate in his series of 144 women with incontinence of different etiologies. In a series of 212 women implanted with the AUS 800 for treatment of type three stress incontinence, Costa *(5)* reported an 88.7% continence rate. Their explantation rate was 4.3% for erosions and infections.

Appell and Abbassian *(2)* in 1988, published their data on 34 patients who had undergone implantation of an AS 800 via a vaginal approach. Their 3-yr follow-up in 19 of these patients revealed total continence. Three of these patients required a revision for mechanical problems. Hadley

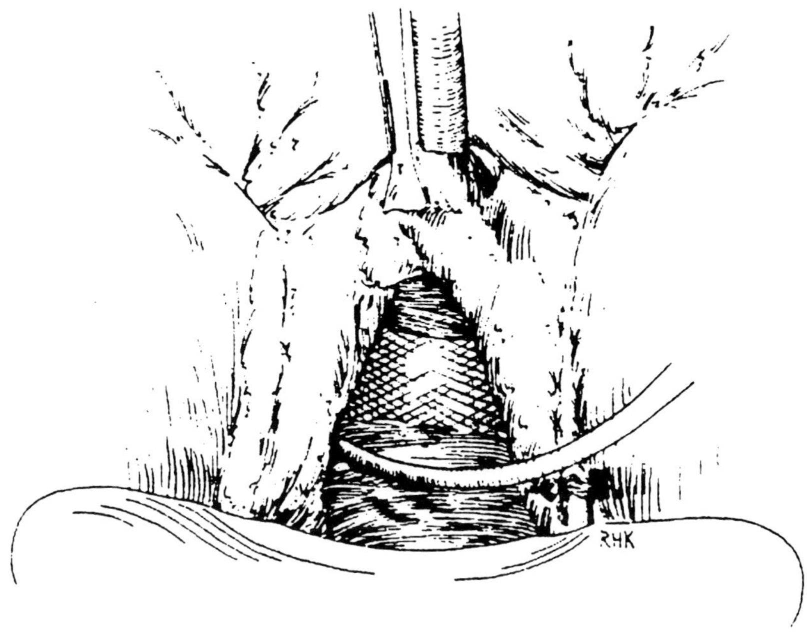

Fig. 12. The cuff is rotated 180° clockwise so the hard snap button ends up lying anterior to the urethra and away from the vaginal wall.

reported that of a series of 14 women, whose implantation was achieved via a vaginal approach, 13 were socially continent *(3)*. The follow-up ranged from 6–24 mo. Thus, no matter which approach is used, it would appear that in most cases of AUS implantation in females with urinary incontinence, the likelihood of success is quite high.

A review of a group of young women who had undergone implantation of the AUS for management of incontinence when they were children (mostly spina bifida or spinal tumors) revealed that sexual activity is not compromised by the presence of an AUS. Seven of the patients conceived and ultimately delivered nine healthy children. The mode of delivery was left to the discretion of the obstetrician, but four were vaginal deliveries without any adverse effects on the mother or baby *(6)*.

CONCLUSION

In summary, women suffering from total urinary incontinence, unresponsive to conventional therapy, can regain continence via implantation of the AMS AS 800 and go on to lead normal productive lives. The implantation may be accomplished via a vaginal or abdominal approach

Table 1
The Etiologies of Incontinence

Etiology	Number of Patients (%)
Myelomeningocoele	18 (26%)
Pelvic fracture	2 (2%)
Spinal cord injury	1 (1%)
Stress incontinence	14 (20%)
Neurogenic bladder	7 (10%)
Exstrophy-epispadias	3 (4%)
Post urethroplasties	8 (11%)
Sacral dysgenesis	2 (2%)
Other	13 (19%)

A total of 239 women have undergone implantation of the different models of the AUS in our facility since 1973. Sixty-eight of these females received the AS 800 model. Patient ages ranged from 5–84 yr.

with equal success depending on the skill and option of the surgeon. As urologists, it behooves us to be familiar with this therapeutic option.

REFERENCES

1. Scott FB (1985) The use of the artificial sphincter in the treatment of urinary incontinence in the female patient. *Urol Clin North Am* 12(2):305.
2. Appell RA (1988) Techniques and results in the implantation of the artificial urinary sphincter in women with Type III stress urinary incontinence by a vaginal approach. *Neurourol Urodynam* 7:613–619.
3. Hadley R (1988) Transvaginal placement of the artificial urinary sphincter in women. *Neurourol Urodynam* 7:292–293.
4. Heitz M, Oliaias R, Schreiter F (1997) Therapy of female urinary incontinence with the AMS 800 artificial sphincter. Indications, outcome, complications and risk factors. *Urologe A* Sep; 36(5):426–31.
5. Costa P, Rabut B, Turret R, Mottet N, Ben Naoum K, Wagner L, Louis JF (1999) Efficiency and Tolerance of the AUS in Females with Medium and Long Term Follow-up. Nimes, France. Abstract P54 , French Congress of Urology (A.F.U. 1999) Nov. 17–21.
6. Fishman IJ, Scott FB (1993) Pregnancy in patients with the artificial urinary sphincter. *J. Urol* 150:340–341.

INDEX

A

AMS 700 CX penile implant,
    characteristics, 181, 182, 186
    failure rate compared with Mentor
        a-1, 192, 193, 195, 198
    modeling procedure for
        Peyronie's disease,
        caveats, 214, 216
        complications, 212–214
        development, 207, 208
        technique, 208, 209, 211, 212
AMS 700 CXM, *see* Penile prosthesis
AMS 700 Ultrex, *see* Penile prosthesis
AMS 800, *see* Artificial urinary
    sphincter
AMS Ambicor, *see* Penile prosthesis
AMS Dynaflex, *see* Penile prosthesis
AMS Hydroflex, *see* Penile prosthesis
Artificial urinary sphincter (AUS),
    AMS 800 features, 265, 266,
        286–288
    double-cuff sphincters, 165
    female patients,
        AMS 800 outcomes, 297–299
        patient selecton and work-up,
            288, 289
        surgical techniques, 289–294,
            296, 297
    history of development, 164,
        263–265, 286
    male patients,
        AMS 800 outcomes, 282, 283
        history of patient, 267
        indications, 266, 269, 270
        Interstim neuromodulation
            program, 268
        laboratory tests, 267–269
        patient selection, 266–268
        physical examination, 267
        postoperative follow-up,
            278, 279
        problems and solutions,
            erosion, 281, 282
            infection, 281
            pump squeezing, 279
            sphincter activation, 279
            urinary incontinene,
                280, 281
            urinary retention, 279, 280
        radical prostatectomy
            incontinence treatment,
            98, 165, 269, 270
        surgical techniques, 270–275,
            277, 278
    operation, 286–288
    reliability, 164, 165
AUS, *see* Artificial urinary sphincter

B

Benign prostatic hyperplasia (BPH),
    prevalence, 117
    transurethral resection of prostate,
        117, 118
    urethral stent,
        clinical trial comparing
            transurethral resection
            of prostate,
            BPH impact index, 133,
                134, 138
            ejaculation, 126, 127
            erection outcomes, 125, 126
            erection pain, 125, 138
            intercourse pain, 125
            IPSS symptom scores, 132
            long-term outcomes, 139
            patient characteristics, 136

peak flow rate, 129, 138, 139
pressure flow studies, 132
procedure, 122, 123, 135
quality-of-life scores, 133
residual urine volume,
129, 131
safety, 123, 124, 137
study design, 121, 122
urethral pain, 124, 125, 137
endoscopic follow-up,
encrustation, 127
epithelialization, 127, 138
hyperplasia, 128
residual hypertrophic
tissue, 128
stent migration, 128
insertion, 120, 121
Urovolume stent studies,
overview, 118–120,
134, 135
Bioglass, injection therapy, 56, 63
Bladder replacement,
grafts, historical perspective, 9
tissue engineering,
beagle studies, 13, 14
cell regeneration, 10
compliance, 14
fetal tissue engineering, 22–24
immunocytochemical
analysis, 14
matrices, 10, 11
strategies, 10
BPH, *see* Benign prostatic
hyperplasia

C

Calcium hydroxylate, injection
therapy, 57, 63
Chondrocyte, penile rod construction,
16, 17
Chondrogel, injection therapy, 59,
65, 68, 74
Collagen, urinary incontinence
treatment with injection,
characteristics, 72, 73
injection technique, 37–39

outcome data, 32, 33
radical prostatectomy patients,
96, 98
Contigen, injection therapy, 58, 65,
66, 67, 68, 70, 71
Corpus cavernosum,
fibrosis, *see also* Peyronie's
disease,
etiologies, 249
implantation surgery,
complications, 259
corporotomy, 254, 255, 258
dilators, 251, 252
downsized prosthesis,
252–254
postoperative care, 259
reconstruction with
synthetic grafts, 258
patient evaluation
for prosthesis,
history, 250
miscellaneous tests, 250
physical examination, 250
penile prosthesis indication,
161, 162, 176, 196
reoperation management in
penile prosthesis
implantation, 235,
237–239
sizing for penile prosthesis, 188
tissue engineering,
cell regeneration, 10
immunocytochemical analysis,
15, 16
matrices, 10, 11
rationale, 15
strategies, 10
tissue harvesting, 16
Cymetra, injection therapy, 58

D

Dacomed Dura II, *see* Penile
prosthesis
Deflux, injection therapy, 57, 65, 68
Detrusor-sphincter dyssynergia
(DSD),
complications, 101, 110

external sphincterectomy, 102,
111, 113
intravesicle pressure minimization,
101, 102
medical management, 102, 113
sphincter ablation, 102
treatment approach, 113
urethral stents,
historical perspective, 102, 103
permanent stents, 103–109
removal, 112
temporary stents, 109, 110, 113
Dextran, injection therapy, 57, 63
DSD, *see* Detrusor-sphincter
dyssynergia
Dura II, development, 5
Durasphere, injection technique, 39
Durasphere, injection therapy, 56,
62, 64

E

ED, *see* Erectile dysfunction
Erectile dysfunction (ED),
historical perspectives, 1, 6
medical treatment, 219
penile prosthesis, *see* Penile
prosthesis
Peyronie's disease association, 202
Ethylene vinyl alcohol, injection
therapy, 57, 68, 69
External sphincterectomy,
detrusor-sphincter
dyssynergia management,
102, 111, 113

F, G

Fat, injection therapy, 59, 65, 67,
68, 73
Flexiflate, development, 5
Gene therapy, tissue engineering,
24, 25

H, I

Hydroflex, development, 5
Hylagel-Uro, injection therapy,
58, 70

Incontinence, *see* Urinary
incontinence
Injectable therapy,
materials,
bioglass, 56, 63
calcium hydroxylate, 57, 63
Chondrogel, 59, 65, 68, 74
collagen, 72, 73
Contigen, 58, 65, 66, 67, 68,
70, 71
Cymetra, 58
Deflux, 57, 65, 68
dextran, 57, 63
Durasphere, 56, 62, 64
ethylene vinyl alcohol, 57,
68, 69
fat, 59, 65, 67, 68, 73
Hylagel-Uro, 58, 70
Macroplastique, 56, 60–62,
64, 66, 68
outcomes by material,
female incontinence, 64, 65
male incontinence, 66, 67
vesicouretal reflux, 68
polyvinyl alcohol, 57, 68
silk-elastin polymer, 58, 70
small intestine submucosa,
58, 71, 72
smooth muscle, 59, 74
table, 56–59
Teflon, 55, 56, 60, 64, 66, 68
Urethrin, 56
Urocol, 56
Urologen, 58
UroVive, 57, 64, 66, 68, 69, 70
Teflon injection following
radical prostatectomy, *see*
Teflon injection therapy
tissue engineering,
testicular functional
replacement, 20, 22
urinary incontinence, 19, 20
vesicouretal reflux, 19, 20
urinary incontinence treatment,
antegrade injection, 33
carbon steel particles, 34

children, 33
collagen,
    injection technique, 37–39
    outcome data, 32, 33
    Durasphere injection
        technique, 39
    female versus male outcomes,
        74, 75
    goals, 47, 48
    historical perspectives, 29,
        30, 90, 91
    patient selection,
        cystoscopy, 47
        history, 45, 46
        men, 35, 37
        physical examination, 46
        urodynamic testing, 46, 47
        women, 34, 35
    postoperative care, 51–53
    silicone microimplants, 34
    type III stress incontinence,
        30–32
    urethral injection techniques,
        females, 48–50
        males, 50, 51
    vesicouretal reflux,
        patient evaluation, 53, 54
        postoperative care, 54, 55
        techniques, 54

K, L

Kidney, tissue engineering,
    approaches, 18, 19
    cell regeneration, 10
    challenges, 18
    matrices, 10, 11
    strategies, 10
Leydig cell, encapsulation
        and testicular functional
        replacement, 20, 22

M

Macroplastique, injection therapy,
    56, 60–62, 64, 66, 68
Mentor α-1,
    autoinflation, 195, 196
    corporeal fibrosis patients, 196

development and design, 192
failure rate compared with AMS
        700 CX, 192, 193, 195, 198
modeling procedure for
        Peyronie's disease,
    caveats, 214, 216
    complications, 212–214
    development, 207, 208
    technique, 208, 209, 211, 212
    patient satisfaction, 196–198
Mentor Saline-Filled Testicular
        Prosthesis, *see* Testicular
        prosthesis

N–P

Neurogenic bladder, *see*
        Detrusor-sphincter dyssynergia
Omniphase, development, 5
Penile prosthesis,
    device classification and types,
        156–158
    erosion,
        etiology, 251, 242
        management, 242, 243
        sites, 241, 242
        urethral erosion, 243
    historical perspectives, 1–6,
        155, 156
    indications,
        corpus cavernosum fibrosis,
            161, 162, 176, 249–255,
            258, 259
        erectile dysfunction, 189,
            198, 231, 232
        Peyronie's disease, 159–161,
            176, 206–209,
            211–214, 216
        priapism, 162
        radical prostatectomy, 162, 163
        reconstruction, 159, 163, 170
        spinal cord injury, 163, 175, 176
    infection,
        incidence, 220, 221
        pathogens, 222
        prevention,
            antibiotics, 222

site preparation, 221, 222
urinary tract infection
treatment, 221
signs and symptoms, 223
treatment,
antibiotics, 223, 225
removal of implant, 223,
225, 226
salvage, 224–226, 228,
239–241
inflatable prostheses,
AMS 700 CX, 181, 182, 186,
192, 193, 195
AMS 700 CXM, 182, 186,
187, 238, 252, 253
AMS 700 Inflatable Penile
Prosthesis, 180, 181
AMS 700 Ultrex, 182–184, 239
AMS Ambicor, 185
AMS Dynaflex, 184, 185
AMS Hydroflex, 184
history of development,
179, 180
ideal implant
characteristics, 186
implantation,
autoinflation avoidance,
188, 189
corporeal sizing, 188
infrapubic approach, 187
penoscrotal approach, 188
indications for implantation,
185, 186
one-piece prostheses, 184, 185
patient expectations, 187
reliability, 232
selection of device, 186
three-piece prosthesis,
Mentor α-1, *see* Mentor α-1
Mentor IPP, 191, 192
Peyronie's disease
management, *see*
Peyronie's disease
two-piece prosthesis, 185

mechanical devices,
American Medical Systems
products, 172, 177,
180–185
anesthesia for implantation, 175
Dacomed Dura II, 173, 174
history of development,
171, 172
Mentor products, 172–173
patient selection, 175, 176
semirigid implant,
advantages, 174, 175
disadvantages, 176, 177
pain evaluation, 245
position problems, 243, 244
reliability, 167, 168
reoperation,
fibrosis management, 235,
237–239
mechanical failure, 244, 245
patient selection, 232, 233
preparation of patients, 233
repair rates, 219, 220
salvage techniques following
infection, 224–226,
228, 239–241
surgery, 233, 234
tissue engineering,
bending studies, 17, 18
cell regeneration, 10
chondrocytes for rod
construction, 16, 17
matrices, 10, 11, 17, 18
strategies, 10
Peyronie's disease,
diagnosis, 203
discovery, 201
erectile dysfunction
association, 202
etiology, 201, 202
medical treatment, 203, 204
pathogenesis, 202
patient evaluation, 203
penile prosthesis,
Mentor α-1, 196

modeling procedure with
inflatable prosthesis,
caveats, 214, 216
complications, 212–214
development, 207, 208
overview, 160
technique, 208, 209,
211, 212
patient evaluation,
history, 250
miscellaneous tests, 250
physical examination, 250
plaque incision, 160, 161
semirigid devices, 176,
206, 207
surgery,
complications, 259
corporotomy, 254, 255, 258
dilators, 251, 252
downsized prosthesis,
252–254
postoperative care, 259
reconstruction with
synthetic grafts, 258
technique, 160
two-piece hydraulic
prosthesis, 207
plaque excision and grafting,
205, 206
prevalence, 202
shortening surgery, 159, 204, 205
straightening surgery, 159,
205, 206
surgery indications, 204
Polyvinyl alcohol, injection therapy,
57, 68
Priapism, penile prosthesis, 162, 196
Prostatectomy, *see* Radical
prostatectomy

R

Radical prostatectomy,
incontinence treatment,
anatomy, 90
artificial urinary sphincter,
98, 165
bulbourethral sling
procedure, 98
chronic urinary
catherization, 99
collagen injection, 96, 98
incidence of incontinence, 89
Teflon injection,
outcomes, 96, 99
patient selection, 91, 92
technique, 92, 95
penile prosthesis, 162, 163

S

Silicone, implant safety, 142,
143, 153
Silimed oval carving block, *see*
Testicular prosthesis
Silk-elastin polymer, injection
therapy, 58, 70
SIS, *see* Small intestine submucosa
Small Carrion prosthesis,
development, 4, 5
Small intestine submucosa (SIS),
injection therapy, 58, 71, 72
Smooth muscle, injection therapy,
59, 74
Sphincter ablation, detrusor-sphincter
dyssynergia management, 102
Spinal cord injury,
causes, 101
neurogenic bladder, *see* Detrusor-
sphincter dyssynergia
penile prosthesis, 163, 175, 176

T

Teflon injection therapy,
characteristics of particles, 56, 91
historical perspective, 90, 91
incontinence outcomes,
females, 64
males, 66
indications, 55, 60
radical prostatectomy
incontinence treatment,
anatomy, 90
incidence of incontinence, 89
outcomes, 96, 97

patient selection, 91, 92
technique, 92, 95
Urethrin, 56
vesicouretal reflux, 68
Testicular prosthesis,
contraindications, 146
follow-up, 153
historical perspectives, 141, 142
ideal characteristics, 141
indications, 145, 146
Mentor Saline-Filled Testicular
Prosthesis, 143, 145
morbidity,
implant deflation or rupture,
151, 152
infection, 151
migration or migration, 152
miscellaneous problems,
152, 153
survey, 150
silicone safety, 142, 143
Silimed oval carving block, 143
surgery,
adults, 149, 150
infants, 147, 149
technique, 146, 147
Tissue engineering,
bladder replacement,
beagle studies, 13, 14
cell regeneration, 10
compliance, 14
immunocytochemical
analysis, 14
matrices, 10, 11
strategies, 10
corpora cavernosa, 15, 16
fetal tissue engineering, 22–24
gene therapy, 24, 25
injectable therapy,
testicular functional
replacement, 20, 22
urinary incontinence, 19, 20
vesicouretal reflux, 19, 20
kidney, 18, 19
penile prosthesis, 16–18
ureter and urethra, 12

Transurethral resection of prostate
(TURP),
benign prostatic hyperplasia
management, 117, 118
Urovolume stent comparative
clinical trial for benign
prostatic hyperplasia,
BPH impact index, 133,
134, 138
ejaculation, 126, 127
erection outcomes, 125, 126
erection pain, 125, 138
intercourse pain, 125
IPSS symptom scores, 132
long-term outcomes, 139
patient characteristics, 136
peak flow rate, 129, 138, 139
pressure flow studies, 132
procedure, 122, 123, 135
quality-of-life scores, 133
residual urine volume, 129, 131
safety, 123, 124, 137
study design, 121, 122
urethral pain, 124, 125, 137
TURP, *see* Transurethral resection
of prostate

U

Ureter, tissue engineering,
cell expansion, 12
cell regeneration, 10
matrices, 10, 11
matrix degradation, 12
strategies, 10
Urethra, tissue engineering,
cell expansion, 12
cell regeneration, 10
matrices, 10, 11
matrix degradation, 12
strategies, 10
Urethral stent,
benign prostatic hyperplasia,
clinical trial comparing
transurethral resection
of prostate,
BPH impact index, 133,
134, 138

ejaculation, 126, 127
erection outcomes, 125, 126
erection pain, 125, 138
intercourse pain, 125
IPSS symptom scores, 132
long-term outcomes, 139
patient characteristics, 136
peak flow rate, 129, 138, 139
pressure flow studies, 132
procedure, 122, 123, 135
quality-of-life scores, 133
residual urine volume,
129, 131
safety, 123, 124, 137
study design, 121, 122
urethral pain, 124, 125, 137
endoscopic follow-up,
encrustation, 127
epithelialization, 127, 138
hyperplasia, 128
residual hypertrophic
tissue, 128
stent migration, 128
insertion, 120, 121
Urovolume stent studies,
overview, 118–120,
134, 135
detrusor-sphincter dyssynergia
management,
historical perspective, 102, 103
permanent stents, 103–109
removal, 112
temporary stents, 109, 110, 113
Urovolume stent development,
118, 119
Urethrin, injection therapy, 56
Urinary incontinence, see also
Artificial urinary sphincter,
continence mechanisms, 44, 45
definition, 285
etiology, 300
injectable therapy,
antegrade injection, 33
carbon steel particles, 34
children, 33
collagen,

injection technique, 37–39
outcome data, 32, 33
Durasphere injection
technique, 39
female versus male outcomes,
74, 75
goals, 47, 48
historical perspectives, 29, 30
materials, see Injectable
therapy
outcomes by material,
female, 64, 65
male, 66, 67
patient selection,
cystoscopy, 47
history, 45, 46
men, 35, 37
physical examination, 46
urodynamic testing, 46, 47
women, 34, 35
postoperative care, 51–53
silicone microimplants, 34
Teflon injection following
radical prostatectomy,
see Teflon injection
therapy
tissue engineering, 19, 20
type III stress incontinence,
30–32
urethral injection techniques,
females, 48–50
males, 50, 51
prevalence, 285
urethral dysfunction subtypes,
30–32
Urocol, injection therapy, 56
Urologen, injection therapy, 58
UroVive, injection therapy, 57, 64,
66, 68, 69, 70
Urovolume, see Urethral stent

V

Vesicouretal reflux,
injectable therapy,
materials, see Injectable
therapy

outcomes by material, 68
patient evaluation, 53, 54
postoperati ve care, 54, 55
techniques, 54
tissue engineering, 19, 20

uretero–vesicle junction
physiology, 53
Vitamin E, Peyronie's disease
management, 203, 204